THE GOLDEN SEVEN PLUS ONE

CONQUER DISEASE WITH EIGHT KEYS TO HEALTH, BEAUTY, AND PEACE

by

C. Samuel West, D.N., N.D.
Chemist and Lymphologist
*Internationally Known as an Authority on the
Causes of Pain, Loss of Energy,
and Disease*

**DISCOVER
THE ART OF LYMPHASIZING**

**LEARN ABOUT
THE BLOOD PROTEIN RESEARCH**

THIS TEXTBOOK WAS DEVELOPED TO MAKE IT
POSSIBLE TO ESTABLISH DR. WEST'S WORLD-WIDE
FAMILY SELF-H.E.L.P. CENTERS AND IS DESIGNED FOR
FAMILY HOME STUDY

First Printing	–	September 1982
Second Printing	–	January 1983
Third Printing	–	June 1985
Fourth Printing	–	October 1985
Fifth Printing	–	August 1986
Sixth Printing	–	August 1987
Seventh Printing	–	April 1988
Eighth Printing	–	January 1989
Ninth Printing	–	April 1990
Tenth Printing	–	December 1992
Eleventh Printing	–	September 1993
Twelfth Printing	–	June 1994
Thirteenth Printing	–	January 1995
Fourteenth Printing	–	September 1995
Fifteenth Printing	–	September 1996

Library of Congress Cataloging in Publication Data

West, C. Samuel
The Golden Seven Plus One

Orem, Ut.: Samuel Publishing Co.
400P8201811207

Library of Congress Catalog Card Number: 81-86099

Printed in the United States of America

DEDICATION

Part I

I dedicate this book to my "angel" wife, Johna May, and our ten children, who have been willing to live most of the time during the last seven years without a husband and father in order to help save the lives of over 240,000 men, women, and children who are being killed by trapped blood proteins every two months in the United States, and to help save hundreds of thousands who are also killed every month by trapped blood proteins in other countries throughout the world.

I dedicate this book to them because they believe, as I do, that the blood-protein research will not only save the above men, women and children from the unprecedented destruction that is now taking place in the United States and throughout the world, but it also reveals what we must do to raise up a posterity who will be able to conquer disease and live in peace.

Part II

I also dedicate this book to the International Society of Lymphology for accepting me as the 379th member in November of 1979, at the 7th International Congress of Lymphology that was held in Florence, Italy. I also give appreciation to this society for inviting me to present "The Basic Formula Showing How the Blood Plasma Proteins Produce the Conditions That Cause Loss of Energy, Disease and Death at the Cell Level" at the 8th International Congress that was held in Montreal, Canada, in September of 1981.

THE POWER BEHIND THIS BOOK

As the result of an invitation from Dr. Raymond W. Belanger, M.D., President of The 8th International Congress of Lymphology, on September 22, 1981, Dr. West presented *The One Basic Formula* upon which this book is based to some of the top medical research scientists and lymphologists in the world. By accepting this invitation, Dr. West put this formula and seven years of his life to the acid test.

As the tapes of this congress will verify, this formula passed the test. The validity of many presentations were challenged; but no one challenged the validity of this basic formula which makes this book and the following certificate priceless.

The power of this basic formula is that it reveals what can and must be done to prevent and if possible reverse the destruction that is now being caused by the crippling and killer diseases.

As Dr. Joe Nichols, M.D. says in his book, *Please Doctor Do Something,* "There is an epidemic of heart disease, diabetes, and cancer in this country that will destroy America unless something is done quickly to stop it."

We do not have time to lose! Cancer is now killing more children between the ages of 3-14 than anything else. It is affecting two out of three families. One out of every five deaths is now caused by cancer. The atomic bomb killed about seventy thousand people. Cancer is killing over four hundred thousand men, women, and children every year in this nation alone. Heart disease is killing over a million a year. One out of every two deaths in the United States is now caused by heart disease. One out of one is everyone!

It is evident that the time is soon coming when the only ones who will be saved from death and destruction by disease are those who *discover* and *obey* the laws of health. *The One Basic Formula* reveals what these laws are.

The One who made the body made the basic formulas for life and death at the cell level. With His help we have finally found them, and *this is the power behind this book.*

(Note: Disease and death were misspelled on the following certificate because the secretaries did not know how to speak English.)

I

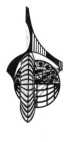

8ᵗʰ INTERNATIONAL
CONGRESS
OF
LYMPHOLOGY
MONTREAL, CANADA

•

SEPTEMBER 20-25, 1981

8ᵉ CONGRÈS
INTERNATIONAL
DE LYMPHOLOGIE

INTERNATIONAL SOCIETY OF LYMPHOLOGY

THIS IS TO CERTIFY THAT

DR. C. SAMUEL WEST has presented a paper entitled
"THE BASIC FORMULA SHOWING HOW THE PLASMA PROTEINS
PRODUCE THE CONDITIONS THAT CAUSE LOSS OF ENERGY,
DESEASE AND DETH AT THE CELL LEVEL" in the
8TH INTERNATIONAL CONGRESS OF LYMPHOLOGY.

RAYMOND BÉLANGER,
President
8th International Congress
of Lymphology

JAMES W. DAVIDSON,
President
of the
Scientific Program Committee
8th International Congress of Lymphology

ALLAN E. DUMONT
President
International Society
of Lymphology

II

TABLE OF CONTENTS

Page

THE POWER BEHIND THIS BOOK I

THE CERTIFICATE which states that on September 22, 1981, Dr. West presented "The Basic Formula" for loss of energy, disease and death at the cell level before some of the top medical research scientists and lymphologists in the world, and there were no objections as to the validity of this formula II

DISCLAIMER XXII

I.   PREFACE XXIV

II. AN INTRODUCTION TO SESSION ONE, THE SEVEN GOLDEN DISCOVERIES, AND THE ART OF LYMPHASIZING WHICH REVEALS WHAT A HEALING ART MUST DO IN ORDER TO WORK . XXV

SESSION I

   A.   THE BLOOD PROTEIN RESEARCH AND THE ART OF LYMPHASIZING ARE THE MOST IMPORTANT HEALTH DISCOVERIES SINCE THE BEGINNING OF MAN 1

   A-1. A promise To Those Who Learn The Principles And Apply The Concepts Contained In This Book . 3

   B.   THE SEVEN GOLDEN DISCOVERIES 4

   B-1. Not Diagnosis Or Prescription 8

   C.   DR. WEST WRITES "THE ONE BASIC FORMULA" WHICH SHOWS HOW THE BLOOD PROTEINS PRODUCE THE CONDITIONS THAT CAUSE LOSS OF ENERGY, DISEASE, AND DEATH AT THE CELL LEVEL 9

D.   "THE ONE BASIC FORMULA" FOR LOSS OF
     ENERGY, DISEASE AND DEATH 10

E.   AT THE 8TH INTERNATIONAL CONGRESS,
     DR. WEST ALSO PRESENTED "THE BASIC
     FORMULA FOR LIFE" WHICH SHOWS THE
     INTERNAL CONDITIONS THAT MUST
     EXIST TO HAVE HEALTHY BODY 13

E-1. The Above Seven Discoveries And This One
     Basic Formula Have Produced A Scientific
     Message For Health and Peace That Will Grow
     To Fill The Whole World 13

F.   THESE SEVEN GOLDEN DISCOVERIES AND
     THIS ONE BASIC FORMULA REVEAL WHAT A
     HEALING ART MUST DO IN ORDER TO
     WORK. THE MIRACLES OF SCIENCE ARE
     NOW REVEALED 14

G.   INTRODUCING A NEW SCIENCE CALLED
     "THE ART OF LYMPHASIZING" WHICH
     REVEALS WHAT CAUSES TRAPPED PLASMA
     PROTEINS (TPP) AROUND THE CELLS 16

G-1. The Mental Laws Of Health And Trapped
     Plasma Protein 17

G-2. The Nutritional Laws And Trapped Plasma
     Proteins 19

G-3. The Physical Laws And Trapped Plasma
     Proteins 22

H.   REVIEW OF SESSION ONE 26

SESSION II--THE COLLEGE OF CAUSE AND SELF-
     HELP PAIN RELIEF 27

A.   INTRODUCTION 27

B.   THE PURPOSE OF THIS SESSION IS NOT
     TO DIAGNOSE OR PRESCRIBE 28

C.   GRATEFUL TO MEDICAL RESEARCH FOR
      MAJOR DISCOVERIES 28

C-1. The Following Medical Research Concerning
      Blood Proteins And Death Will Revolutionize
      The World 29

C-2. Only "A Handful" Know That Our Blood
      Proteins Can Cause Death 31

C-3. It is Not "Just That Simple" 32

C-4. Blood Protein Research Reveals Importance
      Of The Lymphatic System 32

C-5. To Keep The Blood Protein Research From The
      Public Is To Let People Suffer And Die--To
      Ignore It Is To Commit Suicide 37

C-6. The Importance Of The Lymphatic System 37

C-7. What Is Lymph Fluid 38

C-8. How Cells Are Fed 38

D.   HOW MANY TIMES CAN CELLS RE-
      PRODUCE THEMSELVES? 38

D-1. Letter From A Cancer Researcher Who Believes
      Cells Are Meant To Live Forever 39

E.   HOW THE LYMPHATIC SYSTEM
      FUNCTIONS IN DETAIL 40

E-1. What Causes Congestion, Catarrh (Mucous)
      And Inflammation 41

F.   THE ONE AND ONLY FORMULA EXPLAINED
      IN DETAIL 42

F-1. A Different Approach 42

F-2. The Human Body Is An Electrical Being 44

F-3.   Loss Of Energy Is A Sign Of Trapped Protein . . 45

G.   ELECTRICAL SECRETS OF LIFE AND
      DEATH AT THE CELL LEVEL SHOW HOW WE
      CAN PREVENT AND POSSIBLY REVERSE PAIN,
      LOSS OF ENERGY AND DISEASE 45

G-1.   The Secret To The Healing Process 46

G-2.   If You Turn The Electric Generators Off,
      Lights Go Out; If You Turn The Generators
      On The Lights Go On! 47

G-3.   Lack Of Oxygen--The Cause Of Most Pain 48

G-4.   New Research Reveals The Conditions The Body
      Must Be In To Produce A Healthy Cell 48

G-5.   What Causes Smashed Fingers, Turned Ankles,
      And Some People's Bodies To Retain Fluids? . . 51

G-6.   Discovery Six And Seven: Trapped Proteins
      Become Clustered; And Electricity Can
      Dissipate Clustered Proteins 53

G-7.   Why And How The Bio-Electric Self-Help
      Pain Relief Techniques Work! 54

G-8.   Introducing Discovery By Dr. Joseph M.
      Waltz, M.D. 55

G-9.   The Cause Of Headaches, Lower Back, And
      Sciatic Problems And Much More 57

G-10. What Must Happen In The Body For Healing
      To Take Place 57

G-11. A Few Examples To Illustrate The Healing
      Process 57

G-12. The Use Of Pressure Can Heal A Smashed
      Finger In Minutes, Minutes--Not Hours 58

G-13. Masssage And A Light Fast Stroke: Two Other
Self-Help Pain Relief Techniques 60

G-14. What About Swollen And Painful Fingers, Or
Pain In The Neck, Shoulders, Arms, Lower Back,
Hips, Sciatic Nerve, Ankles, Knees, Thighs, Etc. . 60

G-15. The Secret Of The Healing Process 61

G-16. Why It May Be Necessary To Do These
Techniques For Fifteen Seconds Every
Fifteen Minutes 61

H.   ILLUSTRATIONS SHOWING THE BASIC
BIO-ELECTRIC SELF-HELP PAIN RELIEF
TECHNIQUES 62

H-1. To Help Relieve Headaches and Sore Neck
Problems 62

H-2. To Help Relieve My Sore Arms and Legs 63

H-3. To Help Relieve Pain In The Hip, Lower
Back, and Sciatic Nerve 63

H-4. To Help Increase The Circulation In The Liver,
Gall Bladder, Spleen, And Pancreas 63

H-5. To Help Stimulate And Revitalize The Colon . . . 64

H-6. To Help Increase Circulation In The Kidneys . . . 64

H-7. To Help Relieve The Pain In Smashed Or Cut
Finger 65

H-8. To Help Relieve Pain In A Freshly Turned Ankle . 65

I.   THE COLLEGE OF CAUSE 70

I-1. The Cause Of Cancer 70

I-2. Inflammation And The Clustered Protein
Research 71

I-3. The Cause Of Arthritis 72

I-4. The Cause Of Obesity 73

I-5. The Cause of Hypertension (High Blood Pressure) . 74

J. INTRODUCTION TO SESSION THREE 75

SESSION III--THE COLLEGE OF PREVENTION 79

A. FOR MAN TO PREVENT AND IF POSSIBLE
REVERSE DISEASE AND HAVE PEACE ON
EARTH HE MUST MASTER THE NEW
SCIENCE CALLED THE ART OF
LYMPHASIZING 79

B. PREVENTION THROUGH PROPER MENTAL
ATTITUDES, THE MENTAL PART OF THE ART
OF LYMPHASIZING 80

B-1. To Have Health We Must Obey The
Laws Of Peace 81

B-2. Review Of Stress And The Death Process 84

B-3. The Laws of Health Are The Laws of Peace 84

B-4. Mental Attitudes That Cause Death Will Also
Cause War 84

B-5. To Save Your Life, Learn About The Blood 85

B-6. Medical Doctors and The People In The United
States Are In Ignorance As To The Mental,
Nutritrional and Physical Causes Of Death 86

B-7. Knowledge Of Blood Proteins Will Restore Health
And Peace 86

B-8. Why Some Medical Doctors Are Afraid To
Teach The Blood Protein Research 87

B-9. AMA Discipline Boards Keep Medical
Doctors From Practicing Prevention 87

B-10. Why Doctors And The People In The United
States Now Have To Fight For Health Freedoms . 88

B-11. An Age Of Peace And Health That We Have
Never Known Before 90

B-12. "Forgive Them, For They Know Not What
They Do" 91

B-13. To Willfully Cause Stress In Another Person Is
To Cause Their Destruction 92

B-14. The Natural Man, An Enemy To Himself 92

B-15. Medicine And Drugs, Building Ships And
Guns Is Not The Answer 92

B-16. Introducing The World-Wide Golden Family
Self-H.E.L.P. Program 93

B-17. Live Laws of Health; Become Like The
City of Enoch 95

B-18. This Message Must Go To The Nations Of
The Earth 96

C. PREVENTION THROUGH PROPER
NUTRITION, THE NUTRITIONAL PART
OF THE ART OF LYMPHASIZING 96

C-1. Are We Just Dying, Or Are We Being Destroyed? . 97

C-2. Cause Of Death Has Changed Since Early
19th Century. Why? 98

C-3. You Can Know If You Eat A Poison By How It
Makes You Feel 98

C-4. Thirst And Loss Of Energy Are Symptoms Of
Disease And Death. TPP = EX Fl = ▲EE =
Thirst And Loss Of Energy 99

C-5. Why Too Much Salt (Na+ Cl−) Is A Poison
Ex Na+ = TPP = Thirst and Loss Of Energy . . . 99

C-6. Government Document: <u>The Dietary Goals For
The United States</u> Says That Salt, Sugar, Fat,
The High Cholesterol Foods, And Too Much
Meat Are Directly Related To The Destruction
Of Two Hundred Forty Thousand Men, Women
And Children Every Two Months In This
Country Alone 100

C-7. Why The "Simple" Sugars Are Poisons! 101

C-8. Why Fat Is A Poison! 102

C-9. Why The High Cholesterol Foods Are Poisons! . . 103

C-10. <u>The Dietary Goals</u> Calls For A National Health
Education Program To Protect The People
Against The "Interests" Who Are Causing
Their Destruction 103

C-11. The A.M.A., Some Of The Food Processors,
And Others Tried To Discredit Government
Document 104

C-12. Why We Are Publishing A "15 Page Excerpt"
Of The First Edition Of This Government
Document 105

C-13. Government Document Lets You Diagnose
And Prescribe 105

C-14. Government Document States That There Is
Very Little Current Medical Practice Can
Do For The Killer Diseases 106

C-15. Government Document States That Our
Problems Can Never Be Solved By More And
More Medical Care 106

C-16. Government Document Calls For A Nation-
Wide Health Education Program 107

C-17. How To Use The Dietary Goals To Help Get
The Blood Protein Research To Others 108

C-18. We Won't Win The Educational Battle Of Health
And Peace Unless We Take The Offensive 109

C-19. To Take The Offensive, Here Are The Dietary
Goals In More Detail 110

C-20. Dietary Goals Gives Us The Nutritional Diagnosis
For Crippling And Killer Diseases 111

C-21. "Love Is The Desire To Give Everything You
Have To Bless The Lives Of Others." (From a
plaque on the wall of Willard and Catherine
Hunter's home in Ohio.) 112

C-22. Dietary Goals: Nutritionally Prescribes For
Prevention Of Crippling And Killer Diseases . . 113

C-23. Research Supports Dietary Goals: The Public
Must Know That The Body's Requirements For
Calcium Are Low, Not High 114

C-24. More Medical Research Supports Dietary Goals:
The Public Must Know That The Body's
Requirements For Protein Are Low, Not High . . . 115

C-25. Research And The Feb. 1977 Edition of
Dietary Goals Agree 116

C-26. Hypoglycemia--Not Enough Fruits, Vegetables
and Whole Grains 116

C-27. How Hypoglycemia Can Turn Into Diabetes,
High Blood Pressure And Heart Disease 117

C-28. Diabetes Mellitus (Permanent Diabetes) 118

C-29. Medical Research On How To Treat Protein
Deficiency 119

C-30. High Protein Makes You Feel Good, While It
Kills You 119

C-31. Eight Glasses Of Water A Day? Yes, If You Eat
The Wrong Foods 120

C-32. A Transition Program Is Necessary 121

C-33. Why The Transition Process Works 128

C-34. How To Combine Foods 129

C-35. The Transition Concepts In Condensed Form . . 131

C-36. The Basic Transition Diet 132

C-37. Helpful Suggestions To Help Overcome
Addiction 132

C-38. Breathe Deeply Everywhere You Go 133

C-39. What Do I Have To Do To Become A Golden
Family? 134

C-40. What If I Don't Have The Support Of My
Family? 134

C-41. A Sample Food Shopping List, Menu, Recipes
And Dehydrating Techniques To Help You Get
Started On Transition--Your New Way Of Life,
Can Be Found In Appendix B 134

C-42. Dr. West Gives Testimony Of Transition And

The Art Of Lymphasizing Which Is A
"New Way Of Life" 135

D.   PREVENTION THROUGH PROPER EXERCISE:
        THE PHYSICAL PART OF THE ART OF
        LYMPHASIZING 136

D-1.   Dr. West Discovers How To "Run And Not Be
        Weary, Walk And Not Faint!" 136

D-2.   Why The Concepts Of Lymphasizing Are In
        This Book 137

D-3.   The Secret Of The Tarahumara Indians 138

D-4.   About The Tarahumara Indians 138

D-5.   Lymphasizing--The Foundation Upon Which
        Energy In The Body Is Built 139

D-6.   A Complete List Of Lymphasizing Terms 139

D-7.   Definitions And Explanations Of The "a-e"
        Terms Of Lymphasizing 140

D-8.   Activity Is A "Magic" Healer For The Body 144

D-9.   Where Lymphasizing First Began 145

D-10.   Why Babies Love To Be Lymphasized 145

D-11.   Babies Say, "If You Love Me, Lymphasize Me" . 145

D-12.   When Do We Begin To Break The Natural Laws . 146

D-13.   If You Don't Have A Lymphasizer--Get One . . . 147

D-14.   98-Year-Old Woman Saved From Death 148

D-15.   Special Education Children Respond To
        Lymphasizing 148

D-16. The Miracle Of Aerobic Lymphasizing 150

D-17. The Miracle Of Glycogen 151

D-18. Glycogen Can Give You Superhuman Strength . 152

D-19. Two Reasons Why "Miracles" Take Place On
A Lymphasizer 153

D-20. How To Use A Lymphasizer Properly And
Bounce Your Way To Better Health 154

D-21. The Run And Not Be Weary--Walk And Not
Faint Lymphasizing Program 156

D-22. How To Raise Up A Posterity Who Will
Master The Art Of Lymphasizing, Conquer
Disease And Live In Peace 167

D-23. You Are Now Ready To Graduate From The
College Of Cause, The College Of Self-Help
Pain Relief, And From The College Of
Prevention 168

D-24. The Powers Of Hate To Be Replaced By Love.
Golden Families Who Are Willing To
Conquer Disease And Live In Peace And
Harmony Will Be Established 169

D-25. You Can Now Defend Yourselves In The
Battle Of Life And Death 169

SESSION IV--THIS SESSION CONTAINS:
HOW TO DO USE A LYMPHASIZER
ELECTRICALLY AND THE OTHER ADVAN-
CED BIO-ELECTRIC LYMPHASIZING
TECHNIQUES; THE WORK OF DR. JOSEPH
WALTZ, M.D.; DR. DANIEL GRAUPE, M.D.;
DR. FULLER ROYAL, M.D.; TESTIMONIALS;
SPECIAL ACKNOWLEDGMENTS TO THOSE
WHO MADE THIS BOOK POSSIBLE; THE
STORY BEHIND THIS BOOK AND MUCH
MORE 171

A.   NEW MEDICAL DISCOVERIES GIVE
CREDIBILITY TO THE ADVANCED BIO-
ELECTRIC LYMPHASIZING TECHNIQUES . . . 171

A-1. Electricity Used By Medical Doctors To
Diagnose And Prescribe 172

A-2. Eyes, Thoughts And Muscles Work Electrically . . 173

A-3. The Work of Dr. Graupe: "Bionic Arm"
Controlled By Thoughts 174

A-4. Dr. Joseph Waltz Uses Electrical Stimulation
To Help Previously Helpless Cerebral Palsy,
M. S. and Polio Patients 174

A-5. Pictures And Letter Sent By Dr. Waltz 177

A-6. Thanks To Doctors Who Are Willing To Share . . 184

B.   A LIST OF THE ADVANCED BIO-ELECTRIC
LYMPHASIZING TECHNIQUES WHICH CAN
BE DEMONSTRATED BY A QUALIFIED
INSTRUCTOR 185

B-1. Definition Of Bio-Electric Energy 185

C.   EXPLANATIONS WITH PICTURES, AND
STORIES ILLUSTRATING THE ADVANCED
BIO-ELECTRIC LYMPHASIZING
TECHNIQUES 185

C-1. The Story Behind The Bio-Electric Gentle
Bounce For Health, And The Special Bio-
Electric Eye Exercise 186

C-2. How To Do The Bio-Electric Gentle Bounce
For Health 187

C-3. Dr. West's Body Chart 188

C-4. Dorothy Howard Reversed Her Sixty-Five-
Year-Old Crippling Condition Due To Polio, In
Four Months By Using The Bio-Electric Gentle
Bounce For Health 190

C-5. Doors Opened To Other Discoveries 190

C-6. This New Blood Protein Research Teaches
The Cause Of Disease Which Enables Many
People To Know What To Do To Take Care Of
Their Own Problems 191

C-7. Poem, "Bouncy, Bouncy Baby" by Johna May
West 193

C-8 The Special Bio-Electric Eye Exercise 195

C-9. The Breathing And Directed Thinking
Technique 195

C-10. The Bio-Electric Wheelchair Technique 198

C-11. The Bio-Electric Pin-Point Technique 202

C-12. Details Concerning Energy Flow While Doing
The Basic Bio-Electric Self-Help Techniques
Described In Session II 203

C-13. The Bio-Electric Energy Field 204

C-14. The Bio-Electric Energy Field Reverses Injuries . . 204

D. WRITTEN TESTIMONIALS (APPROX. 30
UNNUMBERED PAGES BETWEEEN 207-208)

TESTIMONIAL LETTERS FROM SOME OF
THE PEOPLE WHO HAVE RECEIVED HELP
FROM APPLYING THE SELF-HELP
LYMPHASIZING CONCEPTS 207

E. ADDITIONAL SCIENTIFIC EVIDENCE
WITH TESTIMONIES GIVES VALIDITY

TO THE NUTRITIONAL CONCEPTS AND
THE TRANSITION PROGRAM IN SESSION
THREE 208

E-1.   What About High Protein For Athletes? 208

E-2.   A Very Well-Documented Article Entitled,
       "Top Doctors Reveal . . . Simple Diet Change
       Can Prevent Breast And Colon Cancer"
       Appeared In The National Enquirer,
       September 15, 1979. On Page 20, It States: 208

E-3.   Millions Live--On Low Protein 211

E-4.   Excess Protein--Will Damage Kidneys 212

E-5.   What Dr. Paavo Airola--Says About Protein 212

E-6.   Praise--The Potato 213

E-7.   Disease Results From High Protein--Well
       Documented 214

E-8.   The Following Testimonials Are An Additional
       Witness To The Truth Of Eating Right 215

E-9.   Arnold Ehret--"The Daddy Of Transition" 216

E-10. Ehret Proved--Strength Comes From A Clean
      System 216

E-11. Arnold Ehret Lived On Straight Fruit--For Two
      Years 217

E-12. Teresa Mitchell Follows Ehret--No Fatigue In
      Her Body 218

E-13. Testimony of Teresa Mitchell 220

E-14. Eight Basic Rules For A Disease-Free
      Healthy Life 221

E-15. Dr. Max Warmbrand, M.D., D.O. Confirms
        Above Research And Findings 223

E-16. Complex Carbohydrates -- A Protein Sparer . . . 224

E-17. Protein In The Body Stays High--Even During
        Starvation (Fasting) 226

E-18. What Dr. Otto Buchinger, M.D. Says About
        Fasting In How To Get Well, By Dr. Paavo
        Airola 227

E-19. Vital Organs And Glands Are Not Damaged
        From Fasting 227

F.   "SPECIAL" RECOGNITION GOES TO THE
        FOLLOWING LYMPHASIZER MANUFACT-
        URERS, OTHER COMPANIES AND
        INDIVIDUALS FOR HELPING TO FINANCE
        THE FIRST EDITION OF THIS BOOK 229

G.   MY STORY BEHIND THE GOLDEN SEVEN
        PLUS ONE 232

G-1. Not To Tell Others About This Research--Is
        To Cause Their Destruction 232

G-2. Why I Learned About This Research 234

G-3. "Steel Wall" Number One 235

G-4. "Steel Wall" Number Two 236

G-5. "Steel Wall" Number Three 236

G-6. "Steel Wall" Number Four 237

G-7. "Steel Wall" Number Five 237

G-8. "Steel Wall" Number Six 238

G-9.   "Steel Wall" Number Seven 238

G-10.   How I Learned About Protein And Death 239

G-11.   I Began To Teach About Protein Causing Death   . 240

G-12.   How The Door Opened To Lecture Full-Time   . . 240

G-13.   How I Was Given Help To Write This Book   . . . 241

G-14.   The Day I Knew I Had "THE FORMULA"   242

G-15.   How This Book Was Named 242

G-16.   What Happened When I Tried To Write The
        Original Manuscript 243

H.   "SPECIAL" ACKNOWLEDGMENT AND
        APPRECIATION TO OTHERS WHO HAVE
        HELPED TO MAKE THE GOLDEN SEVEN
        PLUS ONE POSSIBLE 244

APPENDIX A. Excerpts From The Dietary Goals For
        The United States--Dr. West's Statements
        Regarding The Three Page Forward--Senator
        Percy's Three Page Forward To The Second
        Edition Of The Dietary Goals 247

APPENDIX B. Food Shopping List, Sample Lunch
        Menu, Recipes To Help With Transition,
        Directions For Dehydrating Foods 267

APPENDIX C. "The Basic Formula For Death" and
        "The Basic Formula For Life" With
        Definitions Of Terms And Charts 289

APPENDIX D. Bibliography And Additional Reading
        Material 293

GENERAL INDEX 305

SPECIAL INDEX--Charts and Photographs,
        In Order Of Appearance 315

DISCLAIMER

This book is for educational purposes only. It should be fully understood that no information or interpretation of any part of this book is to be used for diagnosis or treatment of disease. The purpose of this book is to teach the cause of disease and what man must do mentally, nutritionally, and physically to prevent and possibly reverse disease. We acknowledge that only a medical doctor has the right to diagnose and treat disease, but we also acknowledge the fact that every human being has the responsibility to do all that is within his power mentally, nutritionally, and physically to prevent and possibly reverse any pain, loss of energy or disease that he may have in his body.

Caution

Because of the nature of the discoveries revealed in this book, anyone who uses any of the information that it contains must do so on his own as a result of his own free agency.

XXII

I. PREFACE

1. The purpose of this book, *The Golden Seven Plus One,* is to help get the *blood protein research* and *the art of lymphasizing* to the nations of the earth.

2. Dr. West has been presenting this research to people in approximately two hundred cities per year. This book is written in very simple terms. It is organized in sessions instead of chapters, and all of the paragraphs are numbered to make this research easy to cross-reference, to study, and to teach.

3. The findings presented in this book will enable every individual and family in the whole world to enjoy the blessings of health along with true inner beauty and peace to a greater degree than ever before. It will help bring to pass a civilization which people have been looking for since the beginning of time—where *love* will rule the emotions and *wisdom* will rule the appetite.

4. Based on the blood protein research, this book teaches the new science called, *The Art of Lymphasizing,* which reveals what man must do mentally, nutritionally, and physically to keep the blood proteins circulating in the body via the lymphatic system.

5. This knowledge will enable those who apply it to help establish a people throughout the world who will exist in peace; and the reason they will exist in peace is because they will know mentally, nutritionally, and physically how to conquer disease.

6. The art of lymphasizing contains discoveries which reveal what the laws of health and peace are. During the seven years it took to write this book, C. Samuel West, D.N., N.D., chemist and lymphologist, came across seven major discoveries pertaining to the life and death processes at the cell level, which only a handful of people in the whole world even know exist.

7. As a result of these seven discoveries, on June 24, 1980, Dr. West wrote the one basic formula that reveals the relationship between the blood proteins and the conditions that must exist for the body to produce a totally healthy cell and how the blood proteins produce the conditions that will damage or kill the cell.

8. With the knowledge that is contained in this book, you will not only learn the cause, but you will also learn how to prevent and if possible reverse pain, inflammation, loss of energy, heart disease, cancer, obesity, multiple sclerosis, polio, arthritis, migraine headaches, lower back and sciatic problems, and every other crippling and killer disease known to man.

9. Also, for the first time in our recorded history, we now have scientific research which reveals that the laws of health are the laws of peace, and the laws of sickness and death are the laws of war.

10. To all who have a desire to benefit from these discoveries, we offer *The Golden Seven Plus One* with the knowledge that the day will come when man will conquer disease and live in peace.

11. In time, this research will be used in World-Wide Family Self-H.E.L.P. (Health Education for Longevity and Peace) Centers, where people can join together in small groups and thereby gain strength from each other as a qualified instructor guides them through this book in detail, session by session.

II. AN INTRODUCTION TO SESSION ONE, THE SEVEN GOLDEN DISCOVERIES AND THE ONE BASIC FORMULA WHICH REVEALS WHAT A HEALING ART MUST DO IN ORDER TO WORK.

1. As you gain a full understanding of the Seven Golden Discoveries and the basic formula presented in Session One, you will understand in detail why doctors are now using electrical devices to reverse previously-helpless patients of cerebral palsy, multiple sclerosis, polio and other spastic diseases.

2. You will be able to understand why doctors are using electricity to reverse the conditions that cause circulation problems and heal bones in weeks that would not heal in years.

3. You will also understand why medical pain clinics are now using electrical devices to reverse the conditions that cause pain in just a short period of time. With the seven golden discoveries and this formula, you will not only understand why these techniques work, but you will also know why and how you can help reverse the conditions that cause most pain by

XXV

yourself with the bio-electric lymphasizing techniques that are presented in Sessions Two and Four.

4. Chiropractors and Naprapaths have known for a long time that the muscles pull the bones out of place, but they have not known why. This book will not only help you understand why the muscles pull bones out of place in the neck and hips causing migraine headaches and lower back and sciatic nerve problems, but it will also help you understand the "self-help bio-electric lymphasizing techniques," which if used properly, will enable you to help reverse the conditions that cause these and other problems that may occur in your body.

5. With the formula which explains how the blood proteins produce the conditions that cause loss of energy, disease and death, we understand how and why herbs are able to help reverse pain and disease and how they speed up healing processes. We can also understand what causes the dark spots and other problems which appear in the iris of the eye which can be detected through Iridology. We can understand why naturopathic and the homeopathic remedies work and why zone therapy, reflexology, and color therapy can be used to reverse the conditions that cause pain and disease. In short, these discoveries help us to understand all of the healing arts. With this knowledge, we can actually teach what a healing art must do in order to work.

6. Most important of all, with this understanding, people will be able to comprehend the importance of the art of lymphasizing which reveals what man must do mentally, nutritionally, and physically to help raise up a posterity who will conquer disease and live in peace.

7. To comprehend the information presented in this book, it is necessary that you study it one session at a time. The paragraphs being numbered make it easy to cross reference and it makes this material easy to refer to and to teach.

SESSION I

A. THE BLOOD PROTEIN RESEARCH AND THE ART OF LYMPHASIZING ARE THE MOST IMPORTANT HEALTH DISCOVERIES SINCE THE BEGINNING OF MAN

1. Modern science deserves a lot of credit for the information contained in this book. As you will learn in this session, some of the newest, most modern medical and scientific discoveries known to man have made it possible for this family health education program to exist. Because of these discoveries, as you learn the concepts and apply the principles contained in this book, you will be taking one of the most important steps that you will ever take in learning what you must do to reverse the conditions that cause disease and to bring health and peace to your body.

2. Until mankind comes to understand in detail the principles and concepts concerning *the blood proteins* and *the art of lymphasizing,* they will remain in partial darkness as far as health and peace are concerned. We will prove through these new scientific discoveries that people can pray for peace from now on; and they will never have peace on earth until they learn to live the laws of health.

3. The laws of nature are the laws of God. Nature is no respecter of persons. No matter how righteous a person is if he breaks the mental, nutritional or physical laws of health, he will cause his own destruction. This new blood protein research will help convince every people on the face of the earth that they must obey the mental, nutritional, and physical laws of health and peace or suffer the consequences which are loss of energy, disease, death and war. If man learns that disobedience to a law will cause loss of energy, disease, and death, and if he willfully disobeys that law without any restraint, he is not only committing suicide, but will probably by his actions be instrumental in destroying others. Generally speaking "misery loves company." If he does not know that breaking a law will destroy him and he breaks it, he will be destroying himself and probably others along with him in ignorance. But either way he is being destroyed and is probably destroying others. Nature is no respecter of persons. If man puts his hand on a hot stove, he

1

gets burned. If he steps in front of a moving car, he gets hit. With an understanding of this blood protein research, anyone can know when they break a law that will cause trapped blood proteins because they will be able to feel it. No one will have to tell them what is right or wrong; they will know when they are being destroyed inside. They can feel it just as sure as they know they get burned when they put their hand on a hot stove.

4. It is interesting that Adam was told that he had to work all the days of his life. The average life span after retirement at present is approximately three to five years. The blood protein research reveals that inactivity will produce the conditions that cause pain, loss of energy, disease and death; and you will know why as you go through this book. We now know that to willfully be physically inactive is to willfully destroy ourselves.

5. These new discoveries also reveal that people are destroying themselves mentally and physically as well. They reveal that certain foods will trap the blood proteins in the spaces around the cells, and by doing so these foods are directly related to the conditions that cause heart disease, cancer, obesity, arthritis and the other crippling and killer diseases which are now slaying over 240,000 men, women, and children every two months in the United States along with thousands of others throughout the world.

6. When they dropped the atom bomb on Hiroshima, it took approximately 70,000 lives—and the people thought that was bad. In the United States alone, people are now being destroyed by the conditions produced from trapped blood proteins at the rate of approximately three atomic bombs every two months—that is eighteen atomic bombs per year.

7. Instead of being so concerned about the destruction that may be caused by war, we ought to be more concerned about the destruction that is now taking place due to trapped blood proteins in the bodies of men, women and children. This destruction is sounding in our ears with a voice loud enough to shake the earth. Those who believe that man can only be destroyed by war are being deceived, and even the best of people will continue to be destroyed by trapped blood proteins unless they pay attention to this research.

8. Before you finish reading this book, you will know why and how certain foods are directly related to the deaths of over 240,000 men, women and children every two months in this

country alone, and what you can do to help prevent this destruction world-wide.

9. These discoveries also reveal that this destruction is
related to the mental attitudes: that man is being destroyed
because he has not yet learned to be big enough to love his
enemies, bless those who curse him, and to do good to those who
hate him. We now know that only our adversary would say,
"Don't love your enemies, don't bless those who curse you,
don't do good to those who hate you, and above all, don't pray
for those who persecute you and despitefully use you."
Everyone will agree that God or good is symbolized by love, and
the adversary or evil is symbolized by hate. Everyone in the
whole world must decide to serve love or hate; and each person
becomes the servant of that which he chooses to obey.

10. As you come to understand these new scientific
discoveries you will come to know that the emotions that
accompany hate will produce the conditions also that cause loss
of energy, disease and death. This is scientific proof that the
same mental attitudes that will cause your death will also cause
war, and the same mental attitudes that are necessary to have
health are also necessary to have peace.

11. You will come to understand more and more as you go
through this course that there is a big difference between just
believing what you should do mentally, nutritionally, and
physically to stay well and *knowing* what you must do! You will
also realize that along with the knowledge and understanding of
these new scientific discoveries comes the faith that will enable
you to do those things mentally, nutritionally, and physically
that you could not do before.

12. Most people truly desire to have health and peace with
all their hearts. But look around and see how many have either
one. You won't have to look far. All you have to do is take a good
look at yourself.

A-1. A Promise To Those Who Learn The Principles And Apply
The Concepts Contained In This Book

1.1. Do you have the optimum health and peace you desire?
Do you have a desire for greater health and peace for your
family? Do you have a desire for greater health and peace in the

world? If you will apply the principles and concepts which you will learn as the result of the seven golden discoveries plus the basic formula, to the best of your ability, you will begin to realize the blessings of health and peace to a greater degree than you have ever dreamed possible. Peace on earth will come as families learn and apply the laws of health.

1.2. As you apply the concepts that you will learn in this course, you will come to know what I say is true because of what you will see taking place in your life and in the lives of your family members who apply them. This promise is too great to ignore, and the witness of whether this promise is true or false lies in what will take place in your life and also in the lives of all those among the nations of the earth who learn the concepts and apply the principles which are taught as a result of this new blood protein research.

B. THE SEVEN GOLDEN DISCOVERIES

1. The Golden Seven refers to these seven discoveries. *The Golden Seven Plus One* is the only book in the world that contains these seven discoveries in one place and it takes these seven discoveries along with the One Basic Formula to fully understand what man must do to conquer disease and live in peace.

2. Knowing that the soft and hard tissues and organs of the body are made up of cells, we also know that to have a crippling or killer disease or any kind of health problem something must produce the conditions in the body that will damage or kill the cells.

3. Listed here are the seven golden discoveries that, together with the formula I have mentioned, reveal the conditions that must exist in the body to produce totally healthy cells and show how the blood proteins produce the conditions that must take place in the body to damage or kill the cells.

I. Every cell generates "an electrical field." It is an actual "electrical generator."

1.1. The thought wave is electrical. The energy coming from the eyes is electrical. Muscles work by electrical impulses from the brain.

1.2. In essence, the human body is an electrical being, and our health, strength and endurance depend upon the energy currents that run through the body.

II. To keep the "electric generators" going, (1) the cells must have oxygen to convert glucose into energy, and (2) the potassium (K+) inside the cells must remain high and sodium (Na+) inside the cells must remain low.

2.1. If too much water gets on a crop, it will damage or kill the crop. The same thing holds true with the cells. Anything that will produce excess fluid and excess sodium (Na+) around the cells will cause them to "drown" from lack of oxygen and will upset the delicate sodium-potassium balance in and around the cells. Excess fluid or excess sodium around the cells will damage or kill the cells and cause the various health problems that man may experience.

III. To have healthy cells, the body must be able to maintain a negative sub-atmospheric pressure condition, or what is called a "dry" state where there is no excess fluid— only enough fluid to fill the crevices around the cells, and that is all.

3.1. Even under normal conditions, the normal pressure in the blood stream causes the blood proteins to *continually* seep through the tiny pores of the blood capillaries into the spaces around the cells.

3.2. There is not enough pressure in these spaces to push the blood proteins back through the tiny pores of the blood capillaries. Therefore, the blood proteins must be *continually* removed and returned to the blood stream via the lymphatic system. If the lymph system completely fails to function and the blood proteins get trapped throughout the body, they will produce the conditions that cause death within twenty-four hours; and trapped blood proteins can cause death in just a few hours.

(For example: The old Indian did not die sick if he could help it. When he felt it was his time to go, he said goodbye to his family and went to the burial grounds. There he found a place where he would sit down, not move, and breathe very shallowly. Within twenty-four hours he would be dead from the conditions caused by trapped proteins in his body. This method of dying works for anyone who tries it.)

IV. Trapped blood proteins attract excess sodium (Na+) and will pull water out of the blood stream to produce (1) excess fluids and (2) excess sodium (Na+) around the cells which are the conditions that will cause a lack of oxygen and will upset the delicate sodium-potassium balance in and around the cells which will cause loss of energy, disease and death at the cell level.

4.1. Lack of oxygen or excess sodium will reduce the electrical energy produced by the cells and will damage or kill them. Trapped blood proteins produce both of these conditions.

4.2. Trapped blood proteins throughout the body on a sudden extreme scale can cause death in just a few hours.

4.3. Death due to shock is actually death due to the conditions caused by trapped blood proteins on a sudden extreme scale.

4.4. Blood plasma is ninety-one percent water. One of the main purposes of the blood proteins, the albumin, the globulin and the fibrinogen, is to keep the water in the blood stream so the blood can deliver oxygen and nutrients to the cells.

4.5. Shock will dilate the tiny pores of the blood capillaries and allow the blood proteins and the water to leave the blood stream so fast that it causes the circulatory system to collapse. Shock can cause trapped proteins and death within just a few hours. Trapped blood proteins are the cause of death which results from traumatic or surgical shock following operations, severe burns, accidental injuries, and are the most common cause of death in modern warfare.

4.6. The research revealing how shock causes death was published in 1953, 1956, and 1960 editions of the Encyclopedia Americana. This was almost thirty years ago. This information is not in the 1970 or later editions. Why aren't we being told that death due to traumatic and surgical shock, etc. is in reality due to trapped blood proteins?

4.7. Trapped blood proteins on a moderate scale will produce the conditions at the cell level that can cause pain, inflammation, the viral infections, the bacterial infections, allergies, parasites, a continual loss of energy, heart disease, cancer, obesity, hypertension (high blood pressure), arthritis, multiple sclerosis, polio, cerebral palsy, and every other crippling and killer disease known to man.

4.8. To prevent and if possible reverse these problems, man must learn how to untrap the blood proteins and keep them circulating in the body via the lymphatic system. To do this he must learn the new science called, *The Art of Lymphasizing.*

V.   The complete Art of Lymphasizing is a new science that reveals the mental, nutritional and physical laws of health which man must obey to keep the blood proteins circulating via the lymphatic system.

5.1. Physical inactivity, poor mental attitudes, and poor nutrition will cause the blood proteins to become "trapped" which will produce any one or all of the above health problems.

5.2. A very important part of this art includes deep breathing and muscular movement, or the equivalent, which is necessary to actively move the lymphatic fluids. The equivalent of deep breathing and muscular movement involves the use of a Lymphasizer. To know how to use a Lymphasizer properly is like having a second set of lungs. To know how to use it bio-electrically, along with the other bio-electric lymphasizing techniques,, enables man to possibly reverse injury and disease. These techniques are explained in detail in Sessions Two, Three and Four.

5.3. A sudden loss of protein and water from the blood stream, as in shock, will cause thirst. Stress causes a shock-like effect on the body and so do certain foods. This is why stress and the "foods" that cause thirst are directly related to loss of energy, disease and death.

5.4. To completely master *the art of lymphasizing* we must know and obey the mental, nutritional, and physical laws that are necessary to keep the blood proteins circulating via the lymphatic system. Those who learn how to do this will help raise up a posterity who will conquer disease and have health, beauty, and peace.

VI. When trapped proteins reduce the energy field produced by the cells, they stick together or cluster which makes them very difficult to be removed by the lymphatic system.

   6.1.   When a person damages their finger or any other area of their body, the poisons from the damaged cells attack the capillaries and dilate the tiny pores and produce a sudden shock-like effect in that area. The result is trapped blood proteins. When they reduce the energy fields produced by the cells, they cluster and cause fluid retention, lack of oxygen, pain, etc.
   6.2.   Anyone who can explain in detail what causes fluid retention or swelling in smashed fingers or other areas of the body is able to explain the cause of pain, loss of energy, and every crippling or killer disease known to man.

VII. Trapped or clustered proteins can be dissipated or removed to help relieve pain, speed up the healing process and possibly reverse injury or disease by proper and correct use of the following: 1) various methods of electrical stimulation; 2) specialized services of a physician or surgeon; 3) various bio-electric lymphasizing techniques; 4) deep breathing techniques on and off of a Lymphasizer; 5) herbs; 6) the naturopathic remedies; 7) the homeopathic remedies; 8) chiropractics and other methods of physical therapy; 9) special diets, colonics, distilled water, fresh juices, or a food supplement that will help eliminate excess fluid along with the poisons and re-establish the delicate chemical balance in and around the cells; 10) color therapy; 11) zone therapy or reflexology and 12) other energy producing therapies.

   7.1.   Iridology, urine, saliva and other tests can be used to tell certain conditions of the body as the result of trapped blood proteins.
   7.2.   To summarize: No "trapped" blood proteins, no lasting pain, no loss of energy, and no diseases!

B-1.   Not Diagnosis Or Prescription

1.1. It is a scientific fact that our blood proteins can cause our death. These seven discoveries are based on seven years of constant research as to why and how the blood proteins cause death. I do not give these seven golden discoveries to diagnose or prescribe but to teach the cause of disease and death and what man must do to prevent and if possible reverse pain, loss of energy or disease in his body.

1.2. Anyone who acts upon these discoveries does so on his own by applying his own free agency. At this point in time these discoveries will not take the place of a surgeon or doctor, for there are times when specialized services are needed. But generally speaking, the doctor of the future, as Thomas Edison said, "will give no medicine but will interest (teach) his patients in the care of the human frame, diet, and in the cause and prevention of disease." And I now know that a person cannot completely fulfill the role of the doctor of the future without a knowledge of how the blood proteins produce the conditions that cause loss of energy and death at the cell level.

C. DR. WEST WRITES THE ONE BASIC FORMULA WHICH SHOWS HOW THE BLOOD PROTEINS PRODUCE THE CONDITIONS THAT CAUSE LOSS OF ENERGY, DISEASE, AND DEATH AT THE CELL LEVEL.

1. After researching for over six years to find the above seven discoveries, on this the 24th day of June, 1980, I, C. Samuel West, D.N., N.D., Chemist, and Lymphologist wrote the one basic formula which reveals how trapped blood proteins produce the conditions that cause loss of energy, disease and death at the cell level.

2. Below is an introduction to this scientific formula. I will start with a square to represent a totally healthy cell and then state the basic conditions that must be present in order to produce a healthy cell. Next, I will explain the basic conditions that will damage or kill the cell and then complete the formula by stating how the blood proteins are not only related, but are the prime cause of basic internal conditions that cause loss of energy, all diseases, and death at the cell level.

3. The formula is written in symbol form. Therefore, to help you read it, once we give the meaning of the symbol, you should say the complete meaning each time you see it. Then you

will be able to follow the steps easily that lead from a healthy cell to a damaged or dead cell. *If you do not fully understand the formula as it is presented here, do not be discouraged because this formula is explained later in the book, in layman's terms, in a manner that anyone of average intelligence can understand.*

D.   THE ONE BASIC FORMULA FOR LOSS OF ENERGY, DISEASE AND DEATH

1.   □ = Perfectly healthy cells = A perfectly healthy body = A peaceful body.

2.   ☒ = Damaged or dead cells = Loss of energy, disease and death.

3.   SCIENTIFIC FACT: If the life process of the cell is functioning properly, the cells will be perfectly healthy.

4.   LP = The normal Life Process of the cell = □

5.   SCIENTIFIC FACT: "The life process has been found to generate Electrical Fields in every organism that has been examined."

6.   EE = The Electric Energy produced by the Life Process of the cell.

7.   LP = EE = □

8.   SCIENTIFIC FACT: "The delicately balanced distribution of inorganic salts (minerals), in and around a living cell, whether plant or animal, accounts for its Electrical properties."

9.   DMB = The Delicate Mineral Balance *in* and *around* the cell.

10. SCIENTIFIC FACT: If we have the delicate mineral balance in and around the cell, the life process will be producing the electric energy necessary to produce a healthy cell.

11. DMB = LP = EE = □

12. SCIENTIFIC FACT: The Sodium-Potassium Pump is the rotation of the sodium single positive ions (Na+) and the potassium single positive ions (K+) in and out of the cell, which generates the Electrical Field produced by the Life Process of the cell. The main purpose of this pump is to bring potassium, calcium, iron, glucose, and other minerals and nutrients *into* the cell, and to pull any excess sodium *out* of the cell. This is the key to the life process and the Electrical Energy produced by healthy cells.

13. Na−K Pump = The Sodium-Potassium Pump = EE

14. Na−K Pump = DMB = LP = EE = □

15. SCIENTIFIC FACT: To keep the life process working, the potassium single positive ions (K+) inside the cell must remain high; the sodium single positive ions (Na+) inside the cell must remain low.

16. Na+, K+ = The delicate mineral balance of the sodium single positive ions (Na+) and the potassium single positive ions (K+) inside the cell.

17. Na+, K+ = Na−K Pump = DMB = LP = EE = □

18. ▲ = To alter, change, or upset.

19. SCIENTIFIC FACT: Anything that will change or upset the delicate balance of Na+ and K+ inside the cell will also change or upset the life processes and the Na−K Pump that brings minerals and nutrients *into* the cell, and this will damage the cell and cause *loss of energy, disease, and death.*

20. Therefore, ▲ Na+, K+ = ▲Na−K Pump = ▲DMB = ▲ LP = ▲EE = ⊠.

21. So in short: ▲ Na+, K+ = ▲ EE = ⊠.
    A change in the delicate sodium-potassium balance in the

cell will alter the electric energy produced by the cell and will damage or kill the cell.

22. Now, what would change the delicate sodium-potassium balance in the cell?

23. SCIENTIFIC FACT: Excess fluid or excess Na+ *outside* or *around* the cell will ▲ Na+, K+ *inside* the cell and will cause loss of energy, disease and death of the cell.

24. EX FL or EX Na+ = Excess fluid or excess sodium single positive ions *around* the cell.

25. Therefore, EX FL or EX Na+ = ▲Na+, K+ = ▲ Na−K Pump = ▲ DMB = ▲ LP = ▲ EE = ☒.

26. In short: EX FL or EX Na+ = ▲ EE = ☒.
Excess fluid or excess sodium single positive ions *around* the cell will alter the electric energy produced by the cell and will damage the cell and cause loss of energy, disease, and death of the cell.

27. Now, what is the basic cause of EX FL and EX Na+ *around* the cells? This is the key to the formula, and to the best of my knowledge, it has been hidden from science from the time of Adam and Eve until now.

28. SCIENTIFIC FACT: The answer is "trapped" plasma proteins *around* the cells. The proteins that make up part of the blood plasma carry a negative charge. If these proteins get "trapped" in the spaces around our cells, they will cause fluid retention and pull the positive sodium ions to them.

29. TPP = Trapped Plasma Proteins around the cells.

30. TPP = EX FL and EX Na+ = ▲Na+, K+ = ▲ Na−K Pump = ▲ DMB = ▲ LP = ▲ EE = ☒.

31. In short, The Basic Formula for loss of energy, disease, and death is:

$$TPP = EX\ FL\ and\ EX\ Na+\ =\ \blacktriangle\ EE\ =\ \boxtimes.$$

32.   I give this basic formula to show that TPP on a *moderate* scale will produce the conditions that will cause pain, loss of energy, and every disease known to man. On an *extreme* scale as in shock, TPP can collapse the circulatory system and cause death within a few hours.

E.   *AT THE 8TH INTERNATIONAL CONGRESS, DR. WEST ALSO PRESENTED "THE BASIC FORMULA FOR LIFE" WHICH SHOWS THE CONDITIONS THAT MUST EXIST TO HAVE A HEALTHY BODY*

1.   On this, the 24th day of June, 1980, I, C. Samuel West, D.N., N.D., Chemist, and Lymphologist, wrote the basic formula for a healthy cell which is:

$$No\ TPP = No\ EX\ FL\ or\ EX\ Na+\ =\ EE\ =\ \square.$$

2.   According to this formula: No trapped blood proteins, no excess sodium, no loss of energy, and no diseases.

3.   Theoretically, the cells could live forever, but every law man breaks, mentally, nutritionally, or physically, will trap the blood proteins and produce the internal conditions that cause loss of energy, disease, and death.

E-1.   *The Above Seven Discoveries And This One Basic Formula Have Produced A Scientific Message For Health And Peace That Will Grow To Fill The Whole World.*

1.1.   With these discoveries and this basic formula we can prove that the same mental attitudes that will cause loss of energy, disease and death will also cause war. We can also prove that the same mental attitudes that are necessary to have health are also necesssary to have peace.

1.2.   The knowledge of these seven golden discoveries and this basic formula have given birth to a new science called, *The Art of Lymphasizing.* This new science reveals what man must do mentally, nutritionally, and physically to conquer disease and have peace on earth.

F. THESE SEVEN GOLDEN DISCOVERIES AND THIS ONE BASIC FORMULA REVEAL WHAT A HEALING ART MUST DO IN ORDER TO WORK. THE MIRACLES OF SCIENCE ARE NOW REVEALED.

1. These seven golden discoveries plus this one basic formula will enable the whole world to understand the cause of every crippling and killer disease known to man and what must happen in the body for healing to take place. Once you understand the cause, you will also understand how to prevent and possibly reverse disease. You will also understand how to help relieve pain and possibly reverse injury.

2. $E = MC^2$ is the formula for the theory of relativity. E is energy. MC^2 is mass multiplied by the speed of light squared. This formula made it possible to create the bombs which can physically *destroy* the world. In contrast, TPP = EX FL and EX Na+ = $\blacktriangle$ EE = $\boxtimes$ is the formula which reveals that T̲rapped P̲lasma P̲roteins in the spaces around the cells will produce E̲xcess F̲luid and E̲xcess S̲odium S̲ingle P̲ositive I̲ons which are the conditions that will cause $\blacktriangle$ EE (loss of energy) and $\boxtimes$ (disease and death at the cell level). This formula will help prevent and if possible reverse the crippling and killer diseases. This will bring health and peace and thus help save the world.

3. These seven golden discoveries and this formula reveal that the human body is an electrical being; that every cell is an actual chemical electrical generator; and they show how trapped blood proteins produce the conditions that will upset the chemical balance, shut the generators off, and damage or kill the cell. They also reveal that electricity and other sources of energy can dissipate the trapped blood proteins and reverse the conditions that cause pain, loss of energy, and disease; and healing can take place faster than we have ever dreamed possible.

4. This knowledge helps us to understand that any healing art that works must somehow be able to dissipate the trapped blood proteins which produce the conditions that shut the electrical generators off to damage or kill the cell.

5. This knowledge has given birth to a new science called *The Art of Lymphasizing.* With the understanding of this new science anyone will be able to know what they can do to prevent and if possible reverse the conditions that cause pain, loss of

energy, and disease. With this knowledge, we can understand why electrical devices are used in some hospitals, medical schools, and pain clinics to help relieve pain, reverse disease, and speed up the healing process. Electricity dissipates trapped blood proteins and turns the generators on at the cell level and healing takes place; and sometimes it happens fantastically fast.

6. Dr. Joseph Waltz at the St. Barnabas Hospital in New York is using Spinal Cord Electrical Stimulation to reverse the conditions that cause cerebral palsy, multiple sclerosis, polio, and other spastic diseases. Three out of four previously helpless patients are receiving dramatic results.

7. Floyd Weston is involved with Dr. Fuller Royal at the Nevada Clinic of Preventive Medicine in Las Vegas where they are diagnosing electrically with the dermatron machine and treating with the homeopathic remedies that work on the principle of energy frequency levels which is a form of electricity. They are having such fantastic results that they are booked months in advanced. I will discuss these centers more later.

8. A woman from China told this author that they have known for thousands of years that herbs work electrically, and that they know exactly which part of the herb goes to which organ; but it is all written in Chinese. This helps to explain why herbs and the naturopathic remedies work.

9. As stated earlier, in order for a healing art to work, it has to have the ability, one way or another, to dissipate the blood proteins and turn the generators on at the cell level. Everything must work on the principle of energy. Where there is no energy, there is no life.

10. Those who practice iridology can tell where the problems are in the body that are being caused by trapped blood proteins in various organs or parts of the body. As the trapped blood proteins produce the conditions that interfere with the life process of the cells and the generators begin to shut off, it shows up in the iris of the eye. This is why those who are skilled in the practice of this art can give the appropriate herb, naturopathic remedy, homeopathic remedy, etc., and over a period of time watch the healing lines appear in the eye.

11. The new knowledge concerning the electrical meridians in the body helps explain how acupuncture, zone therapy, and reflexology work.

12. Knowing that colonics, special enemas, special diets,

distilled water, fresh juices or a mineral supplement will help remove the poisons that will cause trapped blood proteins and also help reestablish the proper chemical balance in and around the cells helps to explain why and how they work.

13. As you come to understand the seven golden discoveries and the one basic formula presented in this book it will help you understand all of the healing arts.

14. One of the most exciting things this research will help you to understand is the *new self help bio-electric* (electrostatic) *lymphasizing techniques* which enables a person to understand how to untrap his own blood proteins and cause healing to take place in his own body in ways which have been impossible to understand until now. With these techniques, people are relieving pain and reversing injury from smashed fingers and turned ankles, etc. within minutes.

15. Details on the cause of disease and the basic bio-electric lymphasizing techniques are presented in Session Two and the advanced bio-electric lymphasizing techniques are presented in Session Three and Four of this book. But to understand them requires the knowledge of the seven golden discoveries and this basic formula.

16. This research also reveals that to have lasting satisfactory results with any of the healing arts requires that we have a complete understanding of *the art of lymphasizing*. This new science explains in detail what man must do mentally, nutritionally, and physically to keep the blood proteins circulating in the body via the lymphatic system. When man masters the art of lymphasizing, he will conquer disease and live in peace. *The art of lymphasizing* is explained in detail in Session Three.

17. To comprehend the information presented in this book, it is necessary that you study it one session at a time. The paragraphs being numbered make it easy to cross reference and it makes this material easy to refer to and to teach.

G. *INTRODUCING A NEW SCIENCE CALLED "THE ART OF LYMPHASIZING" WHICH REVEALS WHAT CAUSES TRAPPED PLASMA PROTEINS (TPP) AROUND THE CELLS.*

1. The most important role that will be played by this new blood protein research is that it will enable man to understand *the art of lymphasizing* which reveals the priceless relationship between health and peace.

2. To completely understand what causes the blood proteins to become trapped around the cells and how to prevent it is the purpose of this course. Once you fully understand the principles and concepts involved in *The Seven Golden Discoveries* and how they apply to this *One Basic Formula*, you will understand in detail what causes the blood proteins to become trapped and what you must do mentally, nutritionally, and physically, to help prevent and possibly reverse the conditions that cause pain, loss of energy, the crippling and killer diseases and other afflictions of the body. In essence you will understand what you must do to master *the art of lymphasizing.*

3. Those who have this knowledge and apply it will be able to help raise up a posterity who can not only "run and not be weary, and walk and not faint," but will also exist in peace.

4. To help prepare you for the next two sessions, where you will learn in detail how trapped blood proteins produce the conditions that cause our various health problems, and what you can do to untrap them and keep them circulating in the body, let's briefly consider the concepts that we have presented in *The Seven Golden Discoveries* and *The Basic Formula.*

5. *The Basic Formula is:*

$$TPP = EX\ FL\ or\ EX\ Na+\ =\ \blacktriangle\ EE\ =\ \boxtimes.$$

According to this basic formula, *anything* that will trap the blood proteins in the spaces around the cells will also cause excess fluid and excess sodium in the spaces around the cells, reduce the electric energy produced by the cells and will damage or kill the cells.

6. With this basic information, you are ready to be introduced to the mental, nutritional, and physical laws of health which man must obey to prevent trapped blood proteins in his body. If he breaks these laws, his problems will begin with loss of energy, but they may progress into one or more of the crippling or killer diseases, death and even war.

G-1. The Mental Laws Of Health And Trapped Plasma Protein.

1.1. Stress will cause loss of energy in your body. In fact, it is well known that stress is one of the main causes of the crippling and killer diseases. Why? Because stress produces a shock-like effect on the body. And so does worry, fear, anger, loss of temper, holding grudges, and resentment.

1.2. The reason these attitudes produce the conditions that cause loss of energy, disease, and death is that they trap the blood proteins in the spaces around the cells. As the blood proteins become trapped, your body goes somewhere between a healthy state and a dead state. Where do you think you are right now? Are you satisfied with the condition you are in, or do you want to improve your condition?

1.3. As you learn what must be done to "untrap" your blood proteins and bring energy and health back into your body, make a commitment to begin right now to *apply what you learn* into your life and into the lives of your loved ones.

1.4. With the knowledge of the seven golden discoveries and the basic formula, if you are not willing to make this commitment, you will continue to not only destroy yourself, but your actions will possibly cause the destruction of others. True or False?

1.5. One of the purposes of this course is to encourage you to make this commitment and then help you keep it. As we go through these sessions, your understanding will become greater and greater, and your commitment to do those things that will bring health and peace to you, and to your friends and loved ones will become stronger and stronger. Let's take another look at the negative emotions that can cause the blood proteins to become trapped in your body.

1.6. If anger, loss of temper, holding grudges, and resentment will trap the blood proteins and cause loss of energy, sickness and death to you and those around you, what are you going to have to learn to do with your enemies? The answer to this question reveals the mental laws of health. You must learn to be big enough to actually *love* your enemies, to *bless* those who curse you, to *do good* to those who hate you, and, if possible, to *pray* for those who persecute you and despitefully use you.

1.7. If you will truly make an effort to do this, it will help establish peace and harmony in your life and the lives of your family. The laws of health are also the laws of peace! To have a truly healthy body, you must learn to live in peace.

1.8. This is a revealing concept. If people throughout the world were to make the commitment to love, bless and do good, *it would be an absolute possibility to conquer disease and establish peace throughout the world.*

1.9. You can now see why we refer to this course as "The World-Wide Family Health Education Program" and why it is also called "The World-Wide Family Self-H.E.L.P. Program," with the H.E.L.P. standing for Health Education for Longevity and Peace.

1.10. Would you like to see every family in the whole world learn what you have learned about health and peace? If this were all there was to this program, it would be worth it. But, you are just beginning to understand the principles and concepts concerning the blood protein research. As we go along, it is going to get better and better. I know that is hard to believe, but the knowledge of these seven golden discoveries and this basic formula has given us a much deeper understanding of the laws of health than ever before.

G-2. *The Nutritional Laws And Trapped Plasma Proteins.*

2.1. You are now ready to be introduced to the principles and concepts concerning good nutrition. As you see how foods fit into the basic formula, for most of you, it is going to revolutionize your whole nutritional program. The beautiful thing of it is that you are going to want to change your nutritional program and you will enjoy it while you do it. Why? Because, as you have learned, when you put stress on your body, it causes trapped plasma proteins.

2.2. Therefore, so as not to cause stress on your bodies, we are going to give you a "transition program." Let's just introduce the nutritional program at this time and then those of you who need to can learn to improve as time goes on.

2.3. If certain "foods" can trap your blood proteins, should they be labeled as a food or as a poison? Now, don't get alarmed with this language. Remember what I said about stress! As you learn that something is a poison, and you find that it has increasingly become your diet, that you are now entrenched with it and that you are completely caught up in using it as though it were a good food, then *you must make whatever adjustments you need to make in a manner that will not cause stress upon your body.*

2.4. We call this process the "transition program," and you will learn more about this in Session Three.

2.5. Now, are you ready to commit yourselves to do whatever you have to, in a transitional way, to stop taking anything into your bodies that you come to know—beyond a shadow of a doubt—will cause trapped proteins, excess fluid and sodium, and the resulting loss of energy that every one of us is experiencing to one degree or another? Are you ready, right now, to make this commitment?

2.6. I know that it's a tough one. When you start talking of food or other things that you have been taking into your body that you enjoy, the very thought of giving them up causes stress. Therefore, we are not going to ask you to give up everything all at one time. Instead, let's do it transitional style.

2.7. Most of you know that certain things such as alcohol, tobacco, certain teas, coffee, cola, and other drinks containing caffeine are not good for your body. As we go along, you will learn that *anything* that damages a cell will cause trapped proteins, excess fluid and sodium, and will produce a deeper state of loss of energy, sickness, and death, in your body; but right now let's look at some substances that most people in our society have been brought up to believe are foods, but instead are deadly poisons to the body.

2.8. When you feed your dog strychnine, the first thing the dog goes for is water. We will go into this in more detail during the next two sessions, but this is enough to get us going in the right direction.

2.9. Remember, water in the blood stream follows the blood proteins. *"Trapped" proteins will pull water out of the blood stream and make you thirsty.* In fact, medical charts show that as a result of "trapped" plasma protein and the resulting fluid retention, people *who have a loose cellular structure* can gain 24-48-72-96 pounds, and more, very quickly.

2.10. You will understand, as we go along, the possible reasons why some people retain more fluid in their body from trapped proteins than others. And when you understand this concept, you will then know what you have believed for a long time: that the thin guy who has a tight cellular structure can have just as much trapped proteins in his body and can be just as sick as the big guy with a loose cellular structure. We will explain this in detail in Session Three.

2.11. With this introduction, let's discuss what foods make you thirsty. What are they? Salt, fats, the red meats, and the high cholesterol foods (such as the animal and dairy products) and sugar. By sugar we mean the simple sugars in cakes, ice cream, and so forth—not the complex sugars in fruits, vegetables and whole grains (seeds and grains are easier to assimilate in sprouted form.)

2.12. Think about it. When you eat that big meal that makes you thirsty, what happens to your energy levels? Are they up or down? With the knowledge of the basic formula showing how trapped proteins cause loss of energy, you realize that you just ate one or more poisons. And further investigation proves that they are actually physically and mentally addicting drugs.

2.13. I now want to emphasize *the transition process* that we talked about where we try to obey the mental laws of health while we improve our nutritional program. Transition requires a lot of wisdom.

2.14. How many of you can commit yourselves, right now, to begin your transition program by staying off salt and sugar during this next week—with the understanding that if you get such a "strong craving" for it that you can't stand it, you will be permitted to have some? Also, in light of *the stress factors,* if you decide to "have a ball" and use a little salt or sugar once or twice this week, *we want you to enjoy it!* Why? Because taking the salt or sugar is bad enough; if eating it causes you stress, it will increase the amount of trapped blood proteins in your body which makes what you are eating more harmful. Therefore, if you are going to eat it, *enjoy it, "lap it up." It may begin to make you sick later, but enjoy it when you do it!*

2.15. Transition is not a diet—it is a "new way of life." Believe it or not, as you begin to stay off the salt, sugar, and other foods most of the time, the trapped proteins, the excess fluid, the excess sodium and the old poisons begin to come out. The sodium-potassium balance becomes reestablished in the cells, the generators begin to turn on, and your energy levels will go up. Therefore, your health, strength and endurance will increase. The more you eat right, the better you will feel; and the better you feel, the more you can eat right. In a few months your whole body chemistry will begin to change and your desire to "have a ball" will come less often and finally your body will begin to reject the foods that make you say, "Yuk, yuk, yuk, water, water, water, trapped protein, excess fluid, and excess sodium shuts my generators off."

G-3. *The Physical Laws And Trapped Plasma Proteins*

3.1. How many of you would like to run and not be weary and walk and not faint?

3.2. You may not believe at this time that this is possible, but before these next two sessions are over, if you will apply the principles and concepts that are taught in this book, as you learn them, you will come to know that this almost impossible dream may be within your grasp.

3.3. To help prepare you for the new "run and not be weary, walk and not faint lymphasizing program" that I am going to teach you in Session Three that makes it possible for people to "run and not be weary and walk and not faint," I want you to begin a basic lymphasizing program now. This is a totally "new approach" to exercise that all of you can do to one degree or another, even if you are in a wheelchair. And you can never tell, with the bio-electric lymphasizing techniques we are going to teach you in Sessions Two, Three and Four, maybe before the race is over the person in the wheelchair could be running longer than anyone else.

3.4. With the things I have seen, it is hard to tell what can or will take place in your body when the "trapped" proteins come out and the excess fluid and excess sodium come out and the generators begin to turn on.

3.5. Muscles work by electrical impulses from the brain. Trapped blood proteins shut our generators off and cause crippling diseases.

3.6. Before this course is over, you are going to understand in detail how Peary Barker, who could not walk for more than two-and-a-half to three minutes at a time for a period of two years, was able to reverse the condition that caused his problem and walked without pain within forty-eight hours after applying the principles and concepts presented in this book. The doctors told him that his condition was incurable; and if they were to operate on him, he would become an invalid.

3.7. You will also come to understand how a lady, who had been on crutches for ten years with arthritis and was on the couch crying in pain when I saw her, was able within thirty minutes to sit up and cross her legs back and forth, shouting for joy, and was able, within the next thirty minutes, to stand up and walk around the house without pain and without crutches. To the amazement of her family, the condition that caused her arthritis was reversed in about one hour right before our eyes.

3.8. The bio-electric lymphasizing techniques that were used to reverse these conditions are almost miracle techniques. They are based upon the knowledge of the principles and concepts contained in the seven golden discoveries and the basic formula. As you go through this text, you will come to know and understand in detail why Peary Barker was able to get himself out of pain in twenty-four hours and why this lady was able to get up and walk without pain in one hour. You will also understand what took place in their bodies that made it possible to reverse the conditions that caused their problems.

3.9. You will also come to understand the story of Dorothy Howard of Seattle, Washington. She had polio when she was about ten months old which left her crippled with pain. Her left leg was paralyzed. When she was sixty-five years old, she attended one of my lectures and learned about the bio-electric lymphasizing techniques and the mental, nutritional, and physical concepts that made it possible for her to reverse these conditions. In about four months she was able to walk with very little pain, if any—with her heel on the floor for the first time in her life. For the first time since her illness, the feeling began to return to her previously-paralyzed leg, and she was able to move her toes—which before had been uncontrollable.

3.10. These stories may sound like miracles to you at this time—but be assured, they are not. All these people did to reverse their disease was to learn what they had to do to get the trapped blood proteins out, the excess fluid and excess sodium out, and get their generators turned on.

3.11. Let me ask you a question: In light of the seven golden discoveries and the formula, if you could get all the generators turned on in all the cells of your body, would you be healthy or sick? Is it that simple? Yes—*it is just that simple!* Yet there is not a college or university in the world teaching it. And if you're truly healthy, you will have peace. Keep this peace concept in mind; we will be expanding on it later.

3.12. Now, in order to prevent disease and to prepare your

body for the things you are going to learn in the following sessions, I want you to begin a basic lymphasizing program. As I said, this is a new approach to exercise and everyone, no matter what condition they are in, can do it to one degree or another. You will come to learn the value of lymphasizing more and more as we go through this course.

3.13. I received the idea for this basic lymphasizing program from Dr. Walker, (the juice man) who lives in Phoenix, Arizona. It is estimated that he is approximately 116 or 117 years old. The reason I do not know exactly how old he is, is because when I asked him, he said, "I'm ageless." And that is all I could get out of him on the subject. However, when my wife and I spent four and a half very choice hours with this wonderful man, he looked good. Many know him as the doctor who writes the "juice books." He is very well known in the health field, and his little wife looks just as sweet and wonderful as he does.

3.14. When we discussed the transition program that we have been talking about, he said, "I like that program! You tell them about transition."

3.15. He gave me a copy of all his books which he personally autographed. Then as we were walking out the driveway to the car, for some reason or other he said, "I want to show you an exercise I do once or twice a day which really invigorates me."

3.16. When he showed it to me, I was thrilled because it contained two parts, and the first part was one of the easiest and simplest that I had ever seen. It was one that everybody could do. Not only that, it was an exercise that I knew would actively move the lymphatic system and help remove the trapped proteins. When I saw him do it, I got so excited that I said, "Dr. Walker, with the knowledge of our blood proteins, I am going to make that walk famous!" I have called this exercise "The Walker-West-Walk Lymphasizing Program." Children like to call it the "Choo-Choo Train Walker-West-Walk."

3.17. This is the way the first part goes: Using the "SHHH" sound, inhale as deeply as you can, exhale as deeply as you can in the following manner: inhale, exhale, inhale, exhale, inhale, exhale, exhale, exhale, completely emptying your lungs by the last exhale. Repeat this process over and over again. You may alternate by doing this: inhale, inhale, inhale, inhale, exhale, exhale, exhale, exhale.

3.18 The second part deals with the arms and legs (for those who are able to do so): swing your arms and step lively and, as you do this, add the first part. Do not do the first part more than once or twice to begin with because some of you may get woozy and light-headed from taking a few deep breaths. If this happens, do not be alarmed. All that means is that you need it badly. You will understand this in more detail as you continue through this text. All you need to understand at this time is that we want you to begin this basic lymphasizing program using the transition approach. As with the nutrition program, you must understand that the more you do it, the better you will feel and the better you feel, the more you will be able to do it.

3.19. Why is this statement true? Because the lungs act as a "suction pump" for the lymphatic system. Deep breathing will help remove the trapped proteins and turn your generators on. In the next session we will go through "The College of Cause and Self-Help Pain Relief," and we will discuss in detail the relationship between our blood proteins and our lymphatic system.

3.20. Let me just ask this question. When Adam and Eve came out of the garden with blood (which included the blood proteins) going through their veins, the Lord told them they had to work—all the days of their lives. Was there a retirement program built in that? Did the Lord say, "Adam, you can go for a certain period of time and then sit in the chair and take it easy? No! With the knowledge of the seven golden discoveries and the basic formula, anyone who goes into retirement is committing willful suicide.

3.21. I will go into this in more detail later. Right now, to help keep the blood protein circulating in the body via the lymphatic system, you must commit yourself to do this basic lymphasizing program until you can do it longer and longer without getting dizzy.

3.22. Okay, Let's try it! Stand up! Get the deep breathing going: inhale, exhale, inhale, exhale, inhale, exhale, exhale, exhale. Now if you can, add the arm and leg movements. Step as lively as you can and swing the arms, but do not get tired or cause any negative stress on your body. If you get tired or cause any negative effects on your body, you are exercising, not lymphasizing. Remember, "the more you are able to do it the better you will feel; and the better you feel, the more you will be able to do it." This concept applies to your commitment to the mental and nutritional programs as well.

H. REVIEW OF SESSION ONE

1. Now, before we end this session, let's review the commitments you have made which will enable you to help reverse pain, loss of energy or disease.

2. Mentally, beginning today, you are going to try to increase your ability to *love* your enemies, *bless* those who curse you, *do good* to those who hate you, and *pray* for those who persecute and despitefully use you.

3. Nutritionally, beginning today, you are going to go off salt and the simple sugars using the transition program. Substitute maple syrup, unsulphured Grandma's Molasses, or honey for regular table sugar; and kelp, Jensen's vegetable seasoning, broth, or Bio-salt for regular table salt. (Note: The Bio-salt label has not been approved by the F.D.A. in the United States. For more information on Bio-salt, contact the following company in Canada: The Biochemic Centre, R.R. No. 1, Anola, Manitoba, Canada, ROE OAO.) Get ready, because as your knowledge and understanding increases, as it will in the next session, you will have a desire to expand your commitment to exclude other foods that will also cause the blood proteins to become trapped.

4. Now, what are you going to begin to do physically? You are going to do the Walker-West-Walk and increase the number of times and the length of time you do it, as you feel like it. This is the basic lymphasizing program, and it must be done as often as possible during the day. But do not cause stress or fatigue. Keep your body feeling like you are sitting in a chair. Remember, the more you apply these mental, nutritional, and physical laws, the better you will feel—and the better you feel, the more you will be able to apply them.

5. According to the formula for loss of energy, disease and death, the key to healing in the body starts with an "E." The word is Endurance! As your endurance increases, you will know that you are reversing disease and healing is taking place in your body.

SESSION II

The College of Cause and Self-Help Pain Relief

A. INTRODUCTION

1. This session presents the theories and concepts based upon the seven golden discoveries and the basic formula, which has developed into what we call "The College of Cause and Self-Help Pain Relief." In this session we go into detail concerning the *cause* of inflammation, pain, loss of energy, and the crippling and killer diseases, and into what must happen in the body to reverse these conditions and cause healing to take place. We also include several illustrations and explanations of the basic bio-electric self-help pain relief techniques, which teaches how you can help relieve pain and speed up the healing processes. As you continue to understand the complete meaning and the importance of the seven golden discoveries, which we have discussed, you will come to know more and more as time goes on that the formula, which reveals the conditions that must exist in the body to produce healthy cells and what must take place to damage or kill them, is correct. And with this knowledge, a change will take place in your life that will be a blessing to you and your loved ones far beyond anything you can now comprehend.

2. Before you go through this session take time to think about and evaluate the emotional, nutritional, and physical concepts that we talked about in Session One.

3. How have you been doing? Have you tried to increase your ability to love, bless, and do good?

4. What have you been doing about salt and the simple sugars? Have you started to make progress in this area? Have you been doing the Walker-West-Walk Lymphasizing Program? If so, have you been able to increase the number of times and the length of time that you have been able to do it? Remember, don't cause stress or fatigue. Do it only as you enjoy it. The more you do it, the better you will feel; and the better you feel, the more you will be able to do it.

5. In this session, you will receive information that will give you a desire to increase your efforts in all of these areas.

B. THE PURPOSE OF THIS SESSION IS NOT TO DIAGNOSE OR PRESCRIBE

1. The information presented in this session is not given to diagnose, treat, or prescribe, nor to take the place of your physician or even suggest that you do anything contrary to his counsel.

2. The purpose of this session is to increase your understanding of the new blood protein research and the new science called The Art of Lymphasizing so you can more fully comprehend the basic principles and concepts of life that deal with the *care* of our human frame; *diet;* the *cause* of disease; and what we must do mentally, nutritionally, and physically to *prevent* and if possible *reverse* disease. And last, but not least, the blood protein research will help establish peace throughout the world, beginning with you and your family.

C.   GRATEFUL TO MEDICAL RESEARCH FOR MAJOR DISCOVERIES

1. We are grateful for the knowledge that has been given to us by medical science and the scientists throughout the world. Without the basic knowledge that has come to them, it would be absolutely impossible for us to be discussing the seven golden discoveries and the basic formula, which enables us to teach blood protein research in its power and simplicity. Without the great doctors and scientists who made the seven golden discoveries, the formula, which is the foundation of this program, would not exist.

2. We would like to thank Dr. Shields of California, for producing the film "The Central Propulsion of Human Thoracic Duct Lymph." This film erases all doubt as to what a person must do to actively move the lymphatic fluids. Unless we engage in an activity that causes us to breathe deeply, we will have trapped plasma proteins in our bodies regardless of whatever else we may do. You will learn more and more as time goes on that deep breathing cannot be replaced by anything as far as the health of your body is concerned.

*C-1. The Following Medical Research Concerning Blood Proteins
And Death Will Revolutionize The World*

1.1. To begin with, let's look at the *Textbook of Medical Physiology* by Arthur C. Guyton. Without the information he has published in this text, this program would not have even had its beginning. (I saw Dr. Guyton in Florence, Italy, in October and November of 1979 at the Seventh International Congress of Lymphology. He is one of the kindest and most gentle individuals I have ever met.)

1.2. I have also been in the home of Dr. H. S. Mayerson in New Orleans. He lectured for Dr. Guyton in his classes on the lymphatic system before 1961. In October 1979 the American Physiology Society held a convention in New Orleans. At this convention several hours were taken to honor Dr. Mayerson. He was one of the first men in the United States to teach information concerning our lymphatic system. He is another man I admire and respect. His report entitled "The Lymphatic System" (found in the June 1963 issue of *Scientific American*) is *priceless*.

1.3. Dr. Guyton published (in 1961) the second edition of the *Textbook of Medical Physiology*, which was put in my hands in 1974 by Mr. Chase, who taught Biology at Westwood High School in Mesa, Arizona. When I opened this medical text, little did I know or realize that I was going to read about some new scientific discoveries that will make it possible for us to eventually conquer disease. The blood protein research will turn the current medical doctors into teachers of health, as well as being able to take care of those who need special attention.

1.4. In June of 1980, I called a doctor in Idaho. I had been conversing with him on several occasions prior to this call concerning some of the principles and concepts pertaining to the lymphatic system and blood proteins. On this occasion, he said that there are many doctors in Germany and Austria who are using the concepts concerning our blood proteins and lymphatic system to help people and that, in the United States, we are about one hundred years behind in this area. In China and other countries doctors are treating cancer with herbs, and with the age of electrical acupuncture, operations are being performed without drugs or anesthetics.

1.5. With this background I am going to quote the medical

research which reveals what I believe is the most important scientific discovery concerning our bodies since the time of Adam and Eve. I learned about it in 1974, and this discovery along with six others that I learned about later enabled me to write *THE ONE BASIC FORMULA* on June 24, 1980.

1.6.   I will now read from page 397 in the fifth edition of *The Textbook of Medical Physiology,* by Dr. Arthur C. Guyton. This discovery will not only revolutionize much of the world, but it is the discovery that the art of lymphasizing is based upon. Here it is:

> The lymphatic system represents an accessory route by which fluids can flow from the interstitial spaces (the spaces around the cells) back into the blood. And, most important of all, the lymphatics can carry (blood) proteins and large particulate matter (dead cells and other toxic materials) away from the tissue spaces, neither of which can be removed by absorption directly into the blood capillary.

Now read this next sentence carefully because this is the statement that is responsible for this entire program:

> We shall see that this removal of (blood) proteins from the interstitial spaces (by our lymphatic system) IS AN ABSOLUTELY ESSENTIAL FUNCTION WITHOUT WHICH WE WOULD DIE WITHIN ABOUT TWENTY-FOUR HOURS!

1.7.   This is the scientific research which states that there is a substance in our blood stream which can cause our death within twenty-four hours. And whether all scientists believe it or not, *this discovery confirms the Biblical account of Adam and Eve.*

1.8.   In the Garden, according to the Bible, Adam and Eve would have lived forever had they not broken the command-ment that was given them that they should not partake of the "tree of knowledge of good and evil." It was eating a food that caused their sorrow and death. Can't you just hear the adversary say, "This food is delicious to the taste and very desirable, but it won't kill you!" After they partook of that food, a change took place in their bodies, and the life-giving substance that was flowing through their veins after that time contained something that caused them to die. They soon received a knowledge of what the blood proteins could do to their body. Life, and now death, were both a part of their blood stream! To have a knowledge of our blood proteins is to have a knowledge of sorrow and death. Anything that will trap the blood protein in the spaces around our cells will cause both.

1.9. The blood, which is 91% water, carries oxygen and nutrients to the cells which they must continually receive without obstruction if they are to remain healthy and strong. Anything that will interfere with this "irrigation" process or the other life processes that take place within the cell will damage or kill the cell and be the cause of inflammation, pain, loss of energy, and all the other discomforts and afflictions that we may experience.

1.10. The only substance that can interfere with the irrigation process where the cells receive oxygen and nutrients and with other life processes within the cell is the proteins that make up part of our blood plasma. The plasma proteins are the albumins, the globulins, and fibrinogens.

1.11. Until this discovery was made, it was believed our blood proteins were too big to come through the tiny pores of the capillary membranes into the spaces around our cells. Therefore, there was no reason for medical science to even concern itself with the idea that man's own blood proteins could be the cause of the afflictions and the misery that he was experiencing in his body.

C-2. Only "A Handful" Know That Our Blood Proteins Can Cause Death

2.1. To this date, there are only a handful of people in the world who know anything about this blood protein research. Therefore, when medical science came across conditions taking place in the body that they could not explain, the conditions were described as "causes unknown." Due to medical science's lack of knowledge concerning our blood proteins, we have many names that have been attached to conditions in the body for which there has been absolutely no explanation given as to why they occur or as to what can be done to prevent them.

2.2. Who would have ever believed that our crippling and killer diseases, and all the afflictions that man is experiencing (which include contention and war), are caused by breaking the mental, nutritional and physical laws that will cause our blood proteins to become trapped in the spaces around our cells?

2.3. You have just learned that once your blood proteins get into the spaces around your cells, they must be removed by your lymphatic system or they could cause your death within about twenty-four hours. The research concerning shock reveals how the blood proteins could cause death in just a few hours.

C-3.   It Is Not "Just That Simple"

3.1. People say to me, "I just can't believe it is that simple." To this I reply, it is not "just that simple." Without the knowledge of the seven golden discoveries and the basic formula the information contained in this book would be impossible to comprehend. And to get these discoveries it took a young man who came into my home in 1958 seven years to become a coach; after which, three years later, he and his wonderful wife came back into my life and made it possible for me to go back to school. Then after obtaining a pre-med background and a degree in chemisty, it took me seven years of teaching chemistry (during which time I obtained a masters degree in Public School Administration and a doctors degree in the natural healing arts) before I learned enough to even come close to comprehend this discovery, even after I had read about it. Then I had to teach the blood protein research for about seven years before I obtained enough information to write this book. I obtained the last two of the seven golden discoveries in February 1980 while training to become a naturopathic physician which took 30 hours a month for a year and a half. With this knowledge, I wrote the formula on June 24, 1980 and developed the concept of lymphasizing on October 19, 1980. I learned how shock could collapse the circulatory system in March of 1981. What makes it simple is the full understanding of *the seven golden discoveries and the one basic formula.*

C-4.   Blood Protein Research Reveals Importance Of The Lymphatic System

4.1. We introduced seven discoveries, the formula and the

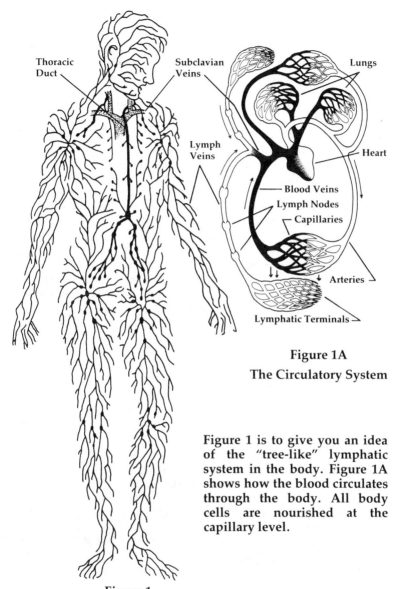

Thoracic Duct

Subclavian Veins

Lungs

Lymph Veins

Heart

Blood Veins
Lymph Nodes
Capillaries

Arteries

Lymphatic Terminals

Figure 1A
The Circulatory System

Figure 1
The Lymphatic System

Figure 1 is to give you an idea of the "tree-like" lymphatic system in the body. Figure 1A shows how the blood circulates through the body. All body cells are nourished at the capillary level.

concept of lymphasizing in brief form in the first session.

4.2. Now let's get into the formula in more detail. On page 401 of Guyton's fifth edition it says: "The importance of this function of the lymphatics cannot be stressed too strongly, for *there is no other route besides the lymphatics through which excess proteins* [which 'seep' out of the blood capillaries into the spaces around our cells] *can return to the circulatory system."*

4.3. To help you understand this, let's take a look at the lymphatic system. See Figure 1 taken from the report called "trapped plasma proteins," by C. Samuel West, N.D.

4.4. About all most people know about their lymphatic system is that they have lymph nodes in the neck, under the arms, and in the groin. As of November 1979, there were only approximately 300 Lymphologists world-wide, and only about 65 in the United States. In February, 1980, I was honored to become the 379th member of the International Society of Lymphology. I believe that this is one of the most important scientific societies in the world! It is made up of surgeons, doctors, physical therapists, naturopaths, and others who are doing research on the blood proteins and the lymphatic system. At the 7th International Congress of this society, held in Florence, Italy, October/November 1979, there were between 250-300 papers presented on the lymphatic system. (One paper every 10 minutes in two different auditoriums for one week). This is where I met Dr. Guyton for the first time and where I saw the film produced by Dr. Shields, which visibly revealed for the first time in history, the relationship between deep breathing and the lymphatic system.

4.5. As you can see, the lymph vessels look like a bunch of tree branches. About the best way to describe this system is as follows: The branches go up into the head; the roots go down into the feet, and the tree trunk is in the chest. The tree trunk is called the thoracic duct. Can you visualize a lymphatic tree inside the body? As you look at Fig. 1, repeat these words in your mind and point to the head, feet and chest as you say it: "The branches go up into the head; the roots go down into the feet, and the tree trunk is in the chest." Memorize that statement so you can explain it to others.

4.6. Let's look now at Figure 2 and try to understand how this system works.

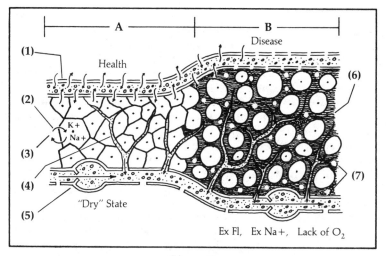

Figure 2
(A) Healthy cells in the dry state.
(B) Unhealthy cells in excess fluid and excess sodium. These are
    the conditions produced by trapped blood proteins. Lack of
    oxygen and excess sodium around the cells will cause pain,
    loss of energy, disease and death.

1. <u>Blood Capillaries</u>: Blood diffuses out of the capillaries to irrigate
   cells with oxygen and nutrients. (3 qts./min. x 80 = 240 qts. or 60
   gal./min.)
2. <u>Every Cell Is An Electrical Generator</u>: Inside the cell the potassium
   level must remain high and the sodium level must remain low. A
   very delicate balance must be maintained. Anything that will upset
   the sodium-potassium balance will damage or kill the cell.
3. <u>Sodium-Potassium Pump</u>: This pump is the rotation of the $Na+$
   and $K+$ in and out of the cell which generates an electrical field. It
   is the key to the life process and the energy produced by the cell.
4. <u>Lymphatic Capillaries</u>: Blood proteins are removed from the tissues
   around the cells through the lymphatic capillaries that carry them to
   the lymphatic vessels.
5. <u>One Way Check Valves</u>: The lymphatic vessels have one way check
   valves that keep the fluids going in one direction.
6. <u>Excess Fluid And Excess Sodium Around The Cells</u>. This is caused
   by trapped blood proteins around the cells.
7. <u>Trapped Plasma Proteins Around The Cells</u>. This is what causes
   pain, loss of energy, disease and death at the cell level.

4.7. Remember, until recently in the United States scientists knew that the blood diffused out of the capillaries to irrigate cells with oxygen and nutrients, but they did not know that the blood proteins continually "seeped" through the tiny pores during this irrigation process. This is what has kept them from finding the cause of disease and death at the cell level.

4.8. Research has now been conducted which confirms the fact that under *the normal pressure in the blood stream* the blood proteins "seep" through the tiny pores of the capillary membranes all the time. Once they seep out into the spaces around the cells, there is not enough pressure out there to push the blood proteins back through the tiny pores of the capillary membranes. Therefore, the *only* way the blood proteins can normally get back into the blood stream is through the lymphatics. Once they "seep" through the *blood* capillaries, they must be picked up by the lymphatic capillaries, which bring them into the *lymphatic* vessels. The lymphatic capillaries are represented in Figure 2 by arrows going down into the lymphatic vessels. The lymphatic vessels have one-way check valves on them that keep the fluids going in one direction. The lymphatic fluids bring the blood proteins up through the muscles in the legs, and up into the big thoracic duct, (which is the tree trunk in the chest), and then the thoracic duct dumps the blood proteins back into the blood stream in the subclavian vein at the base of the neck.

4.9. The main purpose of the blood proteins is to keep the water in the blood stream, but as they get "trapped" in the spaces around our cells, they pull sodium and water out of the blood stream which will cause inflammation, pain and every crippling or killer disease known to man. Are you beginning to understand the importance of this blood protein research? Let's repeat what the medical text said. I believe you will better understand it now.

4.10. "The importance of the function of the lymphatics cannot be stressed too strongly, *for there is no other route besides the lymphatics through which excess [trapped] proteins can return to the circulatory system.*" Now read this next part carefully. "If it were not for this continual removal of protein [from the tissue spaces by the lymphatics] the dynamics of the capillaries would become so abnormal within *only a few hours that life could no longer continue.*" This is just some of the scientific research that *proves* that our own blood proteins can destroy the life processes and cause loss of energy, disease and death in our bodies if they get "trapped" in the spaces around our cells. We are just beginning to prove that the research revealing the cause of heart disease, cancer, and every other crippling and killer disease has already been done. It is hard to believe that this blood protein research could be published in a medical text and in the <u>Encyclopedia</u> <u>Americana</u> for over twenty years without getting any publicity. As far as our health and peace is concerned, this is the most important research on the face of the earth.

C-5. *To Keep The Blood Protein Research From The Public Is To Let People Suffer And Die—To Ignore It is To Commit Suicide.*

5.1. How important is it that every family in the United States, and even the whole world, be given the opportunity to learn about this research? Anyone who would intentionally try to keep this knowledge from the public would be guilty of causing the death of approximately 240,000 men, women, and children every two months. That many people are now being killed every two months from heart disease and cancer alone *because they do not know about this research.* We have never had such destruction of human life since the beginning of this nation.

5.2. Not only does the lymphatic system keep the blood proteins out of the tissue spaces, but it also has the responsibility of helping to keep the poisons and toxic waste out of the body and purify the blood stream. Let us go into this in more detail.

C-6. *The Importance Of The Lymphatic System*

6.1. The tissues of the body which comprise bones, flesh and organs excrete waste products as a result of their daily work. These must be quickly removed, or the tissues involved will suffer damage.

6.2. The cleansing process of the body is performed by a mechanism that is called the lymphatic circulation.

C-7. What Is Lymph Fluid

7.1. All the bones, muscles and organs are interpenetrated by tiny *blood* vessels called capillaries, or arterioles. These are minute offshoots from larger vessels called the arteries. Thus the blood comes to the tissues by way of the arteries and the capillaries.

7.2. After the blood goes through the tiny capillaries, which penetrate all the bones, muscles and organs, they join up again to form larger vessels called veins. Thus, blood is carried away from the tissues by way of the veins.

7.3. The walls of the tiny blood capillaries are very thin and porous and the water along with the dissolved nutrients in the blood stream diffuse back and forth between the capillaries and the spaces around the cells to bathe and permeate the cells of the muscles, organs and the bones to give them the necessary oxygen and nutrients to stay healthy. This clear water, along with the dissolved nutrients, after they have passed the wall of the blood capillaries, is called the lymph fluid. Salt is a solid, sugar is a solid. But when you dissolve them in water you have a colorless solution. All the minerals and nutrients that get to the cells must be dissolved in the water of the blood to get to the cells to nourish them.

C-8. How Cells Are Fed

8.1. Every solid structure in the body is bathed in lymph. There is approximately 12 quarts of lymph in the body compared to three quarts of blood plasma. The lymph in the capillaries is the irrigation water that brings minerals and nutrients to the cells.

8.2. There are about one hundred trillion cells held together by appropriate supporting tissues. These cells in turn are organized into different functional structures; some of which are called organs. Each functional structure plays a part to see that there is a correct amount of fluid with the associated mineral salts around the cells.

D. HOW MANY TIMES CAN CELLS REPRODUCE THEMSELVES?

1. As long as the fluid around the cells remains free of toxic waste and contains the right mineral balance, the cells will continue to live and function normally.

2. How many times can cells reproduce themselves in the body if they function properly? Who knows? *The Medical World News* (October 1974, page 25) stated that two researchers at the Lawrence Berkeley Laboratory in California reported that Vitamin E can more than double the life of human cells cultured in an artificial test tube environment. Normally, these cells in this environment reproduced or doubled about 50 times before dying. But when Doctors Lester Parker and James R. Smith added Vitamin E at about 10 times the normal level in human tissue, the cells reproduced through the one-hundred twentieth generation. This was after the cells had gone two thirds of the way through their life span in that environment.

3. Vitamin E helps to prolong life because it prevents the fats from robbing the oxygen from the red blood cells. When fats combine with oxygen they form "free radicles," which in turn, use up more available oxygen to form toxic peroxides that can damage and destroy cells.

4. Peroxides will cause cells to mutate, and mutated cells are highly cancerous. This helps explain how fats cause lack of oxygen and cancer.

5. Research reveals that if the fluid medium in and around the cells was right, it would be impossible to damage or kill the cells. Scientific research states that there is a continuous automaticity of the body. All the cells will live in a healthy condition until one or more of the functional structures in the body loses its ability to function properly. When this happens, *all* of the cells of the body suffer. Moderate dysfunction of any one of the functional structures leads to sickness, while extreme dysfunction leads to death. Therefore, the main purpose of our body organs is to contribute to the continuous automaticity of the body by keeping the fluid medium in and around the cells right.

D-1. Letter From A Cancer Researcher Who Believes Cells Are Meant To Live Forever.

1.1 The following statements from a letter written by Elisa

Buenaventura will help explain how important this is. She has worked with cell cultures for about ten years as part of her cancer research. She has worked at Boston University Medical School, Tufts Medical School and Southwestern Medical School, conducting research in biophysics, cell biology and biochemistry.

1.2. She says, "Any medical researcher who has worked with tissue cultures knows that cells can be kept alive indefinitely, but you must keep the proper chemical balance in and around the cell and eliminate the waste products of their metabolism."

1.3. She believes that "cells are meant to be eternal. They should not die or degenerate if their environment is kept clean, nutritious and chemically balanced."

1.4. To keep the cell environment clean, nutritious and chemically balanced, the lymph system must play its vital role. When the fluid leaves the blood stream, it becomes lymph. The lymph system begins with the fluid in the spaces around the cells. These spaces gradually become lined tubes called lymphatic capillaries. These capillaries bring the lymph fluid into the lymphatic vessels which have one way check valves and lymph nodes which act as purification plants. These vessels end in one large trunk vessel called the thoracic duct in the chest area. This duct dumps the purified lymph back into the blood stream at the subclavian vein in the region of the neck, and this completes the lymph circuit.

E. HOW THE LYMPHATIC SYSTEM FUNCTIONS IN DETAIL

1. The most important function of the lymphatics is to keep the blood proteins circulating. Other than that, their main function is to drain away the lymph that has lost its nutrients after they have been extracted by the cells. The "dead fluid," along with the dead cells and poisonous waste that have been produced as a result of cell work, must be continually drained away. At rest, the lymph system will drain away about 1.2-2.0 ml. of "dead fluid" per minute. During activity it can drain away about 20 ml. of "dead fluid" per minute.

2. The lymph then is filled with waste products that pass

through the lymph nodes. The lymph nodes fulfill the function of filter beds. These nodes form secretions and possess cells which have the power of neutralizing, dissolving, destroying, or taking up the debris or waste products which may be in the body.

3. The liver which is one of the biggest detoxification plants in the body is loaded with lymphatics. After the lymph system neutralizes or dissolves the toxic wastes and renders the poisons inert, the lymph that is returned into the veins will be in a state of comparative purity. If the lymph system fails to function properly, it can cause hepatitis, (infection of the liver) and every other "itis" you can think about.

4. Even though the lymph system acts like a modern sewage treatment facility, it is literally the tree of life inside the body because when this system fails to function properly, excess blood proteins along with excess fluid and poisons build up in the body and pain, loss of energy, infection and disease will take place.

5. Keep in mind that any mental, emotional, or muscular activity puts cells to work, and working cells put off poisons that must be carried off by the lymph system or they will dilate the blood capillaries and cause "trapped" proteins.

E-1. What Causes Congestion, Catarrh (Mucous) And Inflamation

1.1 When the lymphatic system does not work well, the resulting condition is called congestion. Congestion is a form of lymphatic stagnation.

1.2. If lymphatic stagnation takes place through cells having access to the eliminating organs of the body, such as the skin, bronchial tubes, throat, etc. as well as the digestive tract and internal secreting surfaces, the poisons built up in the lymph system may begin to cause an oozing of the lymph through these open surfaces. This oozing is a common condition known as catarrh or inflammation of the mucous membranes of the nose and throat.

1.3. We say a person has a cold or cough when the lymphatic circulation of that part of the respiratory tract is so retarded that the lymph must be extruded through the lining surfaces of the tissues concerned. If this happens to the skin, it will produce sores or rashes, etc.

1.4. An excessive amount of food, especially of that type which will "trap" the blood proteins such as salt, the simple sugars, fats and the animal and dairy products are the main cause of congestion.

1.5. Eating foods that are of a cleansing nature and lymphasizing will help to restore the lymph circulation to normal.

1.6. Scientific research published in the February 1951 issue of *The Scientific American* by W. Barry Wood, Jr. states that if there is fluid retention in the spaces around the cells (which we now know is due to "trapped" protein) the white blood cells cannot ingest bacteria. Therefore, fluid retention from trapped proteins will make our bodies subject to infectious disease.

1.7. If the body was free of trapped proteins, the body would be in the "dry" state where there is no excess fluid around the cells. In this condition the white blood cells can act, even in the absence of antibody. Therefore, it would be impossible for us to have an infectious disease if we could prevent our blood proteins from becoming trapped.

1.8. As the research says, the importance of the function of our lymphatic system in keeping the blood proteins circulating cannot be stressed too strongly.

F. THE ONE AND ONLY FORMULA EXPLAINED IN DETAIL

1. The next question is, if our blood proteins can cause our death--how do they do it? As we explain in detail how the blood proteins can cause death, you are also going to learn how they are directly related to inflammation, pain, loss of energy, and every crippling and killer disease known to man. The first part of this explanation tells how the blood proteins cause disease and death, and the second part reveals how they cause loss of energy. Let's take a look at the cell. (Refer to Fig. 2 Page 35.)

F-1. A Different Approach

1.1 We are going to approach *the formula* a little differently than we did at the beginning. If you remember, we said that inside the cell the potassium level must remain *high* and the sodium level must remain *low*. That is a very delicate balance; anything that will upset the sodium-potassium balance inside the cell will *damage* or *kill* the cell. Now think about this--you cannot have a crippling or killer disease unless you damage or kill a cell! Therefore, *anything* that will upset the sodium-potassium balance inside the cell will *damage* or *kill* the cell and cause every *crippling* or *killer* disease known to man.

1.2. The big question is: what upsets the sodium-potassium balance inside the cell? Think of *the formula* we gave you at the very beginning. Excess sodium *outside* the cell will upset the delicate sodium-potassium balance *inside* the cell.

1.3. Now, we come to the key to The Formula! What causes excess sodium *outside* the cell? This has been the *hidden* factor in the United States and is the reason doctors in the United States have not been able to understand the cause of our crippling and killer diseases. The answer is, "our blood proteins!" As it states in Number 6 of the explanation in Figure 2, the proteins that make up part of the blood plasma carry a negative charge. If these proteins get trapped in the spaces *around* our cells, they will pull the positive sodium ions to them.

1.4. This combination greatly increases the fluid retention in the spaces around cells to cause a lack of oxygen and nutrients at the cell level. Therefore, if our plasma proteins get "trapped" in the spaces *around* our cells, we will not only have fluid retention, but we will also have excess sodium *around* our cells that will upset the sodium-potassium balance *inside* the cells to further damage or kill the cells. The following, then, is the *first* part of *the basic formula:* Trapped proteins, excess fluid and sodium, will damage or kill the cell. Our blood proteins can collapse our circulatory system and cause death in just a few hours if they get trapped quickly *throughout* the body as in traumatic or surgical shock, severe burns, and accidental injuries. If the blood proteins get trapped slowly, the body will adjust to live in a sick or diseased state.

1.5. Now, I will explain in detail how the trapped plasma proteins cause loss of energy. As you notice in Figure 2, there is a circle going in and out of the cell. This circle represents the constant rotation of sodium and potassium which creates "the electrical field that is generated by the life process of the cell."

Remember, "the life processes have been found to generate electrical fields in every organism that has been examined." And, the delicately balanced distribution of minerals *in* and *around* a living cell, whether plant or animal, accounts for its electrical properties. The energy field that eminates from "finger tips" and "leaves" is shown in Figure 3. The rotation of sodium and potassium in and around the cell is called the sodium-potassium pump. Because sodium continually leaks *into* the cell and postassium continually leaks *out* of the cell, the main purpose of the pump is to pull excess sodium *out* of the cell and bring potassium, calcium, iron, glucose, and other nutrients *into* the cell. This rotation of minerals creates an electrical field. I have come to call the sodium-potassium pump "the electrical generator." This generator is responsible for the electrical fields produced by the cells.

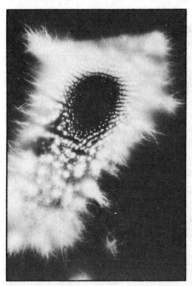 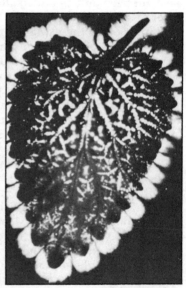

"Finger Tip"   Figure 3   "Leaf Of Plant"

F-2. The Human Body Is An Electrical Being

2.1. Science has proven that the human body is an electrical being. Our thought waves are electrical; the energy coming from our eyes is electrical; and our muscles work by electrical impulses from our brain. If someone is angry at you, they don't have to tell you--you can feel it! Everyone who has fallen in love knows that the energy coming from the eyes is electrical. True? The sodium-potassium pump produces the electric energy that makes it possible for a person to stop, start, and speed up an electric train by thinking about it; turn a wheelchair with electric energy coming from the eyes; activate a typewriter with the electric energy produced by the forehead muscles, and operate a bionic arm. The whole body works electrically off of the energy produced by the sodium-potassium pump. Without these discoveries it is impossible to fully understand the part of the formula that deals with the ▲EE or loss of energy at the cell level.

F-3. Loss Of Energy or ▲EE Is A Sign Of Trapped Protein

3.1. Loss of energy or ▲EE in your body is one of the *first indications* of trapped plasma proteins. To those who have this knowledge, the name or symptom of the problem or disease means nothing anymore. The whole body works electrically off of the energy produced by the sodium-potassium pump. Therefore, they will name the problem or disease according to where the plasma proteins get trapped and how it effects that part of the body.

3.2. Medical schools teach doctors how to treat the symptoms of trapped plasma proteins (TPP). A Certified Lymphologist can teach people how to prevent and if possible reverse the trapped blood proteins. No TPP, no pain, no loss of energy, and no disease.

3.3. With the blood protein research we now know that the one basic formula for the cause of loss of energy, disease and death is: TPP = EX FL, EX Na + = ▲ EE = ⊠. Trapped plasma proteins produce excess fluid and excess sodium around the cells which will alter the electric energy produced by the cells. The result will be a symptom of a disease. And the reverse is also true: No TPP = No EX FL, or EX Na + = EE = ☐. If we have no trapped proteins, we have no excess fluid or excess sodium around our cells and the "generators are on" and "our body is healthy." Review F-1, F-2 and F-3 until you understand it.

G. ELECTRICAL SECRETS OF LIFE AND DEATH AT THE CELL LEVEL SHOW HOW WE CAN PREVENT AND POSSIBLY REVERSE PAIN, LOSS OF ENERGY AND DISEASE

1. This formula not only reveals the secret to the fundamental cause of loss of energy, disease, and death, but it also reveals the secret to the healing processes that will enable us to live one hundred years or more with ease!

2. This research gives us the hidden or previously unknown answers that will help explain every healing art known to man.

3. Therefore, to help you understand the crippling and killer diseases, and how the basic bio-electric self-help relief techniques produce healing in your body, I am going to discuss some concepts that will give you a more detailed understanding of the cause of pain. This will help you understand why doctors are able to relieve pain quickly with electrical devices and heal bones with electricity in weeks that would not heal in years and why a person having a heart attack can be given a "heart attack shot" that brings him *from death to life* in seconds.

4. Then I will end this session by teaching you the cause of the crippling and killer diseases.

G-1. *The Secret To The Healing Process*

1.1. Now that we know that every cell is an electric generator, we are able to think about the body differently than ever before. As George S. White, M.D. said, "The magnetic electrical research field will come to prove that the human body is an electrical being and our health depends on the energy currents which run through the body." If all of your electrical generators are on, you are perfectly healthy. To the extent that they are not on, loss of energy, disease, and death is taking place in your body.

1.2. In 1955 it was reported that Dr. Hans Sellye, a Canadian researcher, believed that all the problems in the body, whether it be a heart attack, a mild case of asthma, or just plain not feeling good is caused from a chemical imbalance in the body. It is reported that the *Journal of the American Medical Association* said at that time, "If future events prove this concept correct, it will become one of the greatest medical advances of this century." *The Lancet*, a leading British medical journal, agreed with that statement. This concept has now been proven to be true.

G-2. If You Turn The Electric Generators Off, Lights Go Out; If You Turn The Generators On, The Lights Go On!

2.1. If you go into a dark house, you flip on a switch and the light goes on. The same principle applies to the cell. If a person is having a heart attack, his generators are going off. With the knowledge of the formula, let us consider what has to happen in the body when a doctor gives a heart attack patient a shot that brings him from death to life in a few seconds. If the generators are being turned off, the shot has to pull the excess fluid and sodium out to turn the generators back on. And that is exactly what the shot does.

2.2. A medical doctor in Utah told me one day of a man who came into his office with a heart attack. He said that he gave the man a shot and pulled him right out of it. I said, "Dr. W., I don't know one thing about that shot, but I know what the shot has to do in order to work."

He asked, "What does it have to do?"

I replied, "It has to pull the excess fluid and sodium out from around the cells."

He answered, "That is exactly what it does!"

Then I said, "Would you like me to explain to you why the shot works so fast?"

2.3. When I explained the formula to him, he got excited. He attended six of my lectures, and he would stand up and tell the people that the discoveries were true, and he sent people to my lectures all over the state.

2.4. I have come to appreciate simplicity. In the beginning of learning anything, it is complicated and difficult to understand. In order to understand something so you can teach it in simplicity, you have to learn a lot. An example of this is: to explain how the heart attack shot works with a knowledge of our blood proteins, all we have to say is, "When excess fluid and excess sodium comes out, the sodium-potassium balance is reestablished and the generators turn on."

2.5. With the knowledge of the formula we can now understand this and every other method of healing known to man. We now know that if anything heals the body or even helps the body--it must remove the "trapped" proteins, the excess fluid and sodium, and turn the generators on!

G-3.   Lack Of Oxygen--The Cause Of Most Pain

3.1. To prepare you for the basic self-help pain relief techniques, you need to understand the cause of most pain in detail. Most pain is caused from lack of oxygen. Medical research states that unoxygenated blood cannot relieve pain. As you sit on a hard chair for a while, you will come to know this is true. As you sit still, you block the circulation, and it begins to hurt. Your natural impulses tell you to move around, and as you do, the oxygenated blood comes in and helps take the pain away. Isn't that exciting? It takes the newest and most modern research to help you understand why you get relief when you move around.

3.2. To help understand the lack of oxygen and pain at the cell level, let's look again at Figure 2 (Page 35). Do you see the statement that says, "3 quarts a minute x 80 = 240 quarts or 60 gallons per minute." Let's understand those figures.

3.3. There are three quarts of blood that go through the blood capillaries every sixty seconds. But, before they go through once every sixty seconds, they diffuse back and forth eighty times to irrigate the cells with oxygen and nutrients. Now think about that. If those three quarts go back and forth eighty times every sixty seconds, they have to go back and forth faster than one time per second. The arrows going ▷ ◁ in Figure 2 represent this diffusion. One thousand and one--they just did it. I don't care how you look at it, those three quarts move back and forth fantastically fast!

3.4. Lack of oxygen and nutrients at the cell level is now becoming clear. If those three quarts diffuse back and forth faster than one time per second, the fluids cannot go out very far from the blood capillaries to irrigate the cells with oxygen and nutrients and still move back and forth that fast! This is why the research states that the cells must remain tight and close to the capillary membranes. It states that if the cells get away from the capillary membranes, oxygen and nutritive damage takes place.

G-4.   New Research Reveals The Conditions The Body Must Be In To Produce A Healthy Cell

4.1. Another major discovery made by Dr. Guyton is the

Figure 4

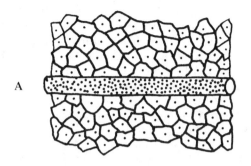

A

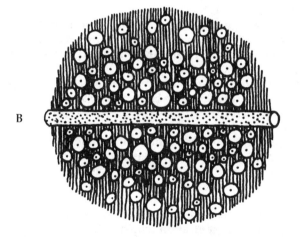

B

(A.) <u>Healthy cells in the dry state</u>. Like a collapsed balloon the pressure is subatmospheric. This condition represents the dry state of perfect health with no excess fluid around the cells, only enough to fill the crevices around the cells and that is all.

(B.) <u>Unhealthy cells, fluid retention, lack of oxygen and nutrients</u>. Like a balloon blown up caused by fluid retention due to trapped blood proteins and excess sodium.

one that reveals what holds the cells tight and close to the capillary membranes. (See Figure 4.) Dr. Guyton discovered in 1961 that to have a healthy body we should have a negative subatmospheric pressure in the spaces around the cells. He calls this condition the "dry" state where there is no excess fluids, only enough fluid to fill the crevices around the cells, and that is all. On page 401 in the 5th edition of his text, he states: "The fact that interstitial fluid pressure is negative [that is, subatmospheric] was discovered only a few years ago, though it has now been confirmed by a number of different independent methods . . . . Even so, it has been difficult for many students and even professional physiologists to understand the significance of the negative pressure." To explain this, the text says we must consider the importance of the tissue fluid (blood) protein concentration because fluid retention in the body is inextricably bound to that of the (blood) protein concentration in the spaces around the cells.

4.2. In other words, "body fluids follow the blood proteins!" Memorize that statement; it is important. The only thing that can cause fluid retention in the spaces around the cell is the blood proteins. Under the normal pressure in the blood stream, the blood proteins "leak" from the capillaries all the time, but because there is not enough pressure in the spaces around the cells to force the blood proteins back through the tiny pores of the blood capillaries, they must be continually removed by the lymphatics, or excess fluid will accumulate around the cells and a lack of oxygen and nutrients will take place. If we put too much water on a crop, it will damage or kill the crop. Likewise, trapped proteins produce excess fluid around the cells, and this will drown the cells. Therefore, by far the most important of all the lymphatic functions is the maintenance of low blood protein concentration in order to maintain the "dry" state and the sub-atmospheric pressure in the spaces around the cells.

4.3. When I was in Italy attending the Seventh International Congress of Lymphology in October/November 1979, Dr. Guyton was there explaining this negative pressure discovery to the lymphologists. To explain this negative pressure condition in the text, Dr. Guyton used a balloon to represent the body. When you suck all the air out of a balloon, you create a negative subatmospheric pressure condition. To have cells that are healthy, this is the condition that must exist throughout our body. Remember, the blood capillaries permeate every solid structure of the body's bones, eyes, organs and everything. It is this sub-atmospheric pressure inside our body that holds the cells tight and close to the capillary membranes so they can get oxygen and nutrients. As the blood diffuses back and forth at the rate of 240 quarts per minute, the blood proteins "seep" out under pressure. Due to lack of pressure in the space around the cells, the blood proteins are the only substances that cannot be immediately returned into the blood stream. Therefore, the only substance in the body that can alter this negative pressure condition and produce the conditions that cause loss of energy, disease and death, is the blood proteins.

G-5. What Causes Smashed Fingers, Turned Ankles, And Some People's Bodies To Retain Fluids?

5.1. When you blow up a collapsed balloon you go from a negative pressure condition to a positive pressure condition. This is what happens in the body when there is fluid retention from "trapped" plasma proteins. The result is excess sodium and lack of oxygen at the cell level.

5.2. When you smash your finger or turn your ankle, they swell up. Why? Because damaged cells produce poisons: histamine (this is why they give antihistamine to counteract it) and bradykinin.

5.3. A poison is a poison because it dilates the blood capillaries (just like shock) which opens up the tiny pores and lets the blood proteins come into the spaces around the cells faster than the lymphatics can pull them out. Memorize that statement because *anything* that will do that *is a deadly poison.*

5.4. Since the lymphatic system is a very slow moving system, anything that will dilate the blood capillaries will cause the blood proteins to come into the tissue spaces faster than the lymphatics can pull it out and cause the proteins to become trapped. Remember, body fluids follow the blood proteins. The blood proteins are what cause the fluid pressure in the blood stream. If they get trapped in the spaces around the cells, they produce fluid pressure in the spaces around the cells. Trapped proteins are the cause of fluid retention in smashed fingers, turned ankles, obesity, etc.

5.5. Medical charts show that it is possible to retain 3, 6, 9, 12, 15 or more gallons of fluid from trapped plasma proteins (See Fig. 5). There are 24 pounds in three gallons. That means that it would be possible for a person to gain weight of 24, 48, 72, 96 or more pounds from trapped blood proteins.

5.6. *This is the cause of obesity.* We will discuss this more later because we now know that the "little" guy can have just as much trapped blood proteins, just as much excess sodium, and his generators can be shut off, and he can be just as sick as the "big" guy. This is additional evidence which proves that over 240,000 men, women, and children are being killed every two months in the United States alone *because they do not know about this research!*

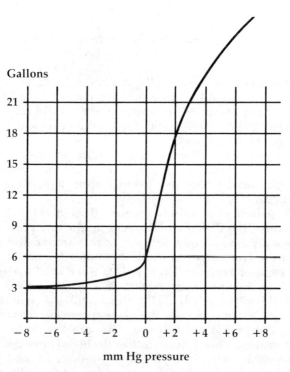

Figure 5

5.7. How many people do know about it? Only a "handful" of people in the whole world, and you are now becoming that handful. You are now beginning to learn the cause of disease and what you must do to heal your body in detail. With this knowledge, in Session Three we are going to teach you how to PREVENT and if possible REVERSE every crippling and killer disease known to man.

G-6.Discovery Six And Seven: Trapped Proteins Become Clustered, And Electricity Can Dissipate Clustered Proteins.

6.1. Now, to help understand the bio-electric self-help pain relief techniques, let's go into the discoveries that I learned in February of 1980 from Professor Doctor Friedrich M. Plog who discovered the Lasar Acupuncture Machine in Germany. After listening to Dr. Plog explain how he could make incisions on the body without pain, extract a tooth without pain, and take pain out of accidents in about 60 seconds, I went up to him and asked, "Dr. Plog, aren't you moving out the blood proteins?" When he answered this question he gave me the last TWO of the Seven Golden Discoveries.

6.2. First, he said, "We have known about the blood proteins for a long time in Germany; they have discovered that when the energy fields are reduced in the spaces around the cells, the blood proteins will *cluster*; and even the lymphatics have a difficult time in removing them." Then he said, "They have also discovered that electricity will dissipate the clustered proteins."

6.3. I had been looking for these two discoveries for 6 years. I know that the blood proteins had the effect of causing a "dam in the ditch" and retaining fluid inside the body and that electric energy and other sources of energy moved the "trapped" proteins out but didn't understand how it all worked until the relationship between clustered proteins and electricity was given to me by Dr. Plog.

6.4. I am sure Dr. Plog did not expect me to understand his statements, but with the knowledge of The Basic Formula we can explain the clustered protein concept in more detail than ever before. Damaged cells produce poisons that cause trapped proteins, and we know that trapped proteins will produce excess fluid and sodium in the spaces around the cells and shut off the electrical generators. Remember, Dr. Plog said, "... when the energy fields are reduced in the spaces around the cells, the blood proteins will cluster." Since the lymphatics have difficulty in removing clustered proteins and the body fluids follow the blood proteins, *it is the clustered proteins that produce fluid retention in the body.* Trapped proteins, excess sodium, shut the generators off; the proteins cluster and cause fluid retention in the spaces around the cells. This will cause a continual lack of oxygen and lasting pain in smashed fingers, turned ankles, and in the joints of the fingers, arms, legs, and so forth. This will also interfere with the healing process.

G-7. Why And How The Bio-Electric Self-Help Pain Relief Techniques Work!

7.1. These discoveries explain why doctors are able to use electrical devices in their pain clinics to relieve pain and speed up the healing process. They also explain why and how they are able to heal bones in weeks with electricity that would not otherwise heal at all (See Fig. *6*).

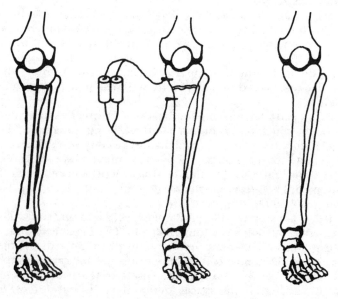

Figure 6

7.2. To my knowledge this was the first experiment where scientists in the U.S. used electricity to heal bones. It was published in the Jan. 1973 issue of the *Science World Magazine*. It was accomplished by a surgeon, Dr. Leroy S. Lavine, of Downstate Medical Center, Brooklyn, New York, and his colleague, Morris H. Shamos, a physicist, of New York University.

7.3. In order to test the theory that an electric current was involved in the healing process, they had to find someone whose bones would not heal by any other means. They finally found a fourteen-year-old boy who had been born with a bone defect in the tibia (the largest of the two bones in the lower part of the leg below the knee). The defect was just below the knee joint.

7.4. Years of treatment had failed to heal the defect in the boy's leg. The doctors made the decision to try the electrical treatment. Using two size D flashlight batteries as a power source, Drs. Lavine and Shamos implanted platinum wires near both ends of the defect. The leg was placed in a cast to keep it from moving. For four months the boy lay in the cast as the current trickled across the "unhealable" area between the electrodes.

7.5. The X-rays were taken; the researchers smiled. They removed the electrodes. They had done their work. The electric treatment was successful.

7.6. To explain what happened in simple terms: the damaged cells produced trapped clustered proteins; the electricity dissipated the clustered proteins; the excess fluid and sodium were removed, the generators turned on, and the life processes were restored. As a result oxygen and nutrients were able to get into the cells, and the bones healed. The Seven Golden Discoveries and the Formula make it possible to explain this healing process in detail. The blood protein research is the most important health message on the face of the earth. As I said before, the research has all been done! Without this research it is impossible to explain the cause and what we might do to prevent and if possible reverse disease.

G-8. Introducing Discovery By Dr. Joseph M. Waltz, M.D.

8.1. With this research we are also able to explain the miraculous work that is being done by Dr. Joseph M. Waltz of

New York City's St. Barnabas Hospital. On December 17, 1980, I called him on the phone to confirm the report that was given in a national newspaper, on July 1, 1980. He not only confirmed all of the accounts given by this newspaper, but he also told me of other cases that had responded to what he calls "the spinal cord stimulator." This electrical device consists of a thin wire containing four electrodes that is implanted, through a needle, in the upper spine near the spinal cord and attached to a portable power pack worn around the waist.

8.2. Three out of four have showed dramatic improvement after being treated with his electrical device. Here are a few wonderful examples of his work that he confirmed over the telephone.

• An 18-year-old girl confined to a wheelchair was able to walk unassisted and feed herself after spinal cord electrical stimulation.

• A 17-year-old palsy victim was suddenly able to control her bladder, speak clearly, and use her hands again.

• A boy was partially cured of uncontrollable gestures and was able to walk again.

• A young woman, once paralyzed, is now getting around on crutches and may soon be walking completely unassisted.

• A 33-year-old woman is able to move her head again and is free of pain.

• A 14-year-old boy is able to use his right hand for the first time in six years.

8.3. To many, the work that is being done by Dr. Waltz would seem like a miracle; and it is truly a scientific miracle. But those who understand the blood protein research appreciate the work that he is doing. (A more detailed account of his work is given in Session IV where we discuss The Advanced Bio-Electric Lymphasizing Techniques.)

8.4. All systems in the body work electrically. Muscles work by electrical impulses from the brain. But as the formula explains, the blood proteins will upset the chemical balance, and this will cause a "short circuit" in the body. When the electrical impulses cannot get from the brain to the muscles as a result of these trapped clustered proteins it will cause multiple sclerosis, polio, and the other spastic crippling and killer diseases.

8.5. The formula, which reveals the conditions that must exist in the body to produce totally healthy cells, is also the formula that reveals the cause of pain and misery in the body and the formula that reveals what must happen in the body for healing to take place.

G-9. *The Cause Of Headaches, Lower Back And Sciatic Problems And Much More.*

9.1. If the trapped clustered proteins and fluid retention take place in the muscles of the neck, it will cause the muscles to pull the bones out of place and make one leg shorter than the other as the whole body adjusts. Also when these muscles are pulled tight, it will block circulation and cause pain going up into the head and in the neck. If it happens in the hip, the muscles will pull that hip forward so that it will be lower than the other. This will pull the muscles tight across the lower back, block the circulation, and cause lower back and sciatic nerve problems.

9.2. If it happens in the fingers, arms, legs, or joints it will cause pain in those areas. If it happens in an organ, it may cause infection, inflammation or disease.

G-10. *What Must Happen In The Body For Healing To Take Place.*

10.1. According to the formula, in order for healing to take place, we must get the trapped clustered proteins out of the damaged area and keep them out. This is the secret. In order to heal the body or even help the body we must keep the blood proteins from becoming trapped. No trapped blood proteins, no excess fluid or sodium: the generators are on, and the cells are healthy, not sick!

10.2. With this information, you are now ready to learn the basic bio-electric self-help pain relief techniques that will help you remove the trapped proteins out of a damaged area to relieve pain and then keep them out so that healing can take place.

G-11. *A Few Examples To Illustrate The Healing Process*

11.1. With this background, you will be able to understand in detail what happened to my mother's sister when she fell on the ice and hurt her hip. The damaged cells caused trapped clustered blood proteins and fluid retention in the muscles of the hip. This pulled the illium (hip) forward and made one hip lower than the other. As the illium was pulled down on one side, it pulled the muscles tight across the lower back and down the sciatic nerve on the other side. This blocked the circulation and caused pain across the back and down the nerve just like sitting for a long time on a hard chair. As a result, my aunt was on crutches for the next thirteen years. She could not stoop down to pick anything off the floor.

11.2. I taught her how to get the blood proteins out of her hip, and at the end of the third treatment, she stooped over, picked up something off my floor, and walked out the door on her own power--without crutches! To learn how to do this, see Fig. 10 on page 67. To keep the proteins out so healing can take place, you may have to do these self-help techniques for fifteen seconds every fifteen minutes the first day; every 30 minutes the second day; and twice a day thereafter for prevention.

11.3. As you know, chiropractors spend four to six years and many thousand of dollars to learn how to relieve pain. They have known for years that the muscles pull the bones out of place, but they have not understood why. With the knowledge of these golden discoveries and this formula, you should now understand this in detail. When chiropractors learn this they are able to teach their chronic patients how to help themselves. Many of them are going into nutrition and exercise and are being a great blessing to many people.

11.4. We are now going to teach you how to untrap the trapped protein to help relieve the pain and speed up the healing process in smashed fingers, turned ankles, swollen arms, legs, joints, etc. The basic bio-electric self-help pain relief techniques that are used to "turn the generators on" and cause healing in your body are pressure, a massage motion, and a light fast stroke.

G-12. *The Use Of Pressure Can Heal A Smashed Finger In Minutes, Minutes--Not Hours.*

12.1. First, let's take a smashed finger. If bones can be healed in weeks that would not heal for years, why can't you heal a smashed finger in minutes, instead of hours? All we have to do to heal a smashed finger very quickly is to keep the blood proteins out. Let us pretend we just smashed our finger. The cells are damaged, poisons are attacking the blood capillaries, and they begin to dilate the tiny pores, which will let the blood proteins flow into the tissue spaces faster than the lymphatics can pull them out. Our first impulse (besides to scream) is to grab it. Right? But most of us are so dumb, that after we grab it, we turn loose to look and see what we did. True or false? Once we turn loose, we don't grab it the second time because when we turn loose, the blood proteins come out and cluster, which causes fluid retention, lack of oxygen, and it hurts so bad that all we do then is shake it, suck it, or put it in ice.

12.2. With the knowledge of these golden discoveries, and the formula, you are not going to turn loose. Let's pretend again that you just smashed your finger. Grab your finger as if you just smashed it, and let's go through the healing process. This time you are not going to turn loose. The same process happens; the poisons from the damaged cells are attacking the blood capillaries; but if you hold on, the proteins can't get through the pores of the capillaries to cause fluid retention, lack of oxygen and slow down the healing process. Think about that. This is why our natural impulses tell us to grab. No trapped proteins, no excess fluid or sodium, the generators are on, and healing begins to take place immediately. If you can keep the generators on, healing will take place very quickly. This means that you can heal a smashed finger while you hold it! Now, how long do you hold on? This is the secret to the healing process. *You hold on until the pain goes away.* What do you have to lose? It feels better while you hold it than it does anywhere else! True or false? Now, I have been saying for years that within five to twenty minutes the poisons will stop attacking the capillaries, the blood capillaries will tighten up, and excess blood proteins can't get into the spaces around the cells to cause lasting pain and slow down the healing process. This was confirmed in Italy. You can time it by the clock. Within twenty minutes the poisons stop attacking the capillaries. If you keep the blood proteins out, there will be no excess fluid or sodium; the generators are on and your finger will heal very quickly. It may be black and blue tomorrow, but no pain. Nine times out of ten you won't even lose your fingernail, and I have even seen the black and blue completely disappear within twenty minutes. People all over the United States and Canada are now proving that this works, which proves again that the formula is correct and the research has been done. If you are going to have a healthy body, you must prevent the blood proteins from becoming "trapped" in the spaces around the cells.

G-13. *Massage And A Light Fast Stroke: Two Other Self-Help Pain Relief Techiques*

13.1. Now I would like to teach you two other self-help pain relief techniques. Both of them require a knowledge of these seven discoveries and the formula in order to know how to use them effectively so as to cause healing to take place in your body. One technique is "a light, fast stroke" and the other is "a massage motion." To help understand them, let's consider the following:

13.2. When you slide across the the carpet, can you generate electricity? Well, we have learned that electricity can help relieve pain whether it be generated from an electrical device or from this new technique of "a light, fast stroke."

G-14. *What About Swollen And Painful Fingers, Or Pain In The Neck, Shoulders, Arms, Lower Back, Hips, Sciatic Nerve, Ankles, Knees, Thighs, Etc.*

14.1. If I had swollen and painful fingers or a pain in the neck, shoulders, arms, lower back, hips, sciatic nerve, ankles, knees or thighs (See Fig. 7, 8, 9), the first thing I would do is use *pressure, a gentle massage motion, and a "light, fast stroke."* The "massage motion" must be used with great care.

14.2 Before you decide to use any of these techniques, you should consult your physician. This is not diagnosis or prescription. We are here to explain how the Self-Help Bio-Electric Techniques work and why they work. *Do NOT* cause stress in the body. Whatever you do, do it as your body enjoys it! Remember, *the lymph system pumps fluid and proteins* out of the tissue spaces each time the tissues are compressed or moved in any other way. Constant pressure, a massage motion, or a light quick stroke will dissipate the clustered proteins, and the more you do it, *without causing* undue stress, the better it will feel; and the better it feels, the more you can do it without causing undue stress. You must remember that if you cause stress, you will cause trapped proteins and produce pain.

14.3. If I had a sore finger that was too tender to hold or massage, then I would use *a light, fast stroke*. This generates energy like sliding across the carpet. It will help dissipate the trapped clustered proteins, turn the electric generators on in the cell, and let the oxygenated blood get to the cells to help relieve the pain and cause the healing process to take place.

G-15. *The Secret Of The Healing Process*

15.1. After using the light, fast stroke for a while, then I would come back and try the massage motion again, finding that I could stand pressure that I could not stand before. "The more you do it, the better it feels; and the better it feels, the more you can do it."

15.2. This is the secret to the healing process, especially if there is a chronic problem. After the pain goes away, many make the mistake of *waiting until the pain comes back*, and then they will say, "Oh, dear! It didn't work!" Be smarter than that! Pay close attention to this next sentence. If a person waits until the blood proteins get back in there and become clustered and cause the return of pain, *he has waited too long!* The secret is this: A person must continue to repeat the self-help techniques while it still *feels good* to keep the blood proteins circulating so healing can take place. This is why deep breathing or using a lymphasizer often is so important. To help speed up the healing process, I combine as many self-help bio-electric lymphasizing techniques as possible.

G-16. *Why It May Be Necessary To Do These Techniques For Fifteen Seconds Every Fifteen Minutes*

16.1. It is easier to blow up a balloon the second time than it is the first time. By the same principle it can take a *lot* of trapped proteins to cluster and blow you up and cause pain the first time. After that, you have what we call "a weak spot in your balloon." You may be able to move the proteins out to relieve pain, but a *small* amount of trapped protein will reduce the energy fields, and "POW!" you get the clustered proteins, fluid retention, lack of oxygen, and the pain comes back again. This is why it may be necessary to repeat these self-help pain relief techniques for fifteen seconds every fifteen minutes to keep the proteins and the excess fluid and sodium out. Anyone can do this. If you can keep the generators on healing will take place, if it can take place. Remember, if all the generators are on in your body, you will be "alive and well," not "alive and sick."

H. ILLUSTRATIONS SHOWING THE BASIC BIO-ELECTRIC SELF-HELP PAIN RELIEF TECHNIQUES

1. Anyone who knows how to apply the self-help bio-electric lymphasizing techniques will be able to relieve pain and cause healing to take place in their body.
2. Those who get a chance to hear Dr. West or receive instructions from a qualified instructor will see these self-help techiques demonstrated. See the Advanced Bio-Electric Lymphasizing Techniques and the testimonial letters in Session Four.
3. The following is not meant to diagnose or prescribe or to take the place of your physician, but to teach how and why certain self-help techniques work. Those who use these techniques do so by their own free will and choice. Their body is their responsibility.

H-1.To Help Relieve Headaches & Sore Neck Problems:
(See Figure 7)

For Headaches and Sore Neck Problems I:

1. Place my left hand on my abdomen.
2. With my right hand I apply pressure behind the left ear down the neck and out across the shoulder. The sore spots tell me where the trapped clustered proteins are. The lymph system pumps fluid and protein out of the tissue spaces each time the tissues are compressed or moved any other way. I may just hold a sore spot like I do a smashed finger.
3. Next, I gently massage the sore spots. I do not cause stress. If I do it right, the more I do it, the better it should feel.
4. I end up by doing the light fast stroke from behind the ear down the neck and out across the shoulder.
5. Then I reverse the hands and repeat for the other side of the neck. I have to work both sides to make it work.
NOTE: When I have a "weak spot," to keep the blood

proteins circulating so healing can take place (like they do with the use of electricity) I *must* continue to do these self-help techniques even after I start to feel good. I may need to do them for fifteen seconds every fifteen minutes the first day, fifteen seconds every thirty minutes the second day, fifteen seconds every hour the third day, and several times a day thereafter, for several months to help the "weak spot" heal.

H-2. To Help Relieve My Sore Arms and Legs:
(See Figures 8 and 9-9A.)

For Sore Arms Or Shoulders I:

1. Use the pressure, the massage motion and the fast stroke as shown in Figure 8.
2. I also do this while I lymphasize on a lymphasizer.

For Sore Knees Or Legs I:

1. Use the pressure, the massage motion and the light fast stroke as shown in Figures 9 and 9A.
2. Always begin by using a very light hand pressure. I do not cause stress. If you have any special problems, you should always consult your physician.

H-3. To Help Relieve Pain In The Hip, Lower Back, and Sciatic Nerve: (See Figure 10 and 10A)

For the Hips, Sciatic Nerve, and Lower Back I:

1. Stand as straight as I can.
2. Place hands high above hips, fingers to the back and thumbs to the front.
3. (a) Stroke the hips one at a time, then both at once. (b) stroke the entire lower back as shown in Figures 10 and 10A.
4. Breathe deeply or use a lymphasizer while I do it.
5. Combine the above with the more advanced techiques in Session Four.

H-4. To Help Increase the Circulation in The Liver, Gall Bladder, Spleen, and Pancreas:
(See Figures 11 and 12.)

For the Liver/Gall Bladder I:

1. Place my left hand on my right shoulder.
2. Cone the fingers on the right hand and start at pit of stomach, just below breast bone, and do the light fast stroke about twenty-one times, following below rib cage all the way out to the right side as shown in Figure 11.
3. Breathe deeply or use a lymphasizer while I do it.
4. Combine the above with the more advanced techniques in Session Four.
4. For the spleen/pancreas I reverse the hands and do the same thing on the other side as shown in Figure 12.

H-5.   *To Help Stimulate and Revitalize The Colon:*
(See Figure 13.)

For the Colon I:
(Descending)
1. Place my right hand on my left shoulder.
2. Stroke or brush *down the left side* along descending colon area with my left hand.
(Transverse)
1. Keep my right hand on my left shoulder.
2. Stroke or brush *across middle* of body along transverse colon area, *right to left,* with my left hand.
(Ascending)
1. Place my left hand on my right shoulder.
2. Stroke or brush *up right side* along ascending colon area with my right hand.
3. Reverse the sequence by doing transverse and descending again.
4. REPEAT the whole process several times.
NOTE: Do descending colon *first* to open up the passage way. Stroke each part 4 or 5 times before going on to the next part.

H-6. *To Help Increase Circulation in The Kidneys:*
(See Figure 14.)

For the Kidneys I:

1. Use the massage motion as shown in Figure 14.
2. Breathe deeply or use a lymphasizer to do it.

3. Combine the above with the more advanced techniques in Session Four.

H-7. To Help Relieve the Pain in Smashed or Cut Finger:
(See Figure 15.)

For a Smashed or Cut Finger I:

1. Hold on until the pain goes away as shown in Figure 15.

H-8. To Help Relieve Pain in a Freshly Turned Ankle:
(See Figure 16.)

For a Turned Ankle I:

1. Take my hurt foot by the arch with the other hand and pull to the inside to limit swelling as shown in Figure 16.
2. Using the hand on the side of the hurt foot I put the middle finger on the painful spot below the ankle bone and massage the fluid and proteins across the top of the foot and down toward the toes. (I am yelling and screaming, but what have I got to lose?) In about five minutes I have been able to run and jump up and down. When the pain disappears, healing begins to take place immediately.

NOTE: To speed up the healing process: I combine as many lymphasizing techniques as possible. I will teach how to lymphasize on a lymphasizer so you can "run and not be weary and walk and not faint," and what you must do to conquer disease, and establish peace in Session Three. In Session Three you will learn how to master the art of lymphasizing. Then in Session Four, I will teach *the advanced bio-electric lymphasizing techniques that can help relieve pain and speed up the healing process. These techniques can help even if a person is in a wheelchair.*

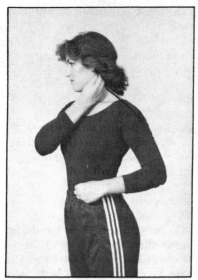

Figure 7
Sore Neck or Migraine Headaches

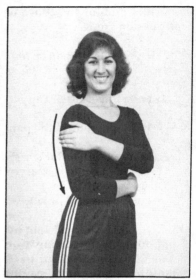

Figure 8
Sore Arms or Shoulders

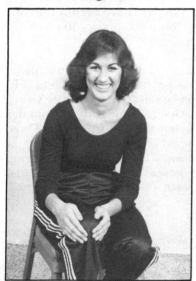

Figure 9
Sore Knees

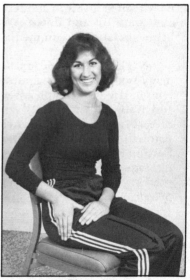

Figure 9A
Sore Legs

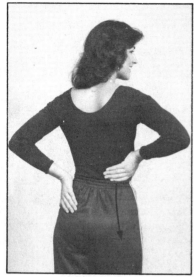

Figure 10
Lower Back or Sciatic Problems

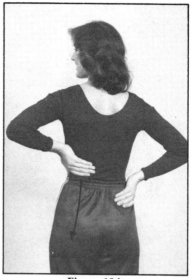

Figure 10A
Lower Back or Sciatic Problems

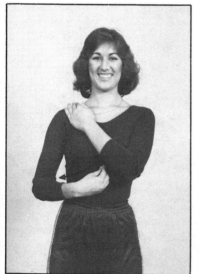

Figure 11
Liver/Gall Bladder

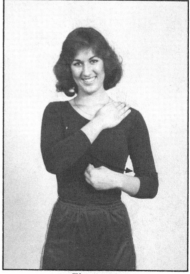

Figure 12
Spleen/Pancreas

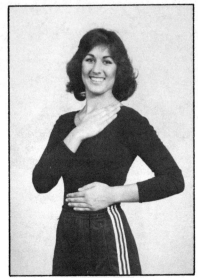

Figure 13
Descending Colon

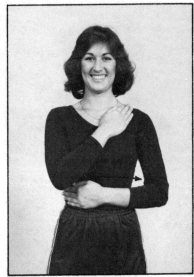

Figure 13A
Transverse Colon

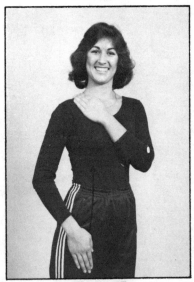

Figure 13B
Ascending Colon

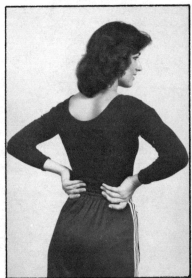

Figure 14
Kidneys/Adrenals

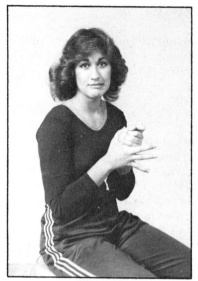

Figure 15
Smashed/Cut Finger

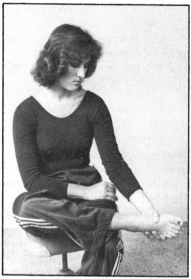

Figure 16
Turned Ankle

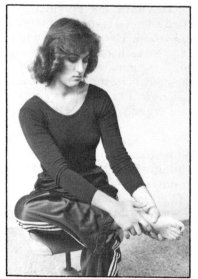

Figure 16A
Turned Ankle

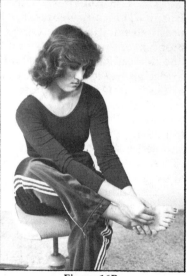

Figure 16B
Turned Ankle

I. THE COLLEGE OF CAUSE

1. Now, let's complete this session by going into the cause of heart disease, cancer, obesity, high blood pressure, arthritis, and the other killer and crippling disease in detail by putting them into *The Basic Formula*.

I-1. The Cause Of Cancer

1.1. First, let's take cancer. Not only is most pain due to lack of oxygen, but lack of oxygen is also the cause of cancer. This has been proven by Dr. Otto Warburg at the Max Planck Institute for Nutritional Research in Germany. He is a Nobel Prize winner. He has taken perfectly healthy cells and has withdrawn oxygen from those cells, and they turn cancerous every single time. Glucose combined with oxygen produces the energy needed for healthy cells. Without oxygen, the glucose will ferment. Cancer cells live on the fermentation of glucose due to lack of oxygen. Trapped plasma proteins is what causes fluid retention and lack of oxygen at the cell level. Dr. Warburg says that no disease is more well-known than cancer.

1.2. Dr. Robert C. Olney, M.D., built the Providence Hospital, Lincoln, Nebraska, a 125 bed hospital owned by a non-profit corporation, The Olney Foundation. He added a broad program of the treatment of cancer and other disease. He wrote a booklet called "Blocked Oxidation." He considered blocked oxidation and toxic substances in the body to be the prime cause of malignant, viral, bacterial and allergic disease. This report states that blocked oxidation in micro-organisms causes them to become pathogenic and parasitic. He says, "With our present knowledge, it should be possible to prevent and wipe out cancer and serious infectious disease." White blood cells can destroy cancer cells, viruses, and bacteria, but in excess fluid and a lack of oxygen, the white blood cells cannot function.

1.3. Cancer is also a "hotspot." To understand how the trapped proteins cause a hotspot, we need to understand the research that explains the cause of inflammation in the body. After Dr. Plog told me about the research concerning clustered protein in Germany, I felt impressed to get back into Dr. Guyton's text and study stress, which is a simple trauma in the body. Stress has a shock-like effect on the body which explains why it can play a major role in causing the killer and crippling diseases. There are burn and trauma clinics in the United States that are awarded millions of dollars to find how and why trauma causes diseases in the body. The research which explains the cause of *all* disease *has already been done!* And it is now being presented in this book.

I-2. *Inflammation And The Clustered Protein Research*

2.1. In May of 1980, I began to do more research on stress, and believe it or not, I came across the clustered protein research that Dr. Plog talked about. This is one of the greatest breakthroughs that has ever been made. It is on page 1,027 of the Fifth edition of the *Textbook of Medical Physiology* by Dr. Arthur C. Guyton. "Almost all tissues of the body respond to tissue damage, whether the damage results from simple trauma or from some cellular disease by the process called inflammation." There is your hotspot! Let's continue: The first stage in the process of inflammation is a "leakage of *large quantities* of plasma-like fluid out of the capillaries into the damaged area followed by a *clotting of the fluids.*" There it is! Simple trauma or damaged cells will cause "leakage" of large quantities of plasma-like fluid out of capillaries. And, as we have already learned, you cannot get "large quantities of plasma-like fluids" out of the capillaries unless you dilate the blood capillaries and open up the tiny pores. Poisons from damaged cells will do this. Here we learn that a simple trauma, such as stress, will do the same thing. Stress, like shock, has the same effect on the body as poisons from a damaged cell. The same process takes place; the tiny capillary pores dilate, and the blood proteins flow into the spaces around the cells faster than the lymphatics can pull them out. The trapped proteins reduce the energy fields, cluster and produce a clotting of the fluids.

2.2 In science, you learn that you cannot destroy energy. You can change its form, but you cannot destroy it. Loss of energy must be converted into heat, light, or sound. When the "energy fields" are reduced at the cell level due to trapped plasma protein, the loss of energy in the body is converted into *heat!* This is the inflammation that comes as a result of trauma or damaged cells. This helps explain why cancer is a "hotspot."

2.3. Now, let's discuss the "clotting of the fluids." Remember, Dr. Plog said that "when the energy fields reduce down in the spaces around the cells, the blood proteins will *cluster*". The body fluids follow the blood proteins. Therefore, clustered proteins will cause a "clotting of the fluids." Without the knowledge of the "clustered protein" concept that we learned from Dr. Plog and The Formula, showing that trapped proteins will "reduce the energy fields" in the body, it would have been impossible to understand inflammation, or the "clotting of the fluids" that is mentioned in Guyton's Text.

2.4. For the first time in history we can make one statement that will tie all these concepts together. Here it is:

> Damaged cells produce poisons that have a shock-like effect on the body. They dilate the blood capillaries and cause trapped clustered proteins along with excess fluid and sodium, which shut the generators off.

2.5. This statement explains why a smashed finger swells up and is the foundation of this entire program. When you gain a complete understanding of why a smashed finger swells up, you will be able to explain the cause of pain, loss of energy, the viral infections, the bacterial infections, allergies, parasites, and every crippling or killer disease known to man and what we must do to reverse and conquer disease and heal our body.

2.6. It should be remembered that shock effects the whole body like damaged cells effect a smashed finger. Shock dilates the capillaries throughout the entire body. When the blood proteins come out with the water, it collapses the circulatory system.

I-3. The Cause Of Arthritis

3.1. When we put arthritis into this formula, it becomes as clear as a bell. Trapped protein, excess sodium, shuts the generator off, and the calcium drops out of solution and forms calcium deposits everywhere it happens. This is the cause of arthritis and hardening of the arteries. This has been proven by Dr. Campbell, who is an Osteopathic physician. he wrote the book *A Doctor's Proven New Home Cure For Arthritis*. This book has been nationally advertised all over the United States for the past several years. He shows pictures in his book of people who have calcified and deteriorated joints. Then, he shows pictures where these same people have perfect joints. They completely rebuild, with no calcium deposits whatsoever. With the knowlege of this Formula and the Seven Golden Discoveries, we can understand this feat. All he does is take the people off salt, sugar, fat, and high cholesterol foods, which we know will trap the blood proteins. No trapped proteins, no excess sodium, the generators are turned back on; the calcium dissolves and the body rebuilds the joints. It's just that simple! All we have to do is obey the mental, nutritional, and physical laws, and we will receive the blessings of health and peace that we all desire. When we break the laws, we find that nature is no respecter of persons. If you put your hand on a hot stove, you get burned. If you step in front of a moving car, you get hit. It doesn't matter if you understand the laws or not, if you break them, you reap the penalty!

3.2. Now, I will put obesity, high blood pressure, and heart disease into The Formula.

I-4. The Cause Of Obesity

4.1. I have already discussed how the blood proteins can cause fluid retention of 3, 6, 9, 12, 15 gallons or more, which is a weight gain of 24, 48, 72, 96 or more pounds. You can blow up some balloons easier than you can others; and we believe some people's bodies are the same way. I believe that some people, for one reason or other, have a loose cellular structure. Just a small amount of trapped protein in their body will cause them to blow up like a balloon.

4.2. Nothing is more exasperating for a person with a loose cellular structure than to sit by a person with the tight cellular structure and watch him eat "like a horse" and nothing happens to him that the observer can apparently see. Yet the other person may only eat half that much and blow up like a balloon. We have known this for a long time, but we could not explain it. We now know that the person with a tight cellular structure can have just as much trapped protein in his body as a person with a loose cellular structure. Having a tight cellular structure, the trapped proteins are not able to pull as much fluid out of the blood stream as they normally would and do under loose structure conditions. It may happen in "pockets", but it will not affect his entire body. These "pockets" are observable in some people. Therefore, trapped proteins are not as observable in a person with a tight cellular structure as they are in a person with a loose cellular structure. However, the trapped proteins will attract the same amount of excess sodium, so the thin person can have just as much trapped protein and excess sodium around his cells which will turn his generators off and make him just as sick as a heavy person.

4.3. Does the thin person get arthritis, cancer, high blood pressure, heart disease, etc.? Yes, he does. Then why does everyone point their finger at the heavy person? Is anyone justified in singling out one particular problem and turning it into one of the highest money making programs in the United States? Is anyone justified in crucifing people because they have a visible problem, when they themselves may be just as sick as those whom they are crucifing? Granted, these people need help, but the person with a loose cellular structure is literally being destroyed in the United States; and we now know that it is not justified. Everyone needs to obey the same mental, nutritional, and physical laws as the heavy person. A loose cellular structure is one of the hardest problems there is to reverse. This person needs a lot of love and understanding.

4.4. Besides that, we cause stress to those we persecute and actively contribute to their problem. We now know that we must learn to be considerate and kind to everyone who has a problem. To do otherwise is to willfully and intentionally harm them.

I-5.The Cause of Hypertension (High Blood Pressure)

5.1. High blood pressure, is directly related to cardio-vascular disease. It strikes thin people as well as heavy people and is a major cause of death in the United States. With the knowledge that the body fluids follow the blood proteins, it is now possible to understand the cause of this killer disease. It is the blood proteins that cause the pressure in the blood stream. If the blood proteins become trapped, they will produce fluid pressure in the spaces around the cells. This increased pressure out in the spaces around the cells will also increase the pressure *in* the blood stream. This is the cause of hypertension.

5.2. There are approximately 24,000,000 people with hypertension and probably another 24,000,000 who have it and don't know it. Hypertension is a key factor in cardiovascular disease which is killing over one million people a year in the United States alone. This is the number-one killer.

5.3. Most lymphologists agree that congestive heart failure is fluid retention in the heart that is characterized by Venous Hypertension (high blood pressure) and Hypertension is directly related to trapped blood proteins.

5.4. Cancer, which is killing between 400,000 and 600,000 per year, is now becoming the number one killer of children and middle-aged women. If you add the victims of the two main killers in the U.S. and divide the number who are being killed by 365 days, you come up with over 4,000 people a day. That's over 120,000 men, women, and children *every month* or 240,000 every two months, who are dying from cardiovascular disease and cancer alone. This is not counting the millions of others who are suffering from some other crippling disease caused by trapped blood proteins.

5.5. As we said before, the A-bomb that was dropped on Hiroshima killed approximately 70,000 people. We are now being killed at the rate of approximately three A-bombs every two months in the United States from the two major diseases caused by trapped blood proteins.

5.6. With the knowledge and understandinng of this Formula and these Seven Golden Discoveries, you now know the cause of inflammation, pain, loss of energy, the allergies, heart disease, cancer, obesity, high blood pressure, arthritis, and every other crippling or killer disease known to man. You also understand the basic bio-electric self-help pain relief techniques. Therefore, you are ready to graduate from The College of Cause and Self-Help Pain Relief and enter into The College of Prevention.

J. INTRODUCTION TO SESSION THREE

1. Can you prevent if you do not know the cause? By learning of The Formula and The Seven Golden Discoveries, you know the *cause* and are ready to learn what you must do to *prevent* the crippling and killer diseases.

2. In the next session, we will go into prevention in detail.

We will also teach you some advanced lymphasizing techniques. Session Three is the most important session of the entire course. There is a big difference in just *thinking* something is right and *knowing* that it is right. As we put the concepts of prevention into The Formula, you will come to understand more clearly than ever before what you must do mentally, nutritionally, and physically to prevent pain, loss of energy, and the crippling and killer disease from taking place in your body. In short, you learn how to master *the art of lymphasizing.*

3. To prepare for this next session, we want you to make an effort to keep salt, sugar, fats, and high cholesterol foods out of the house. If you feel that you "just have to have some," one or two times a week, you are permitted to go out and "have a ball!" When you do it, we want you to enjoy it! This is part of the transition program, which you will come to understand in more detail as we go along. We also want you to continue in your efforts to love, bless and do good. I know that most of you attempt to do these things now, but as we go through this next session, we promise you that you will receive a deeper conviction of their importance than you ever have before.

4. You will also benefit by continuing the deep breathing exercise. See if you can increase the length of time you can do it without causing stress or fatigue.

5. Remember, the key to healing begins with an E. The word is Endurance! The more you make correct principles a part of your life, the better you will feel; and the better you feel, the more you will be able to make them a part of your life.

6. In Session Three you are going to learn how to lymphasize in a way that you will never cause stress on your body and you will never get tired.

7. This next session is actually changing the lives of everyone who goes through it. No one can remain the same when they come to know and understand beyond a shadow of doubt what they are doing mentally, nutritionally, and physically that is bringing pain, loss of energy, and disease into their body. They must be willing to try to change or commit willful suicide.

8. With the understanding that comes from the blood protein research comes faith. With faith you can move

mountains, which means you will be able to do things that will bring health, inner-beauty, and peace into your life and into the lives of others, in ways that have been impossible before.

NOTES

SESSION III

The College Of Prevention

A. FOR MAN TO PREVENT AND IF POSSIBLE REVERSE DISEASE AND HAVE PEACE ON EARTH HE MUST MASTER THE NEW SCIENCE CALLED THE ART OF LYMPHASIZING

1. This session contains principles and concepts concerning the new science called *The Art of Lymphasizing,* which has developed into what we call *The College of Prevention.*

2. In this session we discuss in detail what man must do mentally, nutritionally and physically to *prevent* and if possible *reverse* pain, loss of energy, viral infections, bacterial infections, allergies and the crippling and killer diseases. In short, we are going to teach what you must do to master *the art of lymphasizing.* This new science involves knowing what man must do mentally, nutritionally, and physically to untrap the blood proteins and keep them circulating in the body via the lymphatic system. The individuals and families who learn how to master this science will help raise up a posterity who will conquer disease and establish a civilization on earth that will be one in heart and one in mind, living in peace and harmony with no contention. To help establish a golden civilization where *love* will rule the emotions and *wisdom* will rule the appetite is the purpose of *the blood protein research* and *the art of lymphasizing* which is contained in this book.

3. Toward the end of this session, we will teach you some advanced lymphasizing concepts. By applying the wisdom and the great treasures of knowledge, even hidden treasures, that are found in *the art of lymphasizing,* you will be obeying the laws which enable people to literally *run and not be weary, walk and not faint*; and the destructive forces that are now destroying over 240,000 men, women and children every two months in this country alone *will pass you by as you learn to obey the mental, nutritional and physical laws of health.*

4. Also, as you learn all of the principles involved in bio-electric lymphasizing, you will know how to remove trapped

79

blood proteins from the spaces around your cells faster and easier than ever before. Then as you learn to combine bio-electric lymphasizing with *the art of lymphasizing,* you will cause an increase of healing to take place in your body and know how to reach a state of health and peace that was impossible to obtain before.

5. The individuals and families who take this course (when it becomes available) from a qualified instructor will be able to obtain the strength and understanding that comes from small group participation.

6. The importance of a world-wide family health education program is becoming very evident. Diseases that were rare in the early 1900's are now destroying people throughout the world at a rate which must not be ignored any longer. Until we understand and apply *the art of lymphasizing* the situation is going to get worse.

7. We realize some of the problems you may go through as you try to change your mental, nutritional and physical habits. To help you solve these problems and make these changes is the purpose of this course. For the first time, you are learning about the mental, nutritional and physical concepts of health in light of the basic formula which shows how the blood proteins produce the conditions that cause loss of energy, disease and death at the cell level. As you continue to apply what you learn, you are going to receive strength and courage that you have never had before, and your progress from this day forward will be exciting to say the least.

B. PREVENTION THROUGH PROPER MENTAL ATTITUDES, THE MENTAL PART OF THE ART OF LYMPHASIZING

1. To understand the mental attitudes of people, we must understand history. History records over and over again that it is the nature of man to persecute and destroy those who oppose him in some way.

2. It is very difficult to understand this situation when you consider that if people would only learn to *love* their enemies, *bless* those who curse them, and *do good* to those who hate them, they could bring peace and harmony into their lives. It seems that all people would welcome this. But history records that this is not true.

3. *Yet, the concepts of loving, blessing, and doing good are the basis on which civilizations must be founded, and the concepts which must be obeyed,* if any civilization is going to exist for any period of time in peace, without war and destruction. Love is in the heart of every man as a natural gift, regardless of who he is or where he may be. But the sad thing is that hate, loss of temper, holding grudges, and resentment are natural tendencies that can destroy this gift if they are not controlled. To be able to control these emotions and keep them in their proper place has been the challenge of man since the beginning. One of the main purposes of this session and this entire course is to give all people, regardless of who they are, a greater desire to develop the forces that deal with love until they are able to control the forces that cause hate, loss of temper, holding grudges, and resentment. Only as we learn to do this, will we be able to establish the *peace on earth that all nations are yearning for.*

B-1. To Have Health, We Must Obey The Laws Of Peace

1.1. We are going to scientifically prove that to have health, we must obey the laws of peace. Let's begin by looking at the history, the music, and the words of the song "Let There Be Peace On Earth." (Before this session is through, we hope the words of this song will become a reality in your heart.)

History Behind
"LET THERE BE PEACE ON EARTH"
(Let It Begin With Me)
By Sy Miller and Jill Jackson

One summer evening in 1955, a group of 180 teenagers of all races and religions, meeting at a workshop high in the California mountains, locked arms, formed a circle and sang a song of peace. They felt that singing the song, with its simple basic sentiment — "Let there be peace on earth, and let it begin with me," helped to create a climate for world peace and understanding.

When they came down from the mountain, these inspired young people brought the song with them and started sharing it. And, as though on wings, "Let There Be Peace On Earth" began an amazing journey around the globe. It traveled first, of course with the young campers back to their homes and schools, churches and clubs. Then the circle started by the teenagers began to grow. Soon the song was being shared in all fifty states — at school graduations and at PTA meetings, at Christmas and Easter gatherings and as part of the celebration of Brotherhood Week. It was a theme for Veteran's Day, Human Rights Day and U. N. Day, 4H Clubs and the United Auto Workers began singing it. So did the American Legion, the B'rith, the Kiwanis Clubs and CORE. It was taped, recorded, copied, printed in song books, and passed by word of mouth.

The song spread overseas to Holland, England, France, Germany, Lebanon. To South America, Asia and Australia. The Maoris in New Zealand sang it — even the Zulus in Africa sang it.

Professional singers took it up. Among them, *Ernie Ford, Andy Williams, Danny Kaye, Nat Cole, the Smothers Brothers, Roy Rogers, Dale Evans, Eddie Albert, Edie Adams, John Gary, Pearl Bailey, Roberta Shore, Champ Butler, the King Sisters, Mary Tyler Moore, John Raitt, Robie Lester, Liberace, Bob Crosby, the International Children's Choir, Jack Halloran, Gisele MacKenzie, Richard Summers, Lloyd Bridges, Patti Page, Angela Cartwright, the Young Americans, Carole Wells, Jack Smith, Pat Boone, Johnny Mathis,, Rhonda Fleming, Stan Melton, Norman Luboff, the Bing Crosby, Bob Hope, Lorne Greene and Ted Mack TV Shows and Father Keller's Christopher TV Series.*

The song began to win awards. "Let There Be Peace On Earth" was awarded the George Washington Honor Medal by the Freedoms Foundation at Valley Forge for "Outstanding achievement in helping to bring about a better understanding of the American Way of Life." It also received a Brotherhood Award from the National Conference of Christians and Jews.

This simple thought, "Let There Be Peace On Earth, and Let it Begin With Me" first born on a mountain top in the voices of youth, continues to travel heart to heart — gathering in people everywhere who wish to become a note in a song of understanding and peace — peace for all mankind.

Let There Be Peace On Earth
(Let It Begin With Me)

By
SY MILLER and
JILL JACKSON

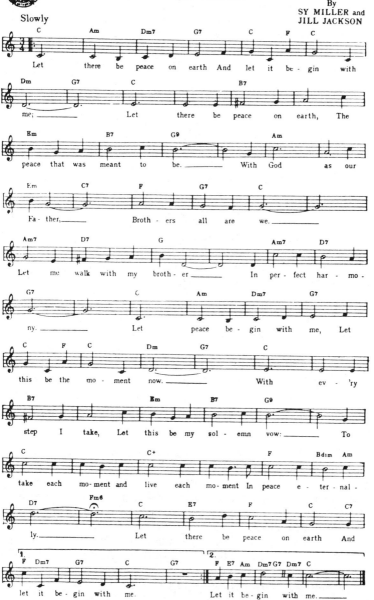

1.2. Where does peace begin? Can you have health if you don't learn to control your emotions of hate, loss of temper, holding grudges, resentment, jealousy, etc.?

B-2. *Review Of Stress And The Death Process*

2.1. Let us review what we have learned regarding stress. Anger, loss of temper, holding grudges, resentment, and jealousy have historically been the cause of murder and war.

2.2. In Sessions One and Two we discussed how a mild trauma such as stress or anger can cause "leakage of large quantities of plasma-like fluids (blood proteins and water) out of the blood capillaries." Stress has a shock-like effect upon the body that will cause *thirst and loss of energy* as it produces trapped plasma proteins and excess fluid and sodium which will reduce the energy fields produced by the cells. This can cause infection, inflammation, and disease in the body. They have known for years that stress was related to the crippling and killer diseases. With the new *Blood Protein Research,* we can now explain why this is true, in detail.

B-3. *The Laws Of Health Are The Laws Of Peace*

3.1. As stress causes loss of energy and disease by producing a shock-like effect upon the body, so does anger, fear, loss of temper, holding grudges, resentment, and jealousy, etc.

3.2. To have health, we must be big enough to *love* our enemies, *bless* those who curse us, and *do good* to those who hate us. In short, we must learn to control our emotions and live in peace.

B-4. *Mental Attitudes That Cause Death Will Also Cause War*

4.1. Cain was the first person to commit murder on this earth. This was the beginning of war! Let's look at the heart of Cain. Did Cain have anger in his heart? Did he lose his temper? Did he hold grudges, and harbor resentment, jealousy and discontentment? He did every single one of them! We have just proven that *the formula for death is also the formula for war.* The same emotions that bring sickness and death in our body are the same emotions that will cause one person to destroy another.

4.2. There was also another major destructive factor in the heart of Cain. This was the uncontrollable desire to get gain. You can put it into the formula and know exactly how desire to get gain is still causing conspiring men to bury the government documents and scientific research which reveals how we are being destroyed. As a result many innocent people are still promoting "foods" and other products that are *slaying* us with killer disease, *torturing* us with crippling disease, and *binding* us down and bringing us into *misery*. Men who have the *heart of Cain* are true enemies to those who desire health and peace. These enemies are truly seeking to destroy our lives, and we had better seek wisdom because the wickedness of these men is now revealing itself unto us in a manner that is speaking in our ears *with a voice loud enough to shake the earth.* If the death of over two hundred and forty thousand men, women, and children every two months in the United States alone is not enough to "shake the earth," then what is? This destruction will continue. It will not pass us by, unless we obtain the *wisdom* and *great treasures of knowledge* that are revealed in the blood protein research and the art of lymphasizing.

B-5. To Save Your Life, Learn About The Blood

5.1. It is very interesting that the children of Israel put blood on their doors to keep the destroying angel from slaying them. It is just as interesting that as we learn more about the blood, we learn what the destructive forces are that are now slaying over 240,000 people every two months in the United States and how they are doing it. It is also interesting that if we use this knowledge *wisely* this destruction will pass us by and not slay us. *This is more than just symbolism, it is reality,* and this fact will become clearer as we go along.

5.2. When Adam and Eve came out of the garden with blood, (which included the blood proteins), going through their veins, they were told that they were going to die. The Lord knew all about our blood proteins, and that they would eventually cause our death. This is why I believe he symbolized the adversary as a serpent. The snake's venom that kills us is *protein*. When it gets into the blood stream, it dilates the tiny pores of the capillary membranes just like the poison from a damaged cell, anger, loss of temper, holding grudges, and resentment. There is the heart of Cain; there is the adversary. The serpent is truly symbolic of our blood proteins. Anyone or anything that will trap our blood proteins will help cause disease and death. All the adversary has to do to destroy us is to get us or someone else to do something that will mentally, nutritionally or physically cause us to trap our blood proteins in our body. He has been achieving his objective, but he can only work in darkness. That is, to destroy us he must keep us in ignorance mentally, nutritionally and physically.

B-6. *Medical Doctors And The People In The United States Are In Ignorance As To The Mental, Nutritional and Physical Causes Of Death*

6.1.   In the United States we are in the "medical dark ages." Just as sure as there was a religious dark ages, we are now in the medical dark ages. The dictators have just changed their suits. This is confirmed by Dr. Harold W. Harper and Michael L. Culbert who wrote the book, *How You Can Beat The Killer Diseases*, and by Dr. Mendelsohm, who wrote *The Confessions Of A Medical Heretic* and *Malepractice*. These books and many others confirm that the AMA, the food and drug bureaucracies, many of the food processors, and the international pharmaceutical monopolies rule this nation with an iron hand. In health matters, medical doctors and the lay public in the United States have been stripped of their freedoms.

6.2.   You can't separate freedom from peace, and the way to peace on earth is through health. Therefore, the way to freedom is also through health.

B-7. *Knowledge Of Blood Proteins Will Restore Health and Peace*

7.1.   The knowledge of our blood proteins will not only help us to become healthy, but it will also help us get our health freedoms back. This research contains the answer to the cause of every crippling and killer disease known to man and what we must do to heal the body. It also gives us a greater knowledge of how the adversary works to destroy our freedoms, and we must have this knowledge to help establish health and peace throughout the world. The adversary also knows this. He knows that this blood protein research along with the art of lymphasizing will give us the knowledge that will enable us to help get our health freedoms back and stop the destruction that is now taking place.

7.2. We now know that when we live the laws that will prevent disease, we will also prevent war and establish peace on earth. Therefore, we must do all that is in our power to restore the freedoms that are necessary for *everyone* to practice prevention in every sense of the word.

B-8.   Why Some Medical Doctors Are Afraid To Teach The Blood Protein Research

8.1. I have known medical doctors who have become interested in this research but are afraid to teach it. One doctor in Arizona, after reading that our blood proteins could cause death in the body in about twenty-four hours, stood up, pounded his fist on the desk and said to me, "I think we have come to an end of our progress. If I tried teaching this blood protein research, they would take my license away from me. I can't teach it, but maybe I can send people to you." I could not believe the words that came out of his mouth. A doctor who was responsible for saving lives was afraid of "someone" taking his license away if he taught the cause of death.

8.2 Another doctor in Utah became very interested until he got a phone call from the head of the discipline board. When I asked him what had happened, he said, "Do you know who 'he' is? He can take my license away from me."

B-9.   AMA Discipline Boards Keep Medical Doctors From Practicing Prevention

9.1. The lights went on and I now saw the adversary clearly. What Dr. Baum, an M.D., in Idaho told us was true. He stood up in one of my lectures and said that the AMA has discipline boards set up in every state, and they watch the doctors like a hawk. The doctors are told by these "medical emperors" that they are to *treat* disease not *prevent* disease. If they step out of line, their hospital privileges go first and their license second.

9.2. Christina Skidmore of Mesa, Arizona, had multiple

sclerosis so badly that she had to concentrate for about thirty seconds before she could get her legs to move. (Muscles work by electric impulses, and trapped proteins shut the generators off until it causes multiple sclerosis.) Over a period of time, she got off the foods that trap the proteins. She did it too fast, but in three weeks she was not only able to walk, she could run! She demonstrated her ability to do this about a year and a half later for a group of Naturopaths in Arizona. When she showed her doctor that she could run and told him what she had done to get well, she said he told her he knew that what she was doing was making her well, but that he could not discuss diet with any of his other patients without risk of losing his license. You will read Christina's testimony later on in this session. Mrs. Coons another M.S. patient told me her neurologist told her the same thing. In effect those doctors said they knew that diet could help their M.S. patients, but they were afraid to talk about it!. If that is not a "medical dictatorship," keeping people in darkness, then what is it?

B-10. Why Doctors And The People In The United States Now Have To Fight For Health Freedoms

10.1. It is reported that Dr. Benjamin Rush, surgeon general of George Washington's Army and a signer of the Declaration of Independence, had this to say about medical freedom. "Unless we put medical freedom into the Constitution, the time will come when medicine will organize into an undercover dictatorship to restrict the art of healing to one class of men (conventional orthodox treatment) and deny equal privileges to others---. All such laws are un-American and despotic and have no place in a republic. The Constitution of this Republic should make special provisions for medical freedom as well as religious freedom." (Source unidentified)

10.2. What Dr. Rush feared has become a reality. Many doctors who have attended my lectures have told me that the doctors and the people in the United States are now being ruled by a medical dictatorship and they are now beginning to rebel.

10.3. Dr. Huls, D.O., the doctor who inspired me to go back to school full time with six children to become a doctor had his hospital privileges taken away because he was using unconventional methods to heal his patients. I saw him take an 18-

year-old-girl who was blind and deaf since birth and restore her eyesight and most of her hearing in four treatments. I knew her before she went to see him. When I walked into his office one day she was there, and with tears rolling down her cheeks she told me how he worked on her bone structure through her mouth and released the pressure that restored her hearing and her eyesight. She could see as good as I could and she only had one hearing aid on one ear. It was after this that they took his license away from him. He continued to practice under a massage license and people came to him from all over the world until he died. What a sad ending for such a great doctor. Dr. Cox studied under him before he died, and as a result they have now taken his license away from him. He graduated from the American University of Natural Therapeutics and Preventative Medicine in Feb. 1980 so he could practice as a Naturopathic Physician.

10.4. Dr. Gambi went into preventive medicine in Utah and he ended up having to leave the state. Dr. Robert Vance in Utah is a member of The International Academy of Preventative Medicine which I understand is the largest organization of prevention oriented doctors in the United States. Dr. Vance has suffered continual harassment from the organized medical establishment. They have literally tried to destroy his practice.

10.5. Dr. John Richardson, a courageous physician in California has challenged orthodox medicine over Laetrile (Vitamin B-17) and Nutrition, which he believes can control and prevent cancer. He has been subjected to four harassment trials. Not to continue his fight would mean to Dr. Richardson "condemning people to death." Therefore, he is fighting not only because he is a fighter, but because he knows it is the right thing to do to preserve our freedoms. When any organization tries to exercise control or dominion upon men in any manner that would violate the rights guaranteed by the Constitution and Bill of Rights, any authority they claim to have should be challenged. This concept is the foundation upon which this nation was built.

10.6. Dr. Richardson, M.D., tells how his battle began: "I knew I could not refuse to treat my nurse's sister without breaking my Hippocratic Oath... What I did not then realize was that I was about to bring down upon myself and my family the vengence of the medical machine..." It is because of the arrest of Dr. Richardson in 1972 that the "Committee for Freedom of

Choice in Cancer Therapy" was formed.

10.7. A few of the other doctors who are now fighting for our health freedoms are: Dr. Mendelsohn, M.D., who wrote, *Confessions of a Medical Heretic,* and *Malepractice*; Dr. Boyd, D.O., who wrote *Stay Out of the Hospital*; Dr. Nittler who wrote *A New Breed of Doctor*; Dr. Harper who wrote *How to Beat the Killer Diseases*; Dr. Manner, M.D., who wrote, *The Death of Cancer*; Dr. Baum, M.D., who stood at one of my Idaho lectures and told the people how they took his license away when he went into preventative medicine. Dr. Julian Whitaker, M.D., in California spoke at the National Health Federation several times voicing his feelings openly. Dr. Fuller Royal, M.D., won his fight in Oregon and moved to Nevada to start The Nevada Clinic of Preventative Medicine where he is now diagnosing electrically and using homeopathic remedies to treat disease. If you try to get into his clinic you have to wait about four months.

10.8. Dr. Stevan Cordas, M. D., in Bedford, Texas, and some of his associates are now using herbs to treat disease. I have talked to medical doctors in Denver, Colorado who are sending their cancer patients to the Naturopaths; and the Naturopaths are not even licenced by the state. It is pathetic that doctors in the United States cannot treat their patients the way they would like to.

10.9 Note: All of the names of doctors that we have mentioned or will mention in this book are supplied in order that you might exercise FREEDOM OF CHOICE in the treatment and cure of disease. Not all of the Doctors employ the same treatment program. Therefore if you decide to see these doctors, you will need to do your own research in finding the particular program that you feel is best for you.

10.10. To get a directory showing the doctors by state who are prevention oriented write to the International Academy of Prevention Medicine, 10409 Town and Country Way, Houston, Texas. Or call (913) 648-8720.

B-11. An Age of Peace and Health That We Have Never Known Before

11.1. The knowledge of our blood proteins is the key to

health and peace! It is also the knowledge that will help restore our freedoms. God rules by the laws of free agency. The adversary rules by the laws of force. As you gain knowledge of your blood proteins, the adversary is brought out into the light, and he loses his power to control you. As you obey the laws that will prevent your blood proteins from causing your death, you can *bind* the adversary and establish health and peace in your life.

B-12. "Forgive Them, For They Know Not What They Do"

12.1. At this point let us discuss the laws of peace in detail. With the knowledge that anger, loss of temper, holding grudges, and resentment can trap your blood proteins and cause sickness and disease, we now know that we must be able to love our enemies. This scientifically proves that the laws of health are the laws of peace and that the laws of sickness and death are the laws of war. The same mental attitudes that will cause death in our body will also cause a man to kill his brother. The one who made this body knew what he was talking about when he told us we had to be big enough to *love* our enemies, *bless* those who curse us, *do good* to those that hate us, and *pray* for those who persecute us and despitefully use us. What does the adversary say? *Don't* love your enemies. *Don't* bless those who curse you. *Don't* do good to those who hate you, and, above all, *don't* pray for those who persecute you and despitefully use you. We become the servants of him whom we choose to obey. Good is represented by love--and evil by hate--and everyone on the earth must learn to serve one or the other. And man becomes the servant of that which he chooses to obey.

12.2. Now we can understand more clearly than ever before why Jesus said to those who had *hatred* in their hearts that their father was the devil. Now we can understand why he said if you say you *love* me and *hate* your brother, *you're a liar.* You cannot serve love and hate at the same time. We can now understand clearer than ever before why Jesus, while on the cross, was able to say, "Father, forgive them, for they know not what they do." He prayed for those who persecuted him and despitefully used him. *He wouldn't serve anger, loss of temper, holding grudges or resentment, even under those circumstances.* Now we can understand that if someone crosses us and we feel like firing back, unless we are going to serve the forces of evil, we are going to have to say the same thing: "Forgive them, for *they* know not what *they do." There is peace* in those words. *Try them!* They will work a miracle in your life. With understanding comes faith, and with faith you can move mountains which means we can do things which we could not do before.

B-13.   *To Willfully Cause Stress In Another Person Is To Cause Their Destruction*

13.1. The next time someone disturbs you and you feel like firing back, ask yourself these questions. *Am I going to give in to anger, loss of temper, holding grudges, and resentment?" "Am I going to serve love or hate?"* This will give you the strength to *say* and *do* that which will bring health and peace to you and to those with whom you are involved. Truly, if they knew what *you know now,* the only way they could intentionally cause undue stress in you *without any restraint,* would be to willfully cause your destruction.

13.2 Now, husbands, wives, and children, are you going to argue and fight and run each other down? If you willfully let anger instead of love rule your home, you are causing your own problems.

B-14.   *The Natural Man, An Enemy To Himself*

14.1. We can talk about the principles which involve loving, blessing, and doing good all day long, but when someone curses you, is it your natural impulse to turn around and bless him or should he stand ten feet back? The natural man is not only an enemy to all those who want health and peace, but he is also an *enemy to himself. By his actions he will cause contention and trapped blood proteins.* TPP = EX FL, EX Na+ = $\blacktriangle$ EE = $\boxtimes$. *He will be a source of destruction to all those around him until he finally destroys himself.*

B-15.   *Medicine and Drugs, Building Ships and Guns Is Not The Answer*

15.1. The subtitle on the cover of this book could have read "Conquer Disease *and War* With Eight Keys to Health and

<u>World</u> Peace!" The Basic Formula for <u>health</u> is The Basic Formula for <u>peace:</u> No TPP = No EX FL, No EX Na + = EE = ☐. This is one of the most important concepts we can learn. This is why we call this session *The College of Prevention.* I believe you understand better than ever before what you are going to have to do mentally to *prevent* pain, loss of energy, heart disease, cancer, obesity, stroke, high blood pressure, arthritis, and the other crippling and killer diseases from taking place in your body. Every family in the whole world needs to hear and understand these concepts. This is why we call this "The Worldwide Golden Family Self-H.E.L.P. Program." The H.E.L.P. stands for: <u>H</u>ealth <u>E</u>ducation for <u>L</u>ongevity and <u>P</u>eace! The knowledge of our blood proteins gives us the scientific answer to health and world peace for the first time in history. Medicine and drugs, building ships and guns are not the answer. That is treatment, not prevention. To prevent war, sickness, and death *and to help* establish peace on the earth, *the knowledge and understanding of The Basic Formula For Health and World Peace must grow until it fills the whole earth.*

B-16. Introducing The World-Wide Golden Family Self-H.E.L.P. Program

16.1 Let me introduce you to a health education program that could take forty years to complete unless something takes place to speed it up. We must begin *now* to get the blood protein research to the nations of the earth so they will know what they must do to raise up a posterity who will be prepared mentally, nutritionally and physically to conquer disease and live in peace.

16.2. The purpose of this world wide family health education program is to help establish golden families throughout the world who are one in heart, one in mind, who will learn how to conquer disease and live in peace with no poor among them. To do this may take forty years, working just as fast and as hard as we can beginning right now. Our children's children will be the ones to fully realize the blessings of this program; but for them to enjoy the blessings of health and peace we must begin *now* to get the blood protein research to every family in the whole world. To have a knowledge of the blood proteins is to have a knowledge of the causes of pain, sorrow, disease, death, and war to a greater degree than we have ever known before. We now know that the way to peace on earth is through health. The laws of health are the laws of peace. People can cry for peace and pray for peace from now on, and they will never obtain peace in their homes, in their nation or on earth until they learn to live the laws of health.

16.3. It has taken seven years to learn about the seven discoveries concerning life and death at the cell level and to gain the understanding necessary to write the One Basic Formula which made it possible to write this book, *The Golden Seven Plus One, Conquer Disease with Eight Keys to Health, Beauty and Peace.* And it is interesting that right now people in all nations are becoming more interested in health than ever before in history.

16.4. We have been told that in the last days the time would be cut short or the very elect would be deceived. Well, the very elect on the earth today are being destroyed, not by war but by disease. People all over the world are now being destroyed *in a manner* that should speak in our ears with a voice that should shake the earth. I repeat what I have said many times in this book. We have never had a war that has killed 240,000 men, women, and children every two months. *People are being deceived if they think destruction will come only by war; or if they believe it is possible to obtain peace on earth without living the laws of health.* One out of two who are now dying in the United States are dying of heart disease. Cancer is getting one out of four. Wars may be delayed, they come and go; but this destruction is going on every day and it will never cease until people wake up and learn that to have peace and to stop the human sacrifice that is now taking place on the earth, they must live the laws of health as given in detail in this session.

16.5 *Everyone who learns about the blood protein research and thereby obtains the knowledge that will help restore health and peace to the earth has a responsibility to get this research to their families and loved ones first, and then to others just as fast as their time and talents will allow.*

16.6 Everyone who reads these words and feels in their heart that they are true should start using The Dietary Goals for the United States in a way that will help to get the knowledge of the blood proteins and the art of lymphasizing into as many homes as possible. Those who have a desire to conquer disease and live in peace will want to start immediately to help educate others. Section C-17 on page 108 will explain how to use the "Dietary Goals". As you give, so shall you receive. As you attempt to help others, the most important family that you will help bring health and peace to will be your own. How much is health and peace worth? It is priceless. *"Many people spend their health to gain their wealth; they toil, they work, they slave, then they spend their wealth to regain their health, and all they get is the grave."* Which is the most important in the long run, wealth or health? As you get involved in saving lives you will be performing one of the greatest services that can be rendered. Remember, without this knowledge, even the very elect will continue to be destroyed throughout the world. We can now teach them on a scientific basis that if they do not learn to apply the art of lymphasizing, they will cause their own sickness and death and that of their families and loved ones. As we get this knowledge to the nations of the earth, the righteous of the earth, wherever they may be, will be able to raise up a posterity who can "run and not be weary, walk and not faint;" who will, by their actions "bind the adversary" and help establish peace throughout the world.

B-17. Live Laws of Health; Become Like The City of Enoch

17.1. The people who will live these laws of peace will be taking a major step in becoming like the people who lived in the city of Enoch. Most people today would like to see peace on the earth but how many are *ready* for it? Are you ready? Can you bless someone if he curses you and do good to someone who hates you? Let's consider the words of the song again that says "Let There Be Peace On Earth," and see if they mean more to you now than they did before. These words were truly inspired.

> Let there be peace on earth
> And let it begin with me.
> Let there be peace on earth,
> The peace that was meant to be.
> With God as our father,
> Brothers all are we.
> Let me walk with my brother,
> In perfect harmony.

> Let peace begin with me,
> Let this be the moment now,
> With every step I take,
> Let this be my solemn vow,
> To take each moment,
> And live each moment,
> In peace - - - eternally.
> Let there be peace on earth,
> And let it begin with me.
>
>   Sy Miller
>   Jill Jackson

B-18. *This Message Must Go To The Nations Of The Earth*

18.1. We have scientifically proven that to have a truly healthy body, we must have a peaceful body; that to have a truly healthy family, we must have a peaceful family; and that to have a healthy nation and a healthy world, we must have a peaceful nation and a peaceful world!

18.2. Every nation on earth right now is open for a health message. The blood protein research is designed to help bring health and peace into your life and into your home.

18.3. To those who understand this research, it becomes their solemn duty and moral obligation to help get this knowledge to as many others as possible. Those who love, bless, and do good will do all they can to apply these principles and spread this knowledge to others. *The blood protein research has given birth to the most important scientific message for health and world peace on the face of the earth.*

C. PREVENTION THROUGH PROPER NUTRITION, THE NUTRITIONAL PART OF THE ART OF LYMPHASIZING

1. Our mental attitudes are related to health and are probably the most important part of the whole program, but they only represent one third of The College of Prevention. To complete this college we must discuss the need for *good* nutrition and *proper* physical exercise.

2. If there are certain "foods" we are now using that can trap our blood proteins, instead of being called a "food" it should be regarded as a deadly poison. Remember, anyone, or anything that can trap our blood proteins will cause our destruction. We in the United States have been led down the primrose path as far as foods are concerned.

C-1. Are We Just Dying, Or Are We Being Destroyed?

1.1. We now know that our enemies in their secret chambers are seeking our lives. There are those with *evil designs in their hearts* who, for gold, silver, material possessions, and the praises of the world, will take our freedoms from us and promote "foods" and products that will *slay* us with killer diseases, *torture* us with crippling diseases, *bind* us down, and bring us into *misery*. As a nation, we had better seek wisdom. The wickedness of these men is now being revealed unto us *in a manner* that is truly *shaking the earth*. The "foods" they are now promoting, which are actually physically and mentally addicting drugs, are playing a major role in destroying us in the form of heart disease, cancer, obesity, stroke, high blood pressure, hypoglycemia, diabetes, arthritis and the other killer and crippling diseases. Just think about it: from heart disease and cancer alone, there are over two hundred and forty thousand men, women, and children being slain every two months in the United States alone. This does not count the millions of others who are suffering from other killer and crippling diseases. We have never had such destruction of human life since the beginning of this nation. The wars we have had are nothing compared to what is now taking place as a result of the death and suffering that is now being caused by trapped blood proteins.

1.2. Today, most people seem to accept this destruction as a normal part of life. They are told that the causes are unknown, and that there is no cure. Therefore, since they are scared of these problems, and they don't know what to do to prevent them, they just put their hands over their heads and go around hoping that these diseases will pass them by. But, as we discussed earlier, *man cannot be saved from this destruction in ignorance of the causes.* Heart disease is now the cause of one out of two deaths in the United States. Cancer is striking one out of four, and they say it will soon get one out of three. If we desire to escape *the enemies who are now destroying us,* we had better get our hands off our heads, take a good look around, and find out what is going on!

C-2. Cause of Death Has Changed Since Early 19th Century. Why?

2.1. As we said, in the beginning of the early 19th century, these diseases were scarce, and there are some civilizations who don't have them even today. So what are we doing wrong? What has happened to us? We have already discussed how certain mental attitudes can cause disease and death. That is a big problem, but improper diet and lack of exercise each play just as big a part as far as disease is concerned, and disease can effect your mental attitude.

2.2. Let's consider what it would be like to have a body that is really healthy and how we can know when this body is being destroyed. There is a great difference in being alive and well and being alive and sick. According to the formula, if you didn't have any trapped proteins in your body, all your generators would be on and you would be perfectly healthy. You would not have any painful crippling or killer disease, no infections, no allergies and no loss of energy, in your body. It is hard to imagine what a truly healthy body would feel like, but it is easy to remember what it feels like when you put your hand on a hot stove.

C-3. You Can Know If You Eat a Poison By How It Makes You Feel

3.1. There *are* foods that will trap your blood proteins and as you learn how to tell what they are, *you had better also learn how to work with the mental addictions these poisons produce or this knowledge will cause stress* and cause even more problems than you have at this time. To understand this the first thing you need to understand is the symptoms of poison. Once you know the effect that a poison has on the body, you will be able to feel it just like putting your hand on a hot stove. If trapped blood proteins on an extreme scale can cause your destruction within just a few hours, you should be able to feel the symptoms of destruction in minutes--and you can! All you have to do is know what to look for. With the knowledge of the formula we know that one effect a poison would have upon your body as it traps your blood proteins is *loss of energy.* TPP = ▲ EE. A poison effects the body just like shock or stress. *A poison is a poison because it causes trapped blood proteins.* It is the trapped blood proteins that shut the generators off and drain the energy out of the body. The next symptom is *thirst.* The water in the blood stream follows the blood proteins. TPP = EX FL = Thirst.

C-4. *Thirst And Loss Of Energy Are Symptoms Of Disease And Death.* TPP = EX FL = ▲ EE = *Thirst and Loss Of Energy*

4.1. If you feed a dog strychnine, the first thing he goes for is water. A poison, like shock, will cause trapped proteins which pull the water out of the blood stream into the spaces around the cells, and you will feel a need to replace the water in your blood stream immediately. So the two symptoms that tell us we are eating a poison that will cause sickness and death are *thirst* and *loss of energy.*

4.2. Just as sure as you know you have burned your hand when you put it on a hot stove, the next time you eat something that causes thirst or loss of energy, you know you are getting "burned" inside. These "foods" are now helping to destroy 240,000 men, women and children every two months in the United States alone. Our enemies do everything they can to make these poisons *delicious to the taste and very desirable.* And the enemy who would destroy you to get *gain* will try to keep you in *ignorance* by doing everything they can to convince you that these foods are harmless. Many advertisers try to convince people that these foods are delicious to the taste and very desirable and won't hurt us, and because of ignorance many people believe them.

4.3. What are the foods that cause loss of energy and make you thirsty? Salt, simple sugars (candies, cakes, ice cream, etc.), fats, the high cholesterol foods (animal and dairy products), and too much meat. And here is the evidence.

C-5. *Why Too Much Salt* (Na + Cl −) Is A Poison
EX Na + = TPP = *Thirst and Loss of Energy.*

5.1. Let's take a look at salt. As you learned in the formula trapped blood proteins carry a negative charge and they pull the positive sodium ions to them. Not only do the proteins attract the sodium, but evidence verifies that salt will trap the blood proteins, and this combination really pulls the water out of the blood stream. This is why salt makes you *thirsty*. Listen to your body; it will tell you when you are getting "burned" inside. Excess sodium outside the cells will also upset the sodium-potassium balance inside the cells. This is why salt will damage or kill the cells and cause the crippling and killer diseases. When a person has fluid retention, the doctor will take him off salt. If a person has high blood pressure, the doctor will try to eliminate salt from his diet. Salt is not only a poison, it is also a physically and mentally addicting drug, and most Americans are addicted. This is why salt is used so extensively in processed foods. *We are not just dying; we are being destroyed!*

C-6. *Government Document: <u>The Dietary Goals For The United States</u> Says That Salt, Sugar, Fat, The High Cholesterol Foods, And Too Much Meat Are Directly Related To The Destruction Of Two Hundred And Forty Thousand Men, Women And Children Every Two Months In This Country Alone!*

6.1. In February 1977, the U.S. Government published a document telling the people in the U.S. that too much salt, sugar, fat, meat, and cholesterol are directly related to heart disease and cancer; and that six of the ten leading causes of death are related to our diet. This is additional evidence to prove that the formula for loss of energy, disease and death is correct. One out of two who are now dying in the United States are dying of cardiovascular disease. One out of five is dying of cancer.

6.2. Most of the evidence verifies that the only sodium we need is the salt we get in our natural fruits, vegetables, and whole grains or sprouts. If you fail to do something about your salt intake, you are committing willful suicide. You cannot now blame the enemy any longer if you are willing to destroy yourself. If you decide to disregard this evidence, what effect will it have on your children? Are you willing to destroy them too?

6.3. Instead of salt use kelp, spike, vegit, Jensen's vegetable broth and seasoning or Bio-salt. They are good on your baked potatoes, salads, and raw or slightly steamed vegetables that you should eat for lunch and dinner. Raw yams, grated beets, and other vegetables are delicious without any seasoning. The fresh fruits that are good for breakfast and lunch do not need seasoning either. In fact, when you are thirsty, try a juicy fruit; you get the liquid arfd all the nutrients too.

6.4. The blood plasma is 91% water with dissolved minerals and nutrients. The fluid that is diffused back and forth from the blood capillaries is almost all water with dissolved minerals and nutrients. So when you eat food that is mostly water with dissolved minerals and nutrients, you are actually eating the water that must continually be replenished in the blood stream to irrigate the cells. As the cells extract the minerals and nutrients out of the water in the blood, it becomes dead fluid and the body discards it via the eliminative organs. This dead fluid must be replaced with foods that are mostly water with dissolved minerals and nutrients, which are foods that do *not* make you thirsty.

6.5. When you eat foods, that make you thirsty, you have to drink a lot of water to hopefully get enough dissolved minerals and nutrients into the bloodstream; and also to activate the kidneys to help get rid of the poisonous by-products that are produced from eating these kinds of food.

6.6. High protein foods are a poor source of glucose which is the source of energy for the cells. We will discuss this later on. Fruits, vegetables, sprouts, etc. are the primary source of glucose and these foods do not make you thirsty.

6.1. It is interesting that when the children of Israel put blood on their doors *the destroying angel passed them by;* and that when we learn about the blood, we will stay away from the foods that make us thirsty so the diseases that are now causing destruction on the earth will pass us by and not slay us.

C-7. Why the "Simple" Sugars Are Poisons!

7.1. Now, let's take a look at the *"simple"* sugars--the candies, cakes, ice cream, etc. The *complex* sugars in fruits and vegetables and whole grains or sprouts are released very slowly into the blood stream. Your body can handle them just fine. But the simple sugars are released very quicky into the blood stream. Too much sugar in the blood stream will dilate the capillary membranes just like stress, shock, or poisons from damaged cells. Sugar is also a physically and mentally addicting drug, just like alcohol. The simple sugars will *trap* your blood proteins, pull the water out of the blood, make you *thirsty, shut your generators off,* and damage or kill the cells. Yet many people will continue to say, "This food is delicious and very desirable, but it won't hurt you!"

7.2. One of the first places the poisons will hit you is in the head. Many people feel it is sheer "inspiration" to have a clear thought in their head once or twice a year. If they would untrap their blood proteins, they should be able to think clearly all the time.

7.3. If you fail to do something about your simple sugar intake, beginning today, you will be committing willful suicide. Also, are you going to continue to feed it to your children without restraint? Like we said, there is a big difference between *thinking* it is bad and *knowing* it is bad. If you crave something sweet, try fruit.

C-8. Why Fat Is A Poison!

8.1. A body charged with oxygen is a body charged with electrical energy! But too much fat, like sugar and salt, will rob the body of oxygen and reduce the electrical energy produced by the cells. From the seven golden discoveries and the formula we have learned that our bodies run on electricity. The food we eat, if it is the right kind of food, is converted chemically into electricity, which makes it possible for us to function.

8.2. However, without oxygen, it is impossible for the cell to complete its energy cycle. Oxygen is a food for the body and is one of the most important foods we can get. Glucose plus oxygen yields A.T.P. (adenosine triphosphate) which the cell must have to produce energy.

8.3. Deep breathing saturates the blood with oxygen. These oxygen-laden red blood cells carry a negative electrical charge. Like the negative polls of two magnets, two oxygen-laden red blood cells repel each other. The blood actually moves through the body electrically. This is how and why the blood is able to go through the entire body so quickly. Three quarts of blood goes through our capillaries every sixty seconds. That is why *it is better to breathe deeply five minutes a day than walk five minutes without breathing deeply.*

8.4. The red blood cells must travel through the tiny

capillaries single file. *If there are not enough charged oxygen-laden red blood cells, the red blood cells will stick together and cause a microscopic traffic jam.* This blockage will dilate the tiny pores of the capillary membranes and cause "trapped" proteins in the spaces around the cells. "Trapped" blood proteins will produce excess fluid around the cells, and the cells will begin to "drown" and die because of lack of oxygen; we die from lack of oxygen at the cell level.

8.5.   Too much fat in the blood stream will rob the red blood cells of their oxygen and produce the microscopic traffic jam and the resulting trapped blood proteins. When this happens in the brain, the brain cells suffer from oxygen starvation; and senility, dullness, and irritability set in. Lack of oxygen will effect other parts of the body in a similar manner, but the place where we recognize it is in the brain. Your body will tell you when you eat a poison. Just pay attention to it and heed the warnings: *thirst and loss* of *energy. You may also lose the ability to concentrate.*

C-9. *Why The High Cholesterol Foods Are Poisons!*

9.1.   How do the high cholesterol foods (the animal products and dairy products) and red meats "trap" the blood proteins? Cholesterol has been the subject of great debate, but when you learn about "cholesterol epoxide," the debate is over. The body makes its own cholesterol. When you take excess cholesterol into your body, *cholesterol epoxide* and other poisons are formed. In the February 1977 issue of *Scientific American* it states that cholesterol epoxide and other substances formed from cholesterol will *cause cells to mutate* which will cause cancer. That research also states the cholesterol levels correlate with the incidence of *coronary heart disease.* The same principle applies to eating too much or the wrong kind of meat. It is the poisonous by-products produced from the breakdown of meat that dilate the blood capillaries and cause trapped proteins, thirst and loss of energy. *Listen to your body–it will tell you.*

C-10. *The Dietary Goals Calls For a National Health Education Program to Protect the People Against The "Interests" Who Are Causing Their Destruction*

10.1.   To confirm the above findings, let's look at the

Dietary Goals for the United States. This is the most valuable document that has been published by the government for the benefit of the people since the Constitution and the Bill of Rights. It tells that there are "interests" who are "creating our present problems," and it calls for a national health education program to alert families, school teachers, public health nurses, health educators, nutritionists, and physicians so they will know what can cause death. This document was published by the United States Senate Select Committee on Nutrition and Human Needs in February 1977. Before December, this document was attacked by some of the food processors, and the AMA and others; and the first edition was put out of print. (How it ever got published in the first place was a miracle.) This document not only tells who some of our enemies are, but what we must do to keep them from destroying us. Remember, the adversary works in darkness by keeping us ignorant of his ways. When we gain knowledge of how he works we can "bind" him because he loses his power to harm us.

C-11. The A.M.A., Some Of The Food Processors, And Others Tried to Discredit Government Document

11.1. The government formed the committee that published this document to see if there were foods the American people were eating that would cause heart disease, cancer obesity, stroke, and the other killer and crippling diseases. They found that there *were* foods that were directly related to the above diseases, so they published this report to the people of the United States in an attempt to save their lives. It was even advertised on national television, but *something* happened because it only lasted a very short time. Today you hear very little mentioned about this report. In fact, the second edition that was published in December 1977 contained a three page foreward quoting the A.M.A. who said that *to change your diet may be harmful,* and these three pages attempted to discredit the entire document by saying that *science has not proven any connection between diet and disease.* Also, the first edition only cost one dollar, while the second edition cost two dollars and forty cents. (A fifteen page excerpt of the first addition along with discrediting statements in the three page forward of the second edition can be found in the appendix of this book.)

11.2 Comments and quotations from the first edition as given below will help you understand why they (our enemies and our destroyers) tried to discredit one of the most powerful documents published by the government since the Constitution and the Bill of Rights.

C-12. *Why We Are Publishing A "15 Page Excerpt" Of The First Edition Of This Government Document*

12.1. When I received the second edition in December 1977, I called Mr. H. in Washington, D.C., a staff member in charge of this document, and asked, "Why did those senators put those three pages in the front of this second edition?"

He answered "The men who did it are up for re-election."

My reply to Mr. H. was, "I will not have that second edition. I will not buy it, and I will not promote it in the future. I've got to have that first edition. I have been buying them by the thousands to help save the lives of the people of the United States."

Mr. H. responded that he was very sorry about what happened, but that the first edition was out of print and they would not print any more copies.

"Then I will have to print it myself." I told him.

Mr. H. said, "I guess you can; it's a public document."

This is why we are now publishing a "fifteen page excerpt" of this first edition which contains information that together with this blood protein research will expose and destroy our adversaries.

12.2. The entire "fifteen page excerpt" can be obtained from the Samuel Publishing Co., Box 1051, Orem, Utah 84057. ($1.00 per copy; 3-49, 50¢ each; 50-99, 40¢ each; 100 or more, 35¢ each.) Add 5% for postage and handling. Prices subject to change.

C-13. *Government Document Lets You Diagnose and Prescribe*

13.1. Let me ask you a question. If you see a person drowning and you are in a position to save his life by throwing him a lifeline, but instead you just turn away and let him drown, are you innocent or guilty of his death? *The Dietary Goals for the United States* is a lifeline. In printing it, the government has stepped into the doctor business. This is why it is so valuable. Believe it or not, this document *nutritionally diagnoses* and *prescribes* for heart disease, cancer, obesity, stroke, and the other major killer diseases in the United States. The power of this document lies in the fact that *anyone* who has it in their hands has the right, by quoting from it, to nutritionally diagnose and prescribe for the major diseases. As I said, it is a miracle that it ever got printed in the first place.

C-14. *Government Document States That There Is Very Little Current Medical Practice Can Do For The Killer Diseases*

14.1 In the face of three atomic bombs every two months, or over two hundred forty thousand men, women and children who are now being killed every two months from heart disease and cancer alone in the United States, this committee had to tell the truth. On page six this document states, *"Appropriate public education must emphasize the unfortunate but clear limitation of current medical practice in curing the common killing diseases. Once hypertension, diabetes, arteriosclerosis or heart diseases are manifest, there is, in reality, very little that medical science can do to return a patient to normal physiological function."*

14.2. This committee is telling the people in the United States that if they have a crippling or killer disease there is very little current medical practice can do for them, and that the public must become aware of this. They are asking for a nation-wide health education program.

14.3. They say *"As awareness of this limitation increases, the importance of prevention will become more obvious."* In other *words, to prevent we must educate.* Prevention is an educational process and prevention of war and disease is what this Golden Family Self-H.E.L.P. Program is all about!

C-15. *Government Document States That Our Problems Can Never Be Solved By More And More Medical Care*

15.1. This means that those who have a crippling or killer disease better start looking for H.E.L.P. or Health Education for Longevity and Peace. No TPP = No EX FL, No EX Na+ = EE = ☐. Salt, sugar, fats, high cholesterol foods = TPP = EX FL,

EX Na+ = ▲EE = ⊠.

15.2. There are many people who realize that most medical schools teach little if anything about nutrition. Due to the fact that this committee found that poor nutrition is directly related to our crippling and killer diseases, and since they knew that most medical doctors know very little about nutrition, on page six they said, *"There is widespread and unfounded confidence in the ability of medical science to cure or mitigate [help] the effects of such diseases once they occur."*

15.3. With the understanding of this limitation of the medical profession, we can now see why page seven of this document quotes Dr. Phillip Lee, Professor of Medicine and Director of the Health Policy Program at the University of California in San Francisco, as follows: *"As a nation, we have come to believe that medicine and medical technology can solve our major health problems. THE ROLE OF SUCH IMPORTANT FACTORS AS DIET IN CANCER AND HEART DISEASE HAS LONG BEEN OBSCURED (HIDDEN) BY THE EMPHASIS (ENFORCED BY THE A.M.A.) ON THE CONQUEST OF THESE DISEASES THROUGH THE MIRACLES OF MODERN MEDICINE. TREATMENT, NOT PREVENTION, HAS BEEN THE ORDER OF THE DAY."*

15.4. No one can disagree with the fact that this is the supreme order of the A.M.A.

15.5. To use this type of language in a document that was nationally publicized on radio and T.V., Dr. Lee must have known about the medical dictatorship that is now in control of most doctors and most of the people in the United States. Dr. Lee courageously went on to inform the people of the United States that, *"The problems can never be solved merely by more and more medical care."*

15.6. Dr. Lee knew that the way to solve or cure disease is to practice prevention. Therefore he said, *"Finally our greatest bulwark against the interests that helped create the present problems is an informed public."*

15.6. No one can disagree with the fact that *Dr. Lee is, by expressing his views in this document, practicing what he believes.*

C-16. Government Document Calls For A Nation-Wide Health Education Program

16.1. One of the main purposes of this government document is to alert the people in the United States that there are interests, or conspiring men with evil designs in their hearts that are helping to create the present problems that are destroying two hundred and forty thousand men, women, and children every two months. It is calling for a national health education program to make people aware that medical practice cannot help because of the foods we are being encouraged to eat which act on the body as a deadly poison. These foods are destroying more people than any war we have ever been engaged in.

16.2. The uncontrollable desire to get gain, or "the heart of Cain," will cause men to slay us with killer diseases and torture us with crippling diseases and not blink an eye while they do it. This document states that the only way to prevention in the United States is through *"appropriate public education."*

16.3. *It is one of the purposes of this book to help fulfill the objectives that are stated in this great document. As stated earlier, it was a miracle that this document was ever published, and that it was given national publicity by magazines, radio and T.V. This document has given us an educational weapon to help stop the suffering and destruction of human life that is now taking place, and we must not let the courageous efforts of those who published this document come to an end. We must get this document into the hands of all who will read it.*

C-17. *How To Use the Dietary Goals To Help Get The Blood Protein Research To Others*

17.1 Below is a suggested approach to help get this document and this research to thousands of Golden Families who would not listen any other way.

17.2 Let us suppose John was a golden friend or loved one and that I wanted to get this knowledge to him and his family.

17.3. To make it tough, let us say that he and his family believed that the medical profession or someone else had all the answers to health and peace, and that they were just positive that you could never help them with any of their problems.

17.4. Here is a dialogue that you may want to memorize because it may save this family *a lot of suffering and possible destruction.*

17.5. Me: *"Hello, John, I have a government document*

here that tells what is killing two hundred and forty thousand men, women and children every two months in the United States, and as a friend of mine (or a neighbor) I would like you to read it and tell me what you think about it."

John: "Sure, I'll be glad to tell you what I think about it." (I have asked for his advice, and this will give him a chance to maybe tell me a thing or two.)

Me: *"Thank you John, I will check with you in a day or two and see what you think of this document."*

Me: (After a day or two.) *"Hi, John, did you get a chance to read that document?"* (If he didn't, tell him you will see him later. If he says, "Yes, I did," say, *"What did you think of it?"* (He will probably say, "Oh, it was pretty good, but I'm not interested in those things right now.") No matter how he replies, show *The Golden Seven Plus One,* and continue with this dialogue: say, *"John, I've got another book here that tells why those foods cause death. Would you like to read it?"* (The government document will spark their curiosity and nine times out of ten those whom you approach this way will want to know more.) Most people will say, "Yes, I would." At this point, hand the book to him and say, *"I hope you enjoy it! I'll check back in a few days and see what you think about it."*

17.6. If John hesitates to say, "Yes, I would," show the cover and say, *"John, this book contains seven golden discoveries and one basic scientific formula which proves how certain foods will cause disease and death at the cell level. I would like you to read it and tell me what you think about it."*

17.7. You may want to suggest that the whole family study this book and ponder over the information that it contains. Once you get *The Golden Seven Plus One* into their hands, you have accomplished your objective. Once they have read the truth, they will have to decide if they want to become a golden family. After we get The Golden Family Self-H.E.L.P. Centers going, maybe you could encourage them to attend.

17.8. Remember, if you try to save a life and fail, you will be rewarded as if you had succeeded. Hopefully, this family will get excited about the information in this book, and they will want to do for others what you have done for them.

C-18. We Won't Win The Educational Battle Of Health And Peace Unless We Take The Offensive

18.1. Paul Harvey once said, "You don't win a battle unless you take the offensive." In the United States alone, people are now being destroyed with heart disease and cancer at the rate of three atomic bombs every two months. Let us as golden families help get this government document along with the Seven Golden Discoveries and The One Basic Formula to our golden neighbors, friends, and loved ones. Then, once they have The Formula which shows how the blood proteins produce the conditions that cause loss of energy, disease and death in their hands, and they fail to try to get it into the hands of other golden families whom they might be able to save by doing so, how can they honestly say that they are innocent if members of those families die from killer, or crippling diseases that might have been prevented had they been willing to help them. Remember, one out of two people are now dying of heart disease, and cancer is now striking one out of four and will soon reach one out of three in the U.S.; and the only thing that can stop this destruction is the knowledge that is in this government document along with the understanding of The Seven Golden Discoveries and this One Basic Formula.

C-19. To Take The Offensive, Here Are The Dietary Goals In More Detail

19.1. It is a miracle that a document like this would come from the government. All the statements from this document that I am quoting in this book are in italics in "the fifteen page excerpt" we are printing in Appendix A. These excerpts along with this book will open the doors and will save thousands of Golden Families from destruction.

19.2. This document states in the forward that "without government and industry commitment to good nutrition, the American people will continue to eat themselves to poor health." And then it says, "our national health depends on how well and how quickly government and industry respond." Industry responded all right! Many in the food industries and the A.M.A. tried to destroy this document. Why? Because it was nutritionally diagnosing and prescribing for our killer diseases. This research and The One Basic Formula and this government document all have the same purpose—to fight the toughest battle that has ever been fought. It is an educational battle against the powers of darkness that are keeping people in ignorance—and slaying them at the rate of three atomic bombs every two months in the United States alone.

C-20. *Dietary Goals Gives Us The Nutritional Diagosis For Crippling And Killer Diseases*

20.1. Here is the nutritional diagnosis for our killer and crippling diseases. On page one of *The Dietary Goals* it says:

> Too much fat, too much sugar or salt, *can be* and *are* linked directly to heart disease, cancer, obesity and stroke among other killer and crippling diseases . . . six of the ten leading causes of death in the United States have been linked to our diet. Those of us within the government *have an obligation* to acknowledge this. *The public wants some guidance,* wants to know the *truth,* and hopefully today we can lay the corner stone for the building of better health for all Americans, through better nutrition.

20.2. To support this diagnosis, on page three, Dr. D.M. Hegsted, professor of Nutrition of Harvard School of Public Health in Boston, Massachusetts says:

> The diet of the American people has become increasingly rich --- rich in *meat,* other sources of *fat* and *cholesterol,* and in *sugar* [salt, sugar, fat, high cholesterol foods, meat = TPP = EX FL, EX Na+ = $\blacktriangle$EE = $\boxtimes$.]. . . The question to be asked, therefore, is not why should we change our diets, but why not? What are the risks associated with eating less meats, less fat, less saturated fat, less cholesterol, less sugar, and less salt and more fruits, vegetables, unsaturated fats, and cereal products especially whole grain cereals. There are none that can be identified and important benefits can be expected . . . .

Then Dr. Hegsted made this courageous statement:

> "Ischemic heart disease, cancer, diabetes, and hypertension (high blood pressure) are diseases that kill us. They are epidemic in our population. We cannot afford to temporize."

In other words, he says we must tell the truth, no matter what! He emphasized this by saying:

> "We have an obligation to inform the *public* of the current state of knowledge and to *assist* the public in making correct food choices. *To do less is to avoid our responsibility."*

C-21. *"Love Is The Desire To Give Everything You Have To Bless The Lives Of Others." (From a plaque on the wall of Willard and Catherine Hunter's home in Ohio)*

21.1. With our knowledge of the seven golden discoveries and the formula we know more about the deadly effects of these foods than others. Therefore, *our* responsibility is greater than theirs. Some were willing to let their voice be heard throughout the world, and we should be willing to do the same.

21.2. On page seven, Dr. Phillip Lee spells out what we can do to help get this information to the world. In his plea to save lives, he says:

> It is *important* that the *Dietary Goals for the United States* be made widely available because it is the *only* publication of its kind, and it will be invaluable as a resource for *parents* [They want this information in every home in the United States.], *school teachers* [How are school teachers going to be able to teach the students what foods are good or bad if they don't have the correct information in their hands? All that most of them have now is the information published by the "interests" that have helped create the present problems.], *public health nurses, health educators, nutritionists, physicians,* and *others who are involved in providing people with information about the foods we eat. (That includes everyone.)*

21.3. We have designed a new cover for this document so people will have a greater desire to read it. It must fulfill the purpose for which it was intended. We are going to do all we can to make this document widely available, because *it is the only publication of its kind. We have shaded the portions that will bring out the importance of this document.*

21.4. This committee has given us one of the most

important documents that has ever come from the government. We should be willing to give our lives if that is what it takes, to help save over 240,000 men, women, and children who are being destroyed every two months because they do not know about this research.

21.5. We hear of wars and rumors of wars in foreign lands, but we know not the hearts of men in our own land. We have never had a war that killed over 240,000 people every two months. When they dropped the A-bomb on Nagasaki and Hiroshima it killed about 70,000 people and we thought that was bad. The worst destruction of human life that we have ever experienced is now taking place. The war is going on, and because of ignorance, we are being slain at the rate of over 4,000 men, women and children every day.

21.6. It is their money against our lives, and those who have the "heart of Cain" will continue to slay us for money and power.

21.7. We must not become a silent partner and let our destroyers continue to slay people by keeping them in darkness. We must help educate everyone we can so they will know who is destroying them, and how they are doing it. *Our destroyers can only work in darkness. When they are exposed, they lose their power.*

21.8. It took *courage,* or a *miracle,* for these men to make the above statements and to publish the dietary goals for the benefit of all mankind. They exposed those who are destroying us and *they have asked us to educate and inform the public.* To remain silent with the knowledge we now have, we would not be just avoiding our responsibility; we would become a partner to destruction. According to this research, we are *not just dying; we are being nutritionally destroyed.*

C-22. Dietary Goals: *Nutritionally Prescribes For Prevention Of Crippling and Killer Diseases*

22.1. To help prevent the suffering and destruction that is being caused by the food that makes us *thirsty,* which we now know is the first symptom of a poison, in this document is the "nutritional prescription" giving the foods that we must eat in order to *prevent* the killer and crippling diseases. The nutritional prescription which you may now quote without fear is found on page 13. In effect, it says to *increase* consumption of fruits, vegetables, and whole grains and to decrease everything else. It suggests that *if* we are going to eat meat, we should increase consumption of *poultry* and *fish.* In other words, *The Dietary Goals for the United States* tells us to *eat more fruits, vegetables, and whole grains, and to eat meat sparingly.* Fish is probably best because it does not make people as thirsty as the other meats do.

C-23. Research Supports Dietary Goals: *The Public Must Know That The Body's Requirements For Calcium Are Low, Not High*

23.1. The *Dietary Goals* are supported in the 5th edition of *The Textbook of Medical Physiology,* where it states on page 1052 that phosphate is absorbed well most of the time *except* when *excess calcium is in the diet.* It says, that by far the major source of calcium in the diet of the American people is milk or milk products. Then it makes the interesting statement that *"excess calcium . . . tends to form almost insoluable calcium phosphate products that can not be absorbed;* therefore, they pass on through the bowels to be excreted in the feces." *Excess calcium will drain the phosphorous out of the body* which the cell must have to make A.T.P. (adenosin triphosphate). A.T.P. is the source of energy for the cell. Without it the cell dies.

23.2. This may be the reason why, if you have milk products you must eat meat which is high in phosphorous. This would help preserve the phosphorous in the body. To try to balance the diet this way, makes sense, only if you are trying to keep people alive long enough to make money on the crippling and killer diseases this diet will cause--while it slowly but surely destroys them.

23.3. This research states that an average adult on the *current* American diet takes in about 800 mg. of calcium each day. Seven hundred milligrams of which is *excreted* in the feces. Therefore, each day, there is only about 100 mg. of calcium that can be *absorbed;* and all of this 100 mg., *except* for that portion stored in the bones (Vitamin D is necessary to store calcium in the bones) is eventually *excreted* in the urine. *Therefore the body's actual calcium requirements are very low, and the necessary calcium can be easily gotten from fruits, vegetables, and whole grains.* Our need for calcium is not nearly as high as we have been led to believe "by the interests that have helped create our present problems."

C-24. More Medical Research Supports Dietary Goals: The Public Must Know That The Body's Requirements For Protein Are Low, Not High

24.1. The same thing goes for protein. The human body is designed to exist on low percentage of protein, not high! Mother's milk is only 2.38% protein at birth and it reduces down to 1.2% to 1.6% within six months. And babies double and triple in size on mother's milk.

24.2. Remember, fruits, vegetables, and whole grains are the primary source of glucose, which is the fuel for the cells. This fuel is what keeps the electrical generators going. Protein is for the *building* of the cells but it is a very poor source of glucose which, when combined with oxygen, is converted into energy inside the cell. Think about it! *When will a human being ever require more protein to build cells than as a little baby who is doubling and trippling in size on mother's milk.*

24.3. Isn't it interesting that most green leafy vegetables and baked potatoes have about the same percentage of protein as mother's milk! The one who created this earth provided us with foods that supply our glucose, protein, calcium and the other mineral and vitamin needs just like he did the rest of the animals. When a *calf* stops nursing, where does it go for the glucose, protein, and vitamin and mineral requirements? *To plant life!* Where does the *horse* go? *To plant life!* Where does the huge *elephant* go for glucose, protein, vitamins and minerals? Again, *plant life!*

24.5. But there are some who say, "Our bodies are not the same; our digestive systems are different." To this we ask, where does the *gorilla*, the strongest animal pound-for-pound, on the earth go for his glucose, protein, vitamins and minerals? Again the answer is *plant life!* If you take the digestive system out of the gorilla and the digestive system out of a man and put them side by side you can't tell which came out of which. *So all nature verifies that if we were to eat more fruit, vegetables, and whole grains, and eat meat sparingly, we would obtain the glucose, protein, vitamins and minerals needed to build strong healthy bodies.* When you do eat meat, you should have poultry or fish. When you think about it deeply, you will realize that every animal on the face of the earth with a long colon goes to plant life for its nutritional needs. The only animals that live on other animals as a source of their glucose, protein, vitamin, and mineral needs are the *short* coloned animals. They are the "scavengers" of the earth. The "living garbage cans." If we try to get glucose out of a high protein diet, instead of a diet that is high in fresh vegetables, sprouts, etc., the body cannot get rid of the poisonous by-products that will cause putrefaction in the colon. These poisons will cause trapped proteins, excess sodium, pull the water out of the blood, and make us thirsty, shut our generators off, and cause loss of energy. High protein eaters need a *short* colon! *Our colons are two thirds too long and that is the "long and short of it!"*

24.6. Carlson Wade has written a book called *Miracle Protein: Secret of Natural Cell-Tissue Rejuvenation.* Chapter 4 is entitled, "Fruits, Vegetables, Herbs, and other Plant Proteins for Miracle Rejuvenation." Read the whole book; it gives evidence upon evidence that what we are saying here is true!

C-25. *Research And The Feb. 1977 Edition Of Dietary Goals Agree*

25.1. According to the formula and the information we have concerning the effects of poisons in our body, we understand now, beyond a shadow of a doubt, that unless men, women and children want to commit willful suicide, they must greatly reduce and almost eliminate salt, simple sugar, fats, and high cholesterol foods. Also, they must increase the consumption of fruits, vegetables and whole grains. Sprout the seeds and grains because it makes them sweet. They become a *better* source of glucose, and sprouting also makes them a better source of other minerals and nutrients for the cell.

C-26. *Hypoglycemia--Not Enough Fruits, Vegetables And Whole Grains*

26.1. While we are talking about glucose, let's discuss hypoglycemia. Hypoglycemia is "low blood glucose." Since glucose is the fuel for the cell, *loss of energy is the first sign of hypoglycemia. Therefore, the symptoms can be produced by anything that will cause trapped blood proteins.*

26.2. This confirms the information given to us in *The Dietary Goals For The United States* and all that we have learned from the blood protein research. When people eat more fruits, vegetables and whole grains, which are the primary source of glucose, and get off the salt, sugar, fats and high cholesterol foods that trap the blood proteins, these symptoms will begin to disappear. But to have complete success, people also have to obey the mental and physical laws as well.

26.3. Hypoglycemia can turn into adrenal diabetes and pituitary diabetes and can end up in high blood pressure and diabetes mellitis or permanent diabetes.

26.4. Knowing that high blood pressure and diabetes mellitis are two of the known factors of heart disease makes hypoglycemia a very serious matter. Loss of energy is the beginning of diseases. To conquer loss of energy is to conquer disease.

26.5. In the light of the blood protein research, let us explain how hypoglycemia turns into the other more serious diseases.

C-27. How Hypoglycemia Can Turn Into Diabetes, High Blood Pressure And Heart Disease

27.1. If you don't get enough glucose from fruits vegetables, and whole grains to supply the demand for glucose required by your cells, *and you are still not on a high protein diet,* then your adrenal gland will produce cortisol in an attempt to take protein *out* of your cells and convert it into glucose and then return it to the cells to supply this need. Conversion of protein to glucose takes place in the liver. See chart on page 288.

· 27.2. Let's explain the disease-producing process that the body has to go through in order to do this. To break down protein in the liver to get glucose out of it, the body has to get rid of the poisonous by-products. Remember, poisons will dilate our blood capillaries and cause trapped protein, etc. This is what makes protein a poor source of glucose. When your adrenal gland secretes cortisol to pull the protein out of the cell, your pituitary gland secretes the growth hormone that goes into the cell in an attempt to preserve (or hold) the protein in the cell. In effect, the growth hormone says "this protein is mine; I need it for reproduction and the preservation of the cell." This sounds good; however, the growth hormone inside the cell has a dangerous side reaction that will produce adrenal diabetes and pituitary diabetes, which may also end up in high blood pressure and permanent diabetes. This is how it happens: While the growth hormone tries to save the protein in the cell, the serious side effect is that it prevents the glucose from coming into the cell. Not only does this rob the cell of its fuel, but this glucose ends up in the blood stream. Too much glucose in the blood stream is the result of this battle between the adrenal gland and the pituitary gland. This is what they call adrenal or pituitary diabetes.

27.3. Too much sugar in the blood from *any* source will "trap" the blood proteins and lead to high blood pressure, which is directly related to cardiovascular disease. Ninety percent of those who have high blood pressure have been diagnosed as having "essential hypertension," which means high blood pressure of "unknown causes." This has been called the "silent killer" because it can happen in the body without people knowing it is taking place. Especially is this the case in the "little guy" with a tight cellular structure. The basic cause of high blood pressure is not unknown anymore!

C-28. Diabetes Mellitus (Permanent Diabetes)

28.1. The next serious side reaction that takes place when there is too much sugar in the blood is that over a long period of time, it will tax the pancreas and turn into diabetes mellitus. In effect, when the pancreas sees too much sugar or glucose in the blood, it says, "I've got to get that sugar out of the blood and into the cells where it belongs because too much sugar in the blood is deadly." Therefore, the pancreas starts secreting insulin to accomplish this task. If this condition lasts for a long time, the insulin producing cells in the pancreas get "burned out." The pancreas literally kills itself in an attempt to save the body. When the insulin producing cells get burned out, the body no longer gets insulin, and this is how hypoglycemia turns into premanent diabetes or diabetes mellitus. The basic cause, then, of hypoglycemia, adrenal or pituitary diabetes, the resulting high blood pressure, and diabetes mellitus is that we are not eating enough fruit, vegetables, whole grains or sprouts, and we are not eating meat sparingly.

C-29. *Medical Research On How To Treat Protein Deficiency*

29.1. Let us strive now to understand a problem that has been confusing many people in both the natural and the medical fields. Why do doctors put hypoglycemics and diabetics on high protein diets? This has also brought about the high protein industry that is promoted by many even in the natural health field.

29.2. In order to understand the high protein problem, which is widespread, we must understand protein deficiency, which is rare.

29.3. What is the best treatment for protein deficiency? According to the fifth edition of the *Textbook of Medical Physiology* on page 932, the most effective of all therapies for severe acute protein deficiency is an intravenous administration of plasma protein. Within hours, the amino acids of the administered protein become distributed throughout the cells of the body to form proteins where they are needed. This would be a lot better than putting people on a high protein program which we now know will cause crippling and killer diseases.

C-30. *High Protein Makes You Feel Good, While It Kills You*

30.1. The thing that is most confusing, and which is causing more problems than you can imagine is: When people go on a high protein diet for hypoglycemia and diabetes, why does it make them feel better, while it kills them? The doctors do not claim that giving these patients high protein will cure the problem. In fact, they say there is no cure! The only thing they know is that when the patient is given high protein, it seems to arrest or appease the disease and make them feel better until the dangerous side reactions of the high protein program makes them worse or kills them.

30.2. At this point we must take time to remind you again that the high protein program is treatment, not prevention; and treatment, not prevention, as the entire program of the AMA has been very effective. However, in the area of crippling and killer diseases, they are not only ineffective, but dangerous. Until the medical doctors are educated to the importance of nutrition, good mental attitudes, and proper exercise, and demand that AMA put these concepts into their training and give them the right to practice prevention, they will continue to be unable to prevent what is causing the death of most of their patients.

30.3. The doctors must understand, and you must understand, that the reason a high protein diet makes you feel good–while it kills you–is because it by-passes the pituitary-adrenal gland battle. This is how it does it.

30.4. Remember, protein is a poor source of glucose. If a person is not eating enough fruits, vegetables and whole grains for the body's protein and glucose requirements, and still is not eating a high enough protein diet to get the body's glucose requirements from proteins, the adrenal gland will excrete cortisol, which will take the protein in the cells to the liver to get glucose from it; and the battle begins. But if you go on a diet that is high in protein, the body will be able to use the protein that comes in through the mouth and by-pass the adrenal-pituitary gland battle. The growth hormone is not in the cell to keep the glucose from getting into it. Therefore, the body will then be able to take the protein that comes in through the mouth, take it to the liver, and convert it into glucose, and since this is not a fast process, for the next several hours, the glucose that comes from the protein can be used by the cells for energy. This is why the patients think they are getting well. The high protein programs make them feel better–while the putrefaction that takes place in the colon and the poisonous by-products cause trapped proteins in the body that will eventually damage the liver and the kidneys; and when this happens the high protein program will backfire, and the patient will have worse problems than he had before.

C-31. *Eight Glasses Of Water A Day? Yes, If You Eat The Wrong Foods.*

31.1. Just as the high protein concept is false so is the eight-glasses-of-water-a-day theory false. When you eat foods that are not mostly water, you must drink large volumes of water not only to replenish the water in the blood stream that is used up through the life processes, but also to activate the kidneys so they will be able to get rid of the excess poisonous by-products that results from eating wrong. Thirst is a defense mechanism. It is a call for water so the body will be able to survive the stress that you are putting it through.

31.2. Dr. Campbell, in his book, *A Doctor's Proven New Home Cure for Arthritis,* agrees with the *Dietary Goals For the United States.* He also agrees that drinking too much water will eventually damage the kidneys and cause further disease.

31.2. When you eat properly, you are eating foods that are almost all water. Therefore, you may never get thirsty unless you exercise and perspire or do something that will put the body under stress.

31.3. You will prove this for yourself as you begin to eat right. But this idea of eating right is not so easy. As we said before we are living in a society that is used to eating poisons. Therefore it is very important that you understand the principle of transition.

C-32. A Transition Program Is Necessary

32.1. To overcome this addiction and still live in society without causing stress takes wisdom. Therefore, to help you do this we are going to give you a transition program that you may have to follow until you educate all those around you.

32.2. To make the transition from the normal American Diet, which we find is a diet consisting mostly of foods that will cause "trapped" proteins, to more fruits, vegetables whole grains and sprouts requires skill. It is not an easy process, and if a person does not know what he is doing, he will cause more harm, not only to himself but to his family and loved ones, than he could ever dream possible.

32.3. People may not believe this and say, "If salt, sugar, fat and high cholesterol foods can cause our death, then we are getting off them right now!" And when they do, their bodies go into a cleansing state, and the poisons that are stored in the cells and the spaces around the cells begin to come out so fast that these people can become very ill in just a short period of time.

32.4. We have discussed this before, but with the knowledge you have now received, you will be able to understand it even better. Some people eat fruit and get sick as it pulls the poisons out. They eat a hamburger and feel better because it stops the cleansing process. Not understanding what has taken place, these people say, "I can't eat fruit. Hamburgers are better for me." Can you now comprehend why fruit can make you sick while it heals you, and a hamburger can make you feel better while it kills you?

32.5. Trying to come off drugs creates a very serious problem. This is why a transition program is necessary. Both mental stress and the addicting foods can trap your blood proteins! If you don't know how to make the transition, your chance of changing your present diet is very small! Why? Because stress can kill you as fast as the wrong foods can. This is why we told you at the end of the last session that it is permissible once or twice a week to go out and have a ball! Knowing the effect of stress, you should now begin to understand. Whatever you do, do it because you *want* to.

32.6. Think about this situation. You get a strong craving for a hamburger, but you say within yourself–"I want it, but I can't have it. I want it, but I can't have it." That is stress! Now you're dead if you do and you're dead if you don't! So what are you going to do? You're going to go out and "have a ball." Then, when you do it, if you look at that food and say, "I really shouldn't eat this," that is stress also! The food is bad enough; don't add stress and make it worse! If you are going to eat it, enjoy it, lap it up; it may make you sick later, but enjoy it when you do it!

32.7. These two letters from Christinia Skidmore will help you understand why transition is necessary.

Testimonial Letter Number One:

> Dear Dr. West,
>   I have been promising you that I would write down all the things that happened to me once I started the "New Way of Life" program, and I hope that it will be of some use to you.
>   As you know, the summer of '76 was quite difficult for me because of how activated my M.S. was. I finally got *so* tired of being sick all the time and *desperate enough* to try the diet, that in August of that year, I set out to make or break myself–health wise. As Arnold Ehret says, "don't go too fast, good food can kill you." *Well, I was so sure that his advice wasn't meant for me, that I could take anything, so I*

began with straight fresh fruit. I ate nothing but fruit for three weeks, until I got so sick that I couldn't even get off the bed. About 10 days into the diet, I started a low grade fever, but thought that I might be coming down with a cold or something because I had so much mucus in my nose and throat. But I stayed with the fruit, determined to see some type of accomplishment. *During the second week,* my fever went quite high and I tried to contact you to let you know what I was doing, and to see if you could tell me what to do for the fever. (I didn't want to take any aspirin, since I was trying to cleanse myself of all my drugs in the first place.) You were out of town at the time, and I remember talking to Dr. Hill about it. He didn't seem to be too startled that I was on just the fruit, so I figured that all must be going along o.k. He told me to make up some catnip tea and drink it freely, but I didn't have any and I was too sick to go out and buy some, so I just layed on my bed and felt miserable. Just before the fever went up, I started noticing that I was passing mucus from everywhere. It was coming from my nose, throat, chest (coughing a lot), eyes, my ears were draining, my urine was full of it, and whenever I had a bowel movement it *really* scared me, because the whole toilet was *filled* with mucus. This sounds terrible, but it all happened. I didn't know what to think, and I was hoping that you would hurry and get back, but I was determined not to quit what I had started. Little did I know at the time what a dangerous thing I was doing, but I have always been the impatient type and take every short cut possible. I was so sure that by eating just the fruit, I could cut my cleansing time a great deal, but I hadn't studied the diet that much and I really didn't know what I was doing. Since I didn't want to wait until you got back to help me start correctly, I paid for it dearly.

During the third week, I was much sicker than I thought I could ever be, and still be conscious. But I forced myself up to prepare some kind of quick meal for my 5 children. I wanted to make them some homemade potato soup, but I didn't have enough energy to make it all by myself, so I sat in a chair and instructed them on how to make it. Together, we got it made, and they had it for dinner that night. The next day, I was even weaker, and couldn't raise my head off the bed. My husband kept telling me that I should see a doctor or at least go off the fruit, but I was determined to make it work for me. *Finally, by night time, I thought that if I just ate a little bit of regular food, maybe it might help in some small way, so I ate a little bowl of the potato soup. Within 15 minutes, I couldn't believe what was happening to me. I sat up on the bed, my fever was leaving, my strength started to come back a little bit, and I got out of bed and began walking around the room. I was still kind of shaky, but it wasn't long until I was walking all over the house, and my kids couldn't believe the change in me. Just a few minutes before that, I was sicker than they had ever seen me, and now I was up for the duration of the evening.*

I still didn't realize what had happened *to me*, that I had actually stopped the cleansing process. All I knew was that I felt better after having eaten some food, so I decided then that I would at least add some vegetables to my diet. From that time on, I wasn't sick like that again, because I must have been eating more correctly. Of course, you had come back by then too, and could give me some much needed nutritional advice.

Little by little, I was feeling much better, in fact, much better than I had in years. I stayed with my fruits and vegetables, lost 32 lbs., and was quite pleased with my progress. It was then time for my 3 month checkup with Dr. Urrea, my neurologist, but I was feeling *so* good, that I called him and told him that I was feeling too good to come in. I decided to go in and see him anyway, just to show off a little bit, so at the end of September I went to see him. I was in such a good mood that day, and feeling quite spunky, that I really gave him a show. *He came out to the waiting room to call me into the examining room, and I gingerly got up from my chair. He had never seen me get up from a chair without a lot of effort and some help from a sturdy source, so he really began to watch my every step. As I got into the room, I went over to the examining table, and simply jumped up on it like a young child would. He was so startled, that he asked me to do it again.* So I did it again. He asked me what I had been doing to myself, and I told him about Professor Ehret's book. In fact, I had it with me and showed it to him. He began with all the usual reflex tests, doing them over and over until he was satisfied that the readings he was getting were correct. He had me walk on my heels and then my toes, and when he was finished watching that, I asked him if he would be interested in seeing the *new* thing that I could do. Of course he was interested! He was already so amazed with me that he could hardly believe his eyes. *I opened the door and went into the hall of his office and proceeded to show him that I could actually run!! I ran for him twice, and he just stood there with his mouth hanging open, watching in disbelief. He then took me in his office and sat quietly for a minute. Then he told me that all my tests showed completely normal reflex and muscle tone, and that he didn't have any other M.S. patients that had shown the progress I had.*

I asked him if the diet could have had anything to do with it, and *he said that he knew what I was doing was making me well, but that he could not discuss diet with any of his other patients without the risk of losing his license. I couldn't believe what he was saying.* He wouldn't let me pay for the office call, because he said that I had come in just for him, and not myself. *Instead of my regular 3 month visits, he told me to see him in a year, unless I needed to sooner, for some reason.*

I left there feeling on top of the world, but too smart for my britches. Since I felt so good, I was sure that I would always feel that way, no matter what, so I gradually began adding other food to my meals, and some of my problems began again. Three weeks after I started eating some regular food, I got mononucleosis along with my 16-year-old daughter, and then 104 temperatures. Then in January, I got a severe case of the respiratory flu, and was down in bed for 3 weeks. I just started to get up a little, when the end of January, my M.S. became fully activated, and I couldn't walk at all. I was numb from my head to my toes, literally. It has taken almost 3 months to get from my bed to my wheelchair, to my feet again. I hope that I have learned my lesson well, because I know that if I had stayed with my fruits and vegetables, and only "had a ball" occasionally, I wouldn't have gotten so bad again. I don't have the courage to try the plain fruit again, nor should I try it, but by at least eating properly on transition, I have begun to feel much better, and will continue to do so, especially as I can add more fuits and vegetables.

I am a firm believer in the Arnold Ehret way of eating, with your additions to make it less monotonous, and encourage everyone I know, especially those with definite health problems, to try the diet and stick to it.

As a closing note to you personally Corwin, I don't want you to forget about the power of the Priesthood. Because in the blessing that my husband gave me, prior to me having started the fruit fast, I was promised that the day would come when I would be completely healed, as long as I used wisdom in my eating habits, and as long as I obeyed *fully* the Word of Wisdom. I was also promised that it, my return to health, *would happen quickly.* So I do not give the transition diet all the credit. Yes, the diet works, and it works well, but *not* as quickly as it did for me. That was only through the hands of the Lord, Jesus Christ. Please don't lose sight of that very important fact in my case.

I sometimes hesitate telling people of my experience with the fruit and my subsequent visit to Dr. Urrea, because it has actually *discouraged* a couple of other M.S. patients who did not get as rapid results. So be careful, my case is a unique one, and I'm sure that you will not ever come across another one like it. People need to be told that it will take time, and they must have patience with the diet and themselves.

> Christina Skidmore
> 2131 W. DePalma Cir.
> Mesa, Arizona 85202

Testimonial Letter Number Two, Date 1-24-79:

Dear Dr. West,

Let me share with you a couple of things that have been happening to me in the last few weeks.

As you know, during the last year I have been losing my sight due to my M.S. This has been a great concern to me as it would to be to anyone—but I did some strange experimenting, and I'm now *convinced* of how to completely help myself.

I know and believe in my heart that everything you have taught me is true, but once in awhile, mentally, I would tell myself that an *extra* splurge of "having a ball" would be o.k.–because I was doing so much better, but those *extra* splurges started taking their toll with things like numbness from my waist down, unclear thinking, inability to manipulate my fingers quickly, loss of balance, quick mood (temper) changes, insomnia, *extreme* fatigue, and of course, my deteriorating vision.

You see, now all of these symptoms are said to be a part of my Multiple Sclerosis, and *consciously* I was accepting that, but subconciously I knew that I was causing these things myself by my "extra splurges."

It wasn't until after Christmas that I finally won out over my conscious stubbornness. My experiment was with Christmas chocolates–of all things! I don't eat candy, but occasionally would have a cookie or a piece of cake, but I was going to force myself into conscious realization of what I was doing to myself.

At a time when I was feeling pretty good and my vision was finally good, I would eat a chocolate, and maybe another, and in less than 45 minutes, my vision took a extreme "turn for the worst," I couldn't focus at all without covering one eye. And then my back, from my 6-yr.-old car injury, would start hurting quite a bit. After 3 or 4 days of one or two chocolates a day, I had myself down in a real slump physically. It took *great* effort to make myself do anything around the house, or to tolerate my children. I was in a great deal of pain, and a rotten mood, and energy level down to about 1½ on a scale of 0-10.

I kept asking myself out loud "Well, is it worth it?" After the 4th day, I finally had to admit that it wasn't and started back on the program–determined again as I was 4 years ago, to make it work. I'm not foolish enough this time to try a fruit fast, but I've eliminated my "splurges"–and in a few days, started feeling much better.

Being still very concerned about my sight, because my doctor had taken what is called a fundus photo, or a picture of my optic nerves, and showed me how damaged the nerve was and couldn't be restored. I asked my husband for a Priesthood blessing to help me accept whatever was to happen,–and this is what I was told: If I would obey completely the Word of Wisdom, continue in my exercise program, and obey the commandments of our Father in Heaven–my sight would be completely restored, and my M.S. would leave my body.

So Corwin, a building doesn't have to fall on me to know that what you're teaching, and my willingness to follow it, is the only answer to my complete health, and anyone elses.

In four weeks time, my vision is clearing. For about two weeks I felt like my eyes were being purged, as I had steis and chalazians (inward like steis *under* the eyelids) in both eyes on upper and lower lids, and they really hurt. Now they are gone and I can see more clearly than I have in months. My strength is returning, and I'm beginning to feel some of my old "zing." My outlook is great–because I KNOW that what I'm doing is right–and that I will be able to help other people to do the same thing.

It takes alot of courage to give up all the "fun foods" that are killing you–but if you want good health–It's worth it!

Thank you for all you do and teach,

Christina Skidmore

Note: Around Nov. 1979, at the naturopathic college in Mesa, Christina demonstrated how she could dance a jig on a lymphasizer. I realize all M.S. patients do not react the same. I have included both of these letters to show the effect diet can have on the body.

C-33. Why The Transition Process Works

33.1. Why does transition work? Because you go into the healing process. As you stay off the foods that make you thirsty most of the time, the trapped proteins begin to be removed from your body. As this takes place the excess fluid and the excess sodium begin to be removed from the spaces around the cells, and your generators begin to turn on. The healing process in the body starts with an "E". The word is endurance! In about four to six weeks, your whole body chemistry will begin to change, your energy will increase and your body will begin to reject naturally and easily, the foods that make you thirsty. As you progress you will desire to eat better and better, but you will always be doing what you want to do, and that is important.

C-34. *How To Combine Foods*

In time you will want to know how to combine foods. I hope the following chart will be of some help. (See Fig.1.)

34.1. When you eat fruit, eat fruit. It is best not to combine them with other foods. Your body will tell you. Just listen to it. If you combine the wrong foods you will produce poisons. You can eat your vegetables and baked potatoes together. Watch out for the nuts, though, for they contain 40% fat. Too much fat will rob the oxygen from the red blood cells, and red blood cells, will stick together and cause a "traffic jam" that will dilate the capillary pores. Nuts make you thirsty. Eat them in moderation. Almonds are probably the best. The transition process is a "new way of life" that will make it possible for us to raise up a posterity who will enjoy health and peace.

34.2. Transition is necessary for many reasons. What are you going to do if you are invited to a special family event or a special social event? If the other people do not know about the blood protein research, you have a problem. If you say, "I'm not going to eat those poisons," they are going to call you a fanatic and that is going to cause stress. You are going to dilate their capillary membranes, and they are going to dilate yours. That is worse than eating the food. True? You don't have to eat much, but you must use wisdom. You do NOT have a right to *willfully* cause stress in other people. You must not force your children or anyone else. We must become big enough to love, bless, do good, and pray. Transition is not a diet. It is a new way of life. To aid in this new way of life, I am going to give you the transition program in a condensed form. You will be able to use this condensed form to study and to help you stay on transition until the time comes that we can all work together in peace and harmony.

SUGGESTIONS FOR FOOD COMBINING

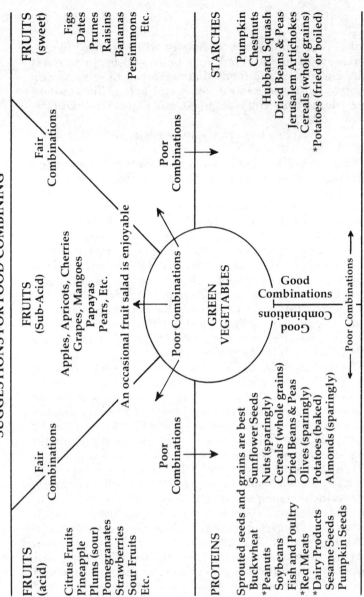

FRUITS (acid)

Citrus Fruits
Pineapple
Plums (sour)
Pomegranates
Strawberries
Sour Fruits
Etc.

FRUITS (Sub-Acid)

Apples, Apricots, Cherries
Grapes, Mangoes
Papayas
Pears, Etc.

FRUITS (sweet)

Figs
Dates
Prunes
Raisins
Bananas
Persimmons
Etc.

STARCHES

Pumpkin
Chestnuts
Hubbard Squash
Dried Beans & Peas
Jerusalem Artichokes
Cereals (whole grains)
*Potatoes (fried or boiled)

PROTEINS

Sprouted seeds and grains are best
Sunflower Seeds
Buckwheat
*Peanuts
Nuts (sparingly)
Soybeans
Cereals (whole grains)
Fish and Poultry
Dried Beans & Peas
*Red Meats
Olives (sparingly)
*Dairy Products
Potatoes (baked)
Sesame Seeds
Almonds (sparingly)
Pumpkin Seeds

GREEN VEGETABLES

Good Combinations

Fair Combinations

Poor Combinations

An occasional fruit salad is enjoyable

Notes: Eat fruit for breakfast, fruit or vegetables for lunch and vegetables with good combinations for dinner. Do not eat fruits and vegetables at the same meal. Avacado is best with acid or sub-acid fruit or green vegetables. Tomatoes may be eaten with non-starchy vegetables and protein. Eat melons alone or leave them alone.

* These foods aren't recommended but are included for clarity.

Figure 1

130

C-35. The Transition Concepts in Condensed Form

35.1. Remember this is *not* a diet, it is a *new way of life.* Study it until you have the concepts memorized. Diets come and go -- a way of life stays with you. However, *conversion* to the following principles is an absolute necessity before you can begin your *new way of life.*

a. The high protein theory is false!

b. Strength and vitality comes directly from a clean system.

c. Poisons cause "trapped" proteins and rob the body of energy.

d. You must eat more fruits, vegetables and whole grains and eat meat sparingly.

e. If good food makes you sick, don't blame the food. You are too full of poisons to handle that food right now.

f. Use wisdom -- *DO NOT eat unless you are hungry!* If you are hungry all the time, you probably have too much poison in your system.

g. Keep fresh fruits and vegetables (or as near fresh as possible) inside the house at all times. To detoxify the body, choose foods according to their cleansing, healing, and eliminating qualities and their mineral values, not according to their caloric values.

h. If you crave the wrong foods, try a fruit *or* a baked potato and a green leafy salad. (Your body craves the poisons it is throwing off, which indicates an addiction.)

i. If you break out in a rash, the body is throwing off the poisons too fast, so slow down. Nothing needs more supervision than eating good food when you are not accustomed to it. Some people say,"Here's good food, come and eat." Arnold Ehret says, *Here's good food; watch out, it can make you very sick if you go too fast.*

j. Remember, at first, fruit may make you sick if it pulls the poisons out too fast. However, in 4-6 months, as your body chemistry changes, *you will be able to eat more fruit,* and then the foods that make you thirsty will begin to make you sick.

k. If you are under a doctor's care, continue until he releases you. *To help speed* up that release date, strengthen the "weak spots" in your body by using the lymphasizing techniques that increase circulation, and increase the ability of the lymph system to keep the blood proteins circulating and to pull poisons and toxins out.

1. *Do not do anything too fast.* It is much better to take your time about this healing business. This is one the most important steps of transition. Follow these principals as you begin your new way of life.

C-36. The Basic Transition Diet

36.1. Fruit for breakfast. A relentless house cleaner.

36.2. Fruit or vegetables and sprouts for lunch. (Once or twice a week add poultry or fish.)

36.3. Vegetables and sprouts for dinner.

36.4. In the beginning, once or twice a week "have a ball!" A spanish dinner, a hamburger, or a nice dinner out is an example. The main thing is that you *enjoy it while you can* because as you transition your desire for food will change; and what you eat to "have a ball" will also change. Even your desire to "have a ball" will decrease as you cleanse your body. Until you cleanse your body, you will need a good vitamin supplement to help fight disease, especially the B vitamin and vitamin C to help fight stress and vitamin E to help fight fats so the cells can get oxygen.

36.5. Eat fruit for in-between snacks.

36.6. When you eat whole wheat bread *toast it* first.

36.7. Don't forget the herbs--they will help you in the transition and cleanse the body.

36.8. Don't ever stuff yourself. Eat little, but well. Better still, eat only when you are hungry--the cleaner the system, the less food you will crave.

36.9. Eat nuts sparingly--they are too high in fats. (Take Vitamin E to help keep all fats from robbing oxygen from the blood and causing disease.)

36.10. Never drink water with meals.

36.11. When thirsty use a mild grain drink. (Let distilled water sit 24 hours over barley or other grains and then drink the water.)

36.12. Make this transition only as fast as you can *enjoy* it.

C-37. Helpful Suggestions To Help Overcome Addiction

37.1. To overcome addiction to salt, sugar, fat, etc., when it comes time to eat say: *"Strength and vitality comes from a clean system."* Then *look* at the food and ask yourself, *"Will this food bring health, strength, and vitality to my body?"*

37.2. If the answer is NO then ask: *"Am I hungry? Do I have to have it?"* If you feel you have a very *strong* craving for it, take a bite and enjoy it; then repeat *both questions.* If a *strong* craving still persists, take another bite and *enjoy* it. Continue this process until you can say, *"O.K., that is enough,"* or the desire to eat only good foods exceeds the desire for the bad foods. Then you will be able to leave it alone and feel proud and good about it. *Until you do that you have not got these addicting foods whipped--they will whip you!*

37.3. Be careful! Do not transition too fast. If you get sick, back off the fruit and steam your vegetables. The cleansing action will stop and you will feel better immediately. This is why fruit can make you *feel* sick while it heals you and a hamburger can make you *feel* better while it kills you!

37.4. On transition you may continue to *"have a ball"* occasionally *until* having a ball stops being desirable. It may take months to reach that point. However, don't feel that you can't *"have a ball"* on special occasions. You must work with the stress factors in you and those of your family and loved ones.

37.5. When you eat fruits and vegetables you will not get thirsty. You will notice that in the morning and during the day you will have a fresh taste in your mouth and a good feeling in your stomach. When you "have a ball" you will have to have water immediately, and the next morning your mouth will be dry with a bad taste. Also, you will probably not feel so good. You will be saying, *"Yuk, yuk, yuk, water, water, water, trapped protein, excess sodium, shuts my generators off!"* I'm afraid that you will have to experience this *many* times as your desire *not* to "have a ball" becomes *greater* than your desire to "have a ball." If a good food makes you sick, don't blame the food. Your body is just too toxic to handle it at this time.

37.6. Keep going. The more you do it, the better you will feel; and the better you feel, the more you can do it.

C-38. Breathe Deeply Everywhere You Go

38.1. This is necessary to keep the blood proteins circulating via the lymphatic system, and to get the necessary oxygen to convert glucose into energy inside the cell.

38.2. Oxygen is the most important food you can get.

38.3. Now, good luck and *ENJOY* your *"new way of life."*

C-39. What Do I Have To Do To Become A Golden Family?

39.1. If you apply the knowledge you have obtained, you will be able to make the mental, nutritional, and physical changes that are necessary to obtain better health and a greater degree of peace! With understanding comes faith, and faith is that *"something within"* that moves people to action which makes it possible for them to become Golden Families.

39.2. This will become a reality in your life as you continue to increase your understanding, and as you increase your ability to love, bless, and do good, and improve your physical and nutritional programs.

C-40. What If I Don't Have The Support Of My Family?

40.1. Remember, if you do not have the full support of your family, this is what transition is for. Do not cause stress, for stress is as bad--and maybe worse--than bad food, and improper exercise.

40.2. Until you can educate all those around you, it may be impossible to do exactly what you would like to do *nutritionally,* but nothing can stop you from doing what you must do *physically* and *mentally.*

40.3. *In fact, when dealing with your family and others, you may need to increase your ability to love, bless, do good, and pray more than ever before in order to prevent TPP* = EX FL, EX Na + = ▲ EE = ☒ from taking place in your body and in the bodies of your family and loved ones.

C-41. A Sample Food Shopping List, Menu, Recipes And Dehydrating Techniques To Help You Get Started On Transition--Your New Way Of Life, Can Be Found In Appendix B

(See Section E in Session Four to obtain additional scientific evidence with testimonials of Arnold Ehret, and Teresa Mitchell to verify that the transition program works.)

C-42. Dr. West Gives Testimony Of Transition And The Art Of Lymphasizing Which is a "New Way of Life."

42.1. Once I obtained all this information, which took many years to accumulate, I remember the time when conversion took place in me. I was at my office at 525 E. Broadway in Mesa, Arizona. It was the middle of the summer of 1975. I can even remember the position I was standing in and the direction I was facing when I said, almost out loud, *"I am going to start a new way of life."* I had weighed between 220 and 230 pounds for almost twenty years. I had tried everything—even water pills—but to no avail. I know what it is like to be on the "weight losers roller coaster. "Well, this time I knew that I was going to lose weight and stay off that roller coaster. I believed in the transition that Arnold Ehret talks about, and I believed that you must enjoy what you do or it is not going to work.

42.2. Therefore, on that day I began my "New Way of Life." Since that time I have lost about 55 pounds and regained strength and vitality that is hard to describe. The best thing is, I have enjoyed it all the way. I am down to approximately 175 pounds for the first time in over twenty-five years. I have been on transition for over six years now, and I enjoy it! I plan to stay on transition until I get the blood protein research to all those whom I am closely associated with so we can live together in peace and harmony.

42.3 One of the greatest things that has happened to me is what I have recently learned about the physical part of the art of lymphasizing. I know now, more than ever before, that it is possible to raise up a people who can live in peace and harmony; and that this people will be able *to run and not be weary and walk and not faint.*

42.4 The art of lymphasizing is a complete science. If I had to study all my life to learn what I have now learned from the blood protein research, it would be worth every minute of it. I know that the basic principles that are being taught as a result of the research are correct. I believe this so strongly that I am willing to give my life if necessary, to help get this knowledge to as many people as I can. The blood protein research contains the scientific answers to disease and war. *I believe with all my heart that the day has come that we must seek out those who are willing to live the laws of health and peace. The strength that will come from people who are united in that effort will make it possible for them to raise up a posterity who will conquer disease and live in peace!* To master the mental and nutritional part of Lymphasizing will take a lot of effort, but the foundation of the art of lymphasizing is the physical part.

D. PREVENTION THROUGH PROPER EXERCISE: THE PHYSICAL PART OF THE ART OF LYMPHASIZING

1. I have given you some new modern concepts concerning the physical part of the art of lymphasizing when I taught the Walker-West Walk and some of the bio-electric pain relief techniques. Of all the things that we have talked about, these advanced lymphasizing techniques are probably the most exciting of all.

D-1. Dr. West Discovers How To "Run And Not Be Weary, Walk And Not Faint!"

1.1. I got hit by a dump truck when I was sixteen, and it left my left ankle with very limited movement. I have not been able to run on a hard surface for any period of time without causing pain in my foot and ankle. However with the wisdom and great treasures of knowledge, even hidden treasures, that are contained in the blood protein research, I have now discovered a way to exercise without *ever* causing undue stress and without *ever* getting tired. When I finish I have absolutely *no fatigue* in my body.

1.2. On October 19, 1980, I named this new approach "lymphasizing". I will never forget the thrill that came over me the first time I said, *"Don't just exercise, lymphasize."* Once or twice a day lymphasize on a lymphasizer, then lymphasize by breathing deeply *everywhere you go.* This is the secret of the Tarahumara Indians." I soon realized that the concept of lymphasizing involved the secret of the healing process and that to become completely effective, lymphasizing had to include proper mental attitudes and good nutrition. The concept turned into a complete science called, *The Art of Lymphasizing.* On December 20, 1980, I used the term bio-electric lymphasizing for the first time. These terms are more descriptive of the principles and concepts contained in the blood protein research than any I had ever used before.

D-2. Why The Concepts Of Lymphasizing Are In This Book

2.1. If I would have had my way this book would have been published in November, 1980, without any mention of lymphasizing. You can thank a man by the name of Bernard Tanner (his friends call him Bernie) that these terms are now contained in this book.

2.2. It was Bernie who convinced me that it was time to write this book. I had tried on many other occasions, but I could not do it. For the last several years I had been lecturing in about two hundred cities on the blood protein research. In July, 1980, with Bernie's help, I cancelled two weeks of my lecture tour. I dictated the original manuscript of this book in fifteen days with the help of a scribe by the name of Billy G. Gonzales. As I dictated to him hour after hour in the manner in which I lecture without notes, he wrote with his own hand the original manuscripts.

2.3. Those who know this story will bear witness that if it were not for Bernie and Bill and the help of the Lord, this book would not exist. I dictated the original manuscript in question and answer form.

2.4. Bill and I wanted to publish the book in November in that form, but Bernie insisted that I change the questions into positive statements. In doing so it delayed the printing of this book; but while I rewrote the manuscript, I learned a lot more about the importance of the blood protein research.

2.5. The blood protein research had to first come from a scientific source, and it has taken the help of many people who have desired to help establish health and peace on the earth for this book to exist.

2.6. *It will yet take the help of everyone who has this desire in their heart to get this book to the nations of the earth so that the message contained in it may fulfill its destiny—which is to help establish a healthy people and a peaceful people in every nation on earth.*

D-3. The Secret Of The Tarahumara Indians

3.1. Lymphasizing is the secret of the Tarahumara Indians who can run one hundred miles or more without rest. A film, called "Coronary Counter Attack," which can be obtained from Brigham Young University in Utah shows these Indians running and tells about them. It shows a mother picking up her baby and walking for several hundred miles to visit relatives. It shows her walking day and night until she gets there. This is what I call being able to "run and not be weary, and walk and not faint."

3.2. Bill McClellan wrote an article about the Tarahumara's entitled, "The Worlds Toughest Runners," in the October 1979 *Runners World Magazine*. In answer to the question of why they run the chief said, "We run because we run. It is necessary. That is all!" The writer's comment was, "Whatever the reasons, they run well." If he could have had the knowledge of the blood protein research, he would have known that the chief gave him the true answer to that question. With the knowledge of the seven golden discoveries and the formula, we know that the chief meant it when he said, *"We run, because we run. It is necessary. That is all!"* When they stop running, they lose the ability to run.

3.3. This very simple statement, "We run because we run," now becomes very profound. Here is another one that takes on more meaning than ever before. *Activity is directly related to health, and inactivity is directly related to death!*

D-4. About The Tarahumara Indians

4.1. Approximately fifty thousand Tarahumara Indians live in Northwest Mexico in a twenty thousand square-mile area. It is the most isolated portion of the vast and forbidding range called the Sierra Tarahumara.

4.2. In this mountain valley that even scorpions avoid, there reside the incredible Tarahumara, a tribe of Indians who are among the most primitive on earth, yet who run distances that are staggering. In their own language, the Indians call themselves Tauramuri, "the footrunners." They are a society of runners. Their diet consists of mainly corn, squash, and beans. They rarely eat meat. The food that is used the most is corn. It is used for tortillas, ground into *vinnole* to make corn meal mush, then broiled and smashed into a gruel. They go to great lengths to protect their fruit from animals.

4.3. They have health and peace. They never inflict pain on their children. There are no jails, soldiers, policemen; and crime is almost non-existent. One could say that they have almost mastered the art of lymphasizing. Women compete in the races as do the children. And the fact is, they hardly walk anywhere. Running is a way of life with them. Why do they run? The Chief gave the answer when he said, "It is necessary. That is all!"

D-5. Lymphasizing-The Foundation Upon Which Energy In The Body Is Built

5.1. The Tarahumara Indians are "naturally" benefiting from obtaining the physical activity that is needed to keep the blood proteins from becoming trapped in the spaces around the cells. This is the secret of the endurance of the Tarahumara Indians. It is the *foundation* upon which energy in the body is built.

5.2. To obtain this endurance, and to learn how to "run and not be weary, and walk and not faint," you will need to understand the total concept of lymphasizing. Therefore, I will first give you a list of *all* the forms of lymphasizing. Then I will give you the definitions along with explanations and examples of all *except* the more advanced bio-electric lymphasizing terms (h-m below). They will be defined and described in Session Four.

D-6. A Complete List Of Lymphasizing Terms

a. The Art of Lymphasizing.
b. The Four *Physical* Laws of Lymphasizing.
c. Lymphasizing or Lymphasize.
d. The Walker-West-Walk.
e. A Lymphasizer.
f. Bio-Electric Lymphasizing.
g. The Basic Bio-Electric Self-Help Pain Relief Techniques. (These techniques involve pressure, massage, and a light fast stroke and were defined and described in Session Two.)

    h. The Bio-Electric "Gentle Bounce for Health."
    i. The Special Bio-Electric "Eye Exercise."
    j. The Bio-Electric "Breathing and Directed Thinking" Technique.
    k. The Bio-Electric "Wheelchair" Technique.
    l. The Bio-Electric "Pin-Point" Techniques.
    m. The Bio-Electric "Energy Field" Technique.

6.1. Generally speaking the principles and concepts behind a-e terms are designed not only to untrap the proteins but also to *keep* them from becoming trapped, which is necessary to build endurance and strength.

6.2. The principles and concepts behind the "f-m" terms are designed to dissipate the trapped proteins out of the damaged areas of the body and to promote healing in these areas.

6.3. As you teach your family to master the mental, nutritional, and the physical parts of the art of lymphasizing, you will begin to conquer disease and live in peace.

D-7. *Definitions and Explanations Of The "a-e" Terms Of Lymphasizing*
(All of the "f-m" terms are defined in Session Four, except the "g" term. It is in Session Two)

a. *The Art of Lymphasizing:*

    (1) Knowing what to do mentally, nutritionally, and physically to keep the blood proteins circulating in the body via the lymphatic system.
    (2) Knowing what to do mentally, nutritionally, and physically to untrap or dissipate the clustered blood proteins to relieve pain and cause healing to take place the body.
    (3) Knowing how to conquer disease and live in peace.

b. *The <u>Four Physical Laws</u> of Lymphasizing:*

    (1) You must lymphasize on a lymphasizer at least once or twice a day, and then continue to lymphasize by doing the Walker-West Walk everywhere you go, or as often as possible. Whether you are on a lymphasizer or

on the ground, a good rule to remember is: Walk-run; walk-run; but do not get tired.

(2) You must never cause negative stress on the body. Negative stress will cause trapped proteins and pain in the ankles, shins, knees, hips, backs, etc. If this happens, you are exercising, not lymphasizing.

(3) You must never get tired. A Tarahumara Indian can run from sun-up to sun-up without fatigue. If you get fatigued, you are exercising not lymphasizing. If you get tired during the day, lie down and breathe deeply. You will feel restored and fresh in 5-10 minutes.

(4) Don't give up! You must understand that "The more you do it (without causing negative stress or fatigue), the better you feel; and the better you feel, the more you can do it." The key to healing in the body starts with an "E". This is the secret of the healing process. Remember, unless you can run one hundred miles without rest, you have trapped proteins in your body. As you lymphasize, you will untrap blood proteins. Therefore, the more you lymphasize, the better you feel, and the better you feel the more you can lymphasize.

NOTE: Laws 2, 3, and 4 also apply mentally and nutritionally as well.

c. *Lymphasizing Or Lymphasize:*

(1) The foundation upon which energy in the body is built.

(2) The mental, nutritional and physical concepts that will untrap or dissipate clustered proteins and keep them circulating in the body via the lymphatic system.

Note: When this term is used alone, it is generally referring to the *physical* part of lymphasizing.

d. *The Walker-West-Walk:*

(1) A form of lymphasizing that utilizes deep breathing and muscular movement. It is named after Dr. Walker, (the juice man) who showed me this walk. He is approximately one hundred and seventeen years

old. It is explained in Session One. To do the Walker-West-Walk: as you walk around, swing your arms and step as lively as you can. While you do this use the "shhh" sound. Breathe in and out through your teeth. With practice, it sounds like a choo-choo train. You inhale-exhale; inhale-exhale; inhale, exhale-exhale-exhale. You can alternate by doing this: Inhale-inhale-inhale-inhale, exhale-exhale-exhale-exhale. The children love it. It is fun and it is good for everyone. You can also do this by breathing in and out through the nose or in through the nose and out through the mouth. If you are in a wheel-chair or confined to a bed, do what you can, as much and as often as you can. The more you do it, the better you will feel; and the better you feel the more you can do it. Endurance without fatigue is the key to healing.

(2) This form of deep breathing must be done everywhere you go, or as often as possible to keep the blood proteins circulating in the body. Get The Walker-West-Walk lymphasizing habit. Until you can run one hundred miles without fatigue, you cannot consider yourself to be in a truly healthy condition.

(d-1) Try An Experiment

1.1. First of all, walk across the floor the way you normally do. Now *lymphasize* across the floor, using the Walker-West Walk. You will find that it is more fun to *lymphasize* across the floor. Obey the four laws of lymphasizing. As you get into the habit of doing it, you will *finish your day with a lot more energy* than you have had before.

1.2. The sooner you teach your children that there is no such thing as retirement, the better off you and you family will be. The average life span after retirement is three to five years. Remember, the Lord admonished us to work all the days of our lives. To continue to walk around all the time the way we normally do is not only a waste of time and energy, it will cause some of the blood proteins to become trapped in the spaces around your cells. You will be able to stay alive, but there is a big difference between being alive and well, and alive and sick.

1.3. If you want to increase your health and strength, you must lymphasize everywhere you go. Begin now to teach your children by precept and example how to become like a Tarahumara Indian.

Note: The Tarahumara Indians have no policemen and no jails, because there is no crime. And the parents inflict no pain upon their children. Wouldn't it be wonderful if the same thing could be said about us?

(d-2) Dr. Van Aaken, M.D., Proves Lymphasizing Principle Works

2.1. Just recently I was given a book written by Ernst Van Aaken, M.D. It is called, *The Van Aaken Method--Finding the Endurance To Run Faster and Live Healthier*. On the back cover he says, "My whole teaching in one sentence is: 'Run slowly, run daily, drink moderately, and don't eat like a pig.'"

2.2. Dr. Van Aaken has coached world record holders. Harold Norpoth won an Olympic silver medal (5000 meters in 1964) and set a world record (2000 meters) while training with Van Aaken. The system includes frequent walking breaks to avoid fatigue. Those who read this book will learn that "only the person who runs daily, lives modestly without touching his reserves, and eats little but well will ever become a good runner," or for that matter, remain truly healthy.

2.3. The reason Dr. Van Aaken's method works is he is teaching his students to obey what we now call the laws of lymphasizing. True health, Dr. Ernst Van Aaken maintains, starts with endurance. And from maximum endurance comes maximum performance. When I began to read this book, I could hardly believe it. Dr. Van Aaken has proven that the *principles of lymphasizing* will enable a person whose body is *conditioned to a hard surface* to actually run and not be weary, and walk and not faint. His whole program is based on a system that does not cause fatigue. He goes for endurance, without fatigue. And when the time comes for the test, his students are breaking the world records and are becoming champions.

2.4. Since most of you are not ready physically or mentally, to do this kind of running on the ground, do The Walker-West-Walk and use a lymphasizer as often as you can.

2.5 Those who know the value of a lymphasizer will spend most of their exercise time on one of these units. *They don't just exercise-they lymphasize!* To really make your time count and speed the healing process in your body, while you lymphasize, breathe deeply and do the light fast stroke on the liver, gall bladder, spleen, pancreas, colon, etc., which you learned about in Session Two.

CAUTION: When you begin to lymphasize, if you get dizzy, don't blame the lymphasizing! If you have too much poison built up in your body, when you untrap your blood proteins, the poisons will go back into the blood stream along with the excess fluid that was being retained by the trapped proteins. Follow the four laws and keep going; if you get dizzy, you need it badly!

e. *A Lymphasizer:*

   (1) A set of lungs. (At the peak of inhalation, the lymph shoots into the blood stream.) Gently moving up and down on a lymphasizer propels the lymph through the body, just like breathing deeply. Thus I call them a lymphasizer. (In D-8 this is explained in detail.)
   (2) A Lymphatic Exerciser.
   (3) A "mini-trampoline" Lymphatic Exercise Unit.

   1. My term *lymphasizer* refers to any "mini-trampoline." I put the term "mini-trampoline" in quotes because it describes what these units look like; but this is where the similarity ends.

   2. Trampolines were built and designed for the purpose of performing acrobatic stunts. It has been called "a trick machine." Some people who should know better think a Lymphasizer is used for the same purpose.

D-8. *Activity Is A "Magic" Healer For The Body*

8.1. Jumping up and down is a form of lymphasizing. As you move up and down, something magical begins to happen in your body. The blood protein research reveals that the lymph system pumps fluid and protein out of the tissue spaces each time the tissues are compressed or moved in any other way.

8.2. At the bottom of the bounce the one-way check valves close. At the top, they open and the lymph fluids are propelled through the system, just like they are when you breathe deeply. If you just walk around without breathing deeply at the same time, it is impossible to get the benefits of lymphasizing. What you will probably get is tired feet and vericose veins. Just walking around will put your body into motion to keep the blood proteins circulating enough to keep you alive–sick, but alive! This is what the doctors in the United States have come to call a normal person. But with the Tarahumara, the Hunza's or other people around the world who are physically active, this is not true. Let's consider where activity for our body first began, and where we began to lose it.

D-9. *Where Lymphasizing First Began*

9.1. Our first experience in lymphasizing was in our mother's womb. That was our first waterbed. After we are born, we cry to be lymphasized just like we cry to nurse. Both of them are necessary to have health and strength.

9.2. When the old Indian felt it was time to die, he would go out and find himself a tree, sit down, not move, and breathe very shallowly. In twenty-four hours he would be dead, just like the blood protein research says. This has also happened to some men who were put in prison camps. They just went into a corner, sat there, and died. This method of dying works for anyone who tries it. That is a fast, easy way to commit suicide. The slow way is to just keep doing what we have been calling "normal" in the United States. (Those who are seeking to have a four day work week are actually going to have more trapped blood proteins, sickness, and death.)

D-10. *Why Babies Love To Be Lymphasized*

10.1. As we have said before, "Activity is directly related to life, and inactivity is directly related to death." Your natural instincts tell you what to do, if you would just listen to them.

10.2. When a baby is born do you just hold it, or do you rock it and bounce it? When a baby cries, do you just hold it or bounce it? Babies will cry to be lymphasized so that they can stay well, and we instinctively lymphasize them for the same reason. Mothers who ignore their babies will have sick babies.

D-11. *Babies Say, "If You Love Me, Lymphasize Me."*

11.1. Babies associate lymphasizing with love. It is a loving experience for them. They are continually saying through their actions, "If you love me, LYMPHASIZE ME!" The back and forth up and down motion experienced riding in a car or being held in a rocking chair is a LYMPHASIZING experience.

11.2. Scientists have tried an experiment with a group of monkeys, using a wire and a cloth mother. The monkeys went to the cloth mother only until the scientists put them both in a rocking chair. Then it didn't even make any difference; they went to both without preference. Even monkeys say it through their actions, "If you love me, lymphasize me."

11.3. That is why a swing, teeter totter, pogo stick, horseback ride, circus ride, jumping up and down in water, and being bounced on daddy's foot or knee is so much fun! We love to do those things that will lymphasize us. Laughing is a lymphasizing experience and so is crying–but either one in excess produces stress.

11.4. When babies are born, the doctor slaps their bottoms to get them to cry. The first cry is truly "the breath of life." That is what a baby has to do to get its lymphatic system moving on its own. It takes "the breath of life" to activate "the tree of life" inside the body. This is why the shallow breather is in serious trouble and why the average life span after retirement is 3-5 years.

11.5. The Lord told Adam and Eve when they came out of the garden that they had to work "all the days of their life." There was no retirement program provided. With this knowledge we now understand why. If a person goes into retirement and sits in that chair and tries to "take it easy," he is committing willful suicide.

D-12. *When Do We Begin to Break the Natural Laws*

12.1. When babies are awake they are continually moving. When they get big enough to stand up in a crib–what do they do? They jump up and down, laughing and yelling for joy. We take them out of the crib, they jump on the bed. We take them off of the bed, and they jump on the couch.

12.2. With a knowledge of this blood protein research, we should get them something else, like a lymphasizer, to jump on. True? Without this knowledge people say, "Get off the bed, get off the couch, sit still, and don't move!" This is where we begin to break the natural laws and cause trapped protein in our children. Our children get their feelings hurt because they do not understand. All they know is that we have deprived them of doing what they instinctively know they must do to feel good.

12.3. In an effort to save the bed, couch, or carpet, we force our children into inactivity and cause trapped proteins in their bodies, and in time many become sick and listless.

12.4. There is a big difference in being alive and well and alive and sick. I'm sure the Tarahumara Indians are not perfect. But if we are to consider them alive and well, we are all, to one degree or another, alive and sick. The "miracle" of lymphasizing is actually the miracle of energy and life, and one of the answers to why many people get sick and die.

D-13. If You Don't Have A Lymphasizer–Get One

13.1. In Session Four, there are many beautiful and seemingly miraculous testimonials of what happens to people when they begin to lymphasize, but there are several personal ones that I would like to share with you at this time. Then I will teach you how to use a lymphasizer so that healing will take place in your body.

13.2. There are many names that manufacturers are putting on these units, but a common name by which they can all be called without offending anyone is a lymphasizer. It is the only name that describes what that unit actually does for the body. It is a lymphasizer.

13.3. Many of you have heard me say, "Forget about selling the lymphasizers. Teach people why they work, and they will get one just as fast as they are able." It is my hope that this book will do the job for which it is designed. For if it does, the number of people who desire to get the blood protein research to the world will increase by the tens of thousands. The manufacturers will be selling units like mad and hopefully will see the importance of helping to get this research to the nations of the earth.

13.4. My mother was over 80 years old when I got her a lymphasizer. She was on a walker and her equilibrium was poor. To get on a lymphasizer she had to put straps around that were attached to the wall, and she had to hold onto something so she would not fall down. She could only bounce about *six* times without getting sick, which you now understand. But she kept going, and now she is able to jog up and down about *one thousand* times. To have energy is to have youth. Therefore, she is becoming younger with the use of a lymphasizer.

D-14. 98-Year-Old Woman Saved From Death

14.1. Malin Lewis had a ninety-eight-year-old mother in Phoenix, Arizona, dying in the hospital. He learned about lymphasizing, brought her home, had her stand up on a lymphasizer with him, with his arms around her to hold her up. As he did a gentle bounce, Malin would say "breathe deeply mother, breathe deeply!"

14.2. I saw that ninety-eight-year-old mother dance and sing on a lymphasizer, and she was still doing it when she was 100 years old. This was truly a miracle of lymphasizing.

14.3. David and Sarah Glick, a beautiful Amish family in Lancaster, Pennsylvania, tell of a little boy who fell in a cesspool. He was under for over five minutes before they got him out. When they released him from the hospital, he was nearly a vegetable. They began to lymphasize him. In a few months, they took him back to the doctors. They would not believe it was the same boy. He was perfectly healthy. Another miracle of lymphasizing. Sarah has literally hundreds of the testimonials she could give of the Amish people who have been helped during the last five years. Frank and Kathy Angelo who live in that area have been instrumental in getting these lymphasizing concepts to thousands. Urias and Marietta Miller have done the same for the Mennonites and others in Ohio. And Richard and Anna Short (my little "Ammonites") are known all over Ohio for their efforts. Scott and Gladys Forsyth have done the same thing with the people in Washington. Jerry and Maple Hinkle have helped get this Blood Protein Research all over the United States. These people, along with others in every state, have many testimonials similar to these I am giving here. "Lymphasizing works."

D-15. Special Education Children Respond To Lymphasizing

(This letter was reproduced in "Rebounding Aerobics")

15.1. Florence Franet, a teacher of special education students at the Mount Diable Unified School District in Concord, California, got the idea of moving the trapped proteins out and turning the generators on when she attended one of my lectures back in 1976.

15.2. She writes, "After attending a lecture and workshop by Dr. C. Samuel West, I purchased a mini-trampoline for my own use and that of my family. I felt so good as a result of using it, I knew I had to share it with my students too."

15.3. Her testimony, which you can read in Session Four, on what happened to these children is two pages long. To make a long story short, she had children from ages 8 to 11 years old. Some of them could not write their name or even speak sentences. Their coordination was so bad, they could not stand on a lymphasizer by themselves for about 3 months. She let them lymphasize as much as they wanted to. As the trapped protein came out of their brains, the excess fluid and the excess sodium came out and the generators began to turn on. Before the year was over, many of these children were able to write their name and speak coherently. *Another Miracle of Lymphasizing.*

15.4. In 1977 and 1978 she did the same thing with high school children who also had brain damage that resulted in the loss of physical coordination, muscle development, self-concept, and language skills. She said, "Some of the better coordinated boys decided to challenge one another to see who could hop on one foot the most number of times. They started out with one hundred, then three hundred, seven hundred, and one thousand! It was getting to be difficult trying to count the number of times accurately (it takes longer to say a number than to take a hop). So we began to use a stop watch and they set five minute periods of time for themselves. Each of these boys could hop on one foot, but not the other, so each was challenging himself to develop his weaker side. One boy did it in three week's time, a second boy did it in seven week's time, and the third is still trying to master that second side. After 6 month's time, he is now very close to mastering it." She said, "I would like to see all of our handicapped students have the opportunity to use a mini-trampoline on a daily basis in order to minimize their handicaps more rapidly."

15.5 Speaking of the younger children she said, "all of the students showed growth in their coordination, language skills, health, and attitudes." This is the miracle of lymphasizing. Mrs. Franet went on to say, "I had expected to see growth for each student during the school year as I had worked with these kind of students for five years previous to working with this group, but this growth far exceeded expectations and I attribute this additional gain to their developments and total stimulation by use of the mini-trampoline."

15.6. Without the knowledge of the *seven golden discoveries and this formula,* it would be impossible to comprehend these testimonials.

15.7 It has taken the newest and most modern scientific discoveries for us to understand in detail the blessings that will come to all who will obey the mental, nutritional and physical laws of health.

D-16. *The Miracle of Aerobic Lymphasizing*

16.1. Now you are ready to learn the difference between *aerobic exercising and aerobic lymphasizing.* There is another miracle that will take place in your body if you can get into the aerobic zone on a *lymphasizer.*

16.2. Without the knowledge you have now obtained, it would be impossible for most people to get into the aerobic zone. Why? Because *aerobic exercise* requires excellent physical condition. You must get your heartbeat in the area of 220 minus your age times 80 percent for a minimum of 12 consecutive minutes. On a hard surface, there are very few of you who could reach that goal; however, if you follow the four laws of lymphasizing while you are in a *LYMPHASIZER,* almost everyone can obtain the benefits of *aerobic lymphasizing* to the point that they will be able to go through a complete lymphasizing program where they will be breathing deeply and perspiring and yet keeping their body feeling like they are sitting in a chair during the entire lymphasizing program.

16.3. The miracle that takes place within the body with the *aerobic lymphasizing* is this: Every cell has the ability to convert glucose into glycogen, especially muscle cells. And glycogen can be stored in the cells as extra energy when it might be needed. Since you do not lose energy *on a lymphasizer* at the bottom of the bounce, I believe the body can convert glucose into glycogen much faster and easier on a lymphasizer than it can on a hard surface. Aerobic exercise on a hard surface puts a person under stress. With aerobic lymphasizing there is no stress and no fatigue. The more you do it, the better you feel; and the better you feel, the more you can do it. And I believe glycogen is involved in this good feeling. When you lymphasize on a lymphasizer, you keep your body feeling like you are sitting in a chair all the time.

16.4. Maybe this helps explain the endurance of a Tarahumara Indian. The fruits, vegetables, and whole grains (the complex carbohydrates) are the primary source of glucose, and the body is able to convert this glucose to glycogen in every cell especially muscle cells.

D-17. *The Miracle of Glycogen*

17.1. Glycogen is a miracle substance. There are very few people who can even comprehend it; but I will explain it to you, and you try.

17.2. Glucose is 180 *grams* per *mole*. To help make it easier to understand, forget about the *moles*. Just think about the *grams*. Glycogen is 5,000,000 *grams* per mole or more! The first time I saw this, my brain said "*misprint, impossible.*" Water is 18 *grams* per mole. Glucose is 180 *grams* per mole. Glucose is ten times heavier than water. To pick up a gallon of glucose would be like picking up ten gallons of water. If glycogen was five million grams per mole, it would be 27,000 times heavier than glucose. Therefore, to pick up a gallon of glycogen would be like picking up 27,000 gallons of glucose or 270,000 gallons of water.

17.3. I went to another source to check out the molecular weight of glycogen, and there it was printed *five million grams per mole or more!* I couldn't believe it! I said to myself, if the body could form that kind of substance within the cell, it would have the ability of producing unbelievable energy within the body. This is exactly what takes place when the body converts glucose into glycogen. Glycogen is so heavy that once it is formed, it drops out as a solid mass inside the cell. Scientists used to think that the little dark spots in the cell were bad. But they found that the healthier the cell, the more dark spots it had. The dark spots have now been identified as glycogen. Glycogen makes it possible for a person to exhibit super human strength and perform seemingly impossible tasks.

17.4. Let me explain how this happens. Divide 180 into 5,000,000 and you find that it takes approximately 27,000 molecules of glucose to make one molecule of glycogen. The secret to the super human strength that comes from glycogen is this: The *first* phase of the energy cycle within the cell *takes place in the absence of oxygen*. Four molecules of ATP (energy) is produced from glucose *without any oxygen* in the first phase. The *second* phase *requires oxygen to convert glucose into energy*. There are 28 molecules of ATP produced in the second phase where oxygen is used in the process. (This brings out another reason why it is important to breathe deeply everywhere you go.)

17.4. Just think about this for a minute. If the *first* phase of the energy cycle can convert glucose to energy in the absence of oxygen, think what would happen if *ONE* molecule of glycogen in every cell of the body would turn loose of 27,000 molecules of glucose all at the same time within every cell of the body, especially the muscle cells, where glycogen is more easily stored.

17.6. If every cell in the muscles were to receive that much glucose at one time, knowing that the first phase of the energy cycle takes place in the cell in the absence of oxygen we can easily understand *how the body could actually produce a small earthquake inside*. The energy produced would simulate *a small volcano* inside the body. Samson probably had an extraordinary ability to convert glucose into glycogen in his muscle cells. What his hair had to do with it is unknown. It could be that he was given this special gift and was told that if he ever allowed anyone to cut his hair he would lose it. But there is no question that in the temple he was given that gift one more time.

D-18. Glycogen Can Give You Superhuman Strength

18.1. This is exactly what happens when the mind calls for a *sudden* demand of strength. The adrenal gland excretes adrenaline (epinephrine), which causes glycogen to turn loose of the glucose inside the cell. This is why you hear the story about Samson and about the little old lady who stepped out of the house and saw a little boy under a car, and she was able to pick up the car to free the boy. This scientifically is *what can take place in the body* when stored glycogen is released under certain conditions.

18.2. In the aerobic zone you are breathing deeply and flooding the cells with oxygen which enables them to convert glucose into A.T.P. and also into glycogen. Some believe that athletes have learned how to get the body in a condition where they can store glycogen with aerobic exercise and have it released when they need it for a sudden burst of energy.

18.3.   The importance of breathing deeply everywhere you go is here established and on a *lymphasizer* almost everyone, in a year's time or less, will have the ability to do aerobic lymphasizing and receive some of the benefits that come from increasing their ability to convert glucose into glycogen inside their muscle cells, and that is something to work for.

18.4.   I would now like to give you a poem that was written by my angel wife, Johna May. It is called: BOUNCY, BOUNCY BABY.

> Bouncy Bouncy Baby
>> We don't rock anymore
> We just get on a *LYMPHASIZER*
>> And bounce from shore to shore.
> Bouncy Bouncy Baby,
>> We don't rock anymore,
> We just get on a *LYMPHASIZER*
>> And bounce forever more.
> *Lymphasizers* are magic,
>> *Lymphasizers* are grand;
> When you learn how to use one,
>> You will understand.
> Rocking chairs are super,
>> Rocking chairs are great,
> But when you get on a *LYMPHASIZER*
>> Old age will have to wait!
> Now you can jump on the bed,
>> And you can jump on the couch,
> But when you buy new furniture
>> Your husband will say OUCH!
> So if you love your family,
>> You know what you can do,
> Go out and get a *LYMPHASIZER*
>> And tell them, *"I love you."*
>> By Johna May West
>> (Wife of Dr. West)

D-19.   Two Reasons Why "Miracles" Take Place on a Lymphasizer

19.1. The first reason that miracles are taking place in the bodies of people who use a *LYMPHASIZER* is this: *The lymph system pumps fluid and protein out of the tissue spaces each time the tissues are compressed or moved in any other way.* Therefore, just a very gentle movement up and down on a *LYMPHASIZER*, will propel the lymph fluids up through the body and pull some of the trapped proteins out the same as if you were running around a track and breathing deeply. People who have a lot of poisons and trapped proteins built up in their body may feel sick after just three gentle bounces. Other people may get sick after bouncing a minute or two. A *LYMPHASIZER* is not a play toy. It will pull the trapped proteins out of the body faster and easier than anything else you can do. But if you have a lot of toxic waste stored in the body, when the lymph system pulls the proteins out, all the excess fluid and toxic waste goes directly into blood stream. Therefore, some people get sick in just a few bounces, and many have to run to the bathroom to empty their bladders. Just keep it up. Follow the Four Laws. *The more you lymphasize the better you will feel; and the better you feel, the more you will be able to lymphasize.*

19.2. The second reason miracles are taking place on a *LYMPHASIZER* is *you don't lose energy at the bottom of the bounce.* This is why many people can get on a *LYMPHASIZER* and gain *endurance* and *strength* where they can't even get started on a hard surface.

19.3. These two facts explain what is happening to people who learn how to use a *LYMPHASIZER*. And we now know that what is taking place in their bodies are not miracles at all. People are just getting the trapped proteins out of their body so that healing can occur.

D-20. How to Use a Lymphasizer Properly and Bounce Your Way to Better Health

20.1. Because a *LYMPHASIZER* plays such an important role in the art of lymphasizing, it is very important that you know how to use it properly.

20.2. To know how to use this unit properly has not been an easy task. I discovered the concepts of lymphasizing as the result of teaching and demonstrating how to use a lymphatic exercise unit almost five days a week for about five years.

20.3. It was around the middle of 1980 when I began to ask this question to the audience, *"How would you like to learn how to go through a complete exercise program without stress or fatigue?"* I was showing people how to do this for months before it finally began to dawn on me that I was doing something that I had never done before and that I had discovered a *TOTALLY NEW APPROACH TO EXERCISE* that is now called *lymphasizing*. By following the four laws of lymphasizing, and by using the lymphasizing program below, you will always keep your body feeling like you are sitting in a chair. On a *lymphasizer*, anyone who can walk can learn how to "run and not be weary, and walk and not faint."

20.4. By following this program, I am now able to demonstrate at every lecture I give how I can go through a complete lymphasizing program without ever getting tired. When I finish, even though I have been breathing deeply and perspiring, I have done so without any fatigue in my body. In effect, with the knowledge contained in the *seven* golden discoveries and the *one* basic formula, I have discovered how to *"run and not be weary and walk and not faint"* on a *lymphasizer*. And the same laws that must be obeyed to do this on a lymphasizer must be obeyed to do it on a hard surface.

20.5. To know how to use a lymphasizer properly, you must know what to look for when you do it. It took me over five years to recognize it. The secret of lymphasizing is *endurance*. Endurance is hard to recognize because it happens so gradually that you take it for granted. Therefore, let endurance, without causing negative stress such as pain or fatigue at any step in this lymphasizing program, be the key to your progress.

20.6. This is contrary to almost every other physical fitness program you have ever heard about. Most of them force you to go to the point of stress. Therefore, people have been conditioned to think, "If I don't feel any bad effects, it isn't doing me any good."

20.7. With the new *lymphasizing* program below, you will feel good all the time. You will *never* get tired. The main thing to remember is this: Follow the Four Laws of Lymphasizing as long as you live. You will soon be lymphasizing your way to better health and don't be satisfied until you can "run and not be weary, and walk and not faint."

20.8. This new lymphasizing program will revolutionize

the whole exercise industry. It is designed to help raise up a posterity who will conquer disease and live in peace. It is appropriately called:

D-21.   *The Run and Not Be Weary - Walk and Not Faint Lymphasizing Program*

Step One: To begin with, just do the *Gentle Bounce* as shown in these pictures (See Fig. 2 and 2A). Directions on how to do the gentle bounce are on page 161. Later, you can substitute *The Bio-Electric Gentle Bounce for Health* as explained on pages 186-188. This makes a lymphasizer priceless. The Bio-Electric Gentle Bounce for Health will immediately increase circulation in the body and make it possible for the cells to receive more oxygen and nutrients. The body that is able to reverse disease will do so if the cells can get enough oxygen and nutrients.

Step Two: Do the Soft Walk (See Fig. 3 and 3A). Directions are on page 162. To speed up the healing process, combine the other *lymphasizing* techniques described in Sessions One and Two. Stay with Steps One and Two until you can do them for at least one half-hour without getting tired before going on to Step Three. The key to healing is endurance.

Step Three: Do the Low Jog (See Fig. 4). Be sure to follow the directions on page 163.

Step Four: Do the basic LYMPHASIZING VARIATIONS below. See the directions on pages 163-165
(a) The Front Kick (See Fig. 5),
(b) The Side Kick (See Fig. 6),
(c) The Seat Bounce (See Fig. 7),
(d) Turning the Other Cheek (See Fig. 8),
(e) The Pony Trot (See Fig. 9), and
(f) The Bronco Buster (See Fig. 10).
(Other variations include the Back Kick, the Front and Back Jump Rope, the Body Twist, etc., etc.)

Step Five: Do AEROBIC LYMPHASIZING (See page 165).

Step Six: Do the Medium Jog (See Fig. 11), and advance slowly, without causing stress or fatigue until you get into a High Jog (See Fig 12). The second you feel any stress or fatigue, go back to Step Two. Now, repeat Step Six

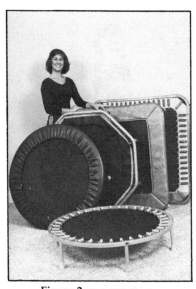

Figure 2 Natalie Witt showing
Different Styles of Lymphasizers

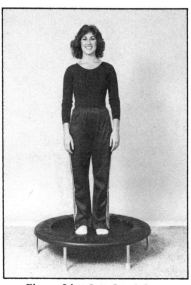

Figure 2A   Step One & Seven
The Gentle Bounce

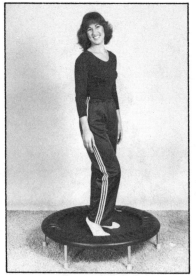

Figure 3   Step Two & Seven
The Soft Walk

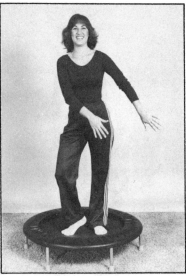

Figure 3A   Step Two & Seven
A Variation Of The Soft Walk

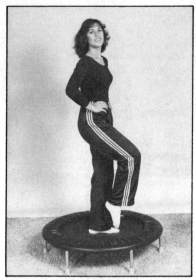

Figure 4   **Step Three & Six**
The Low Jog

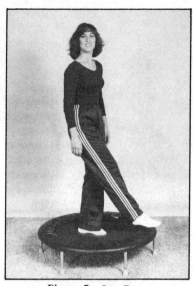

Figure 5   **Step Four**
The Front Kick

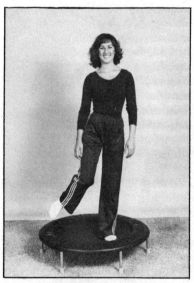

Figure 6   **Step Four**
The Side Kick

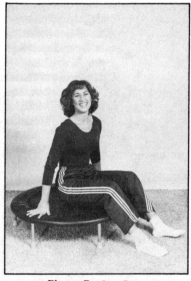

Figure 7   **Step Four**
The Seat Bounce

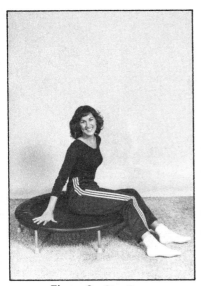

Figure 8   Step Four
Turning The Other Cheek

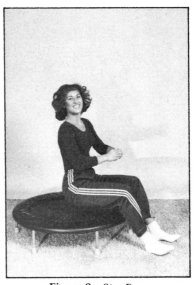

Figure 9   Step Four
The Pony Trot

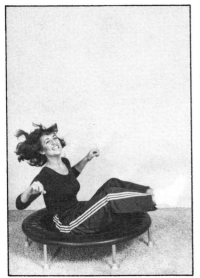

Figure 10   Step Four
The Bronco Buster
"A Kick With Every Buck"

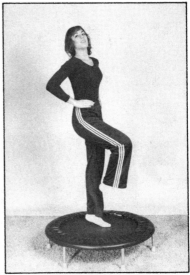

Figure 11   Step Five & Six
The Medium Jog

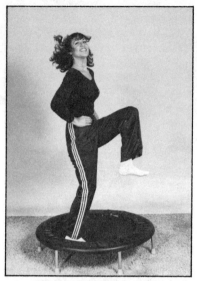

Figure 12   Step Five & Six
The High Jog

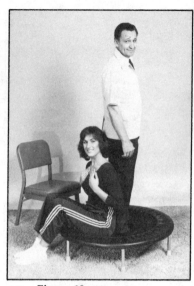

Figure 13 For Those Who Can't
Stand or Sit By Themselves

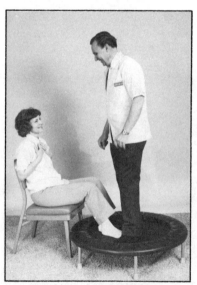

Figure 14 The Bio-Electric Wheel-
Chair Technique — Dr. West With His Wife

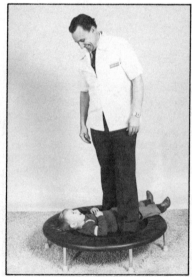

Figure 15 On A Bed Or Lymphasizer
Dr. West With His Youngest Son, Daniel

over and over. Remember the key to healing starts
with an "E"! The word is *Endurance.* How *long* can
you do it without causing stress or fatigue?

Step Seven: When you want to stop, be sure to slow down
properly so you will be able to end up with Gentle
Bounce or preferably The Bio-Electric Gentle Bounce
for Health with no fatigue in your body.

DIRECTIONS FOR STEP ONE

Note: There are several different styles of lymphasizers (See
Fig. 2). Some like one, some like the other, but all good quality
units work! The main thing is, if you don't have a lymphasizer, get
one with a bounce that "feels good" to you and use it.

1. If you have never been on a *LYMPHASIZER* before and
you are not used to doing very much exercise, then gently step on
to the mat, while keeping your feet on the mat, do a *gentle bounce*
for about fifteen seconds and stop and see how you feel. Keep
your body feeling as good as if you were sitting in a chair.
Remember, this is not a play toy. If you cause stress or fatigue,
you're exercising, not lymphasizing. If you feel good, then go on
to 30 seconds and check your response again. If you still feel
good, do it for one minute, then two, three, five, ten, fifteen and
thirty minutes or longer.

2. Remember, what we are after is endurance without stress
or fatigue at each step. If you follow The Laws of
LYMPHASIZING, your body will always feel like you are sitting
in a chair. You will never cause any negative stress, and you will
never get tired. You may be able to keep this feeling for only a
few bounces to start with. But the exciting thing is, the more you
do it, the better you will feel; and the better you feel, the more
you will be able to do it. Are you beginning to understand the
healing power of *LYMPHASIZING?*

3. Anybody can start with Step One. If you can't stand on a
lymphasizer, sit on it. If you can't sit alone, then have someone
stand on the mat and hold you up with their hands, or they can
stand with their back to you and you lean against the back of
their legs (See Fig. 13).

4. If you are in a wheelchair and can't stand or sit on a

lymphasizer, then do the Bio-Electric Wheelchair Technique as explained in Session Four (See Fig. 14).

5. If you are confined to a bed, then if necessary, check with your doctor and if possible do the deep breathing as described in the Walker-West-Walk as often as possible without causing stress. Then combine it with the bio-electric breathing and directed thinking technique as explained in Session Four. You can also have someone stand over you and bounce you up and down, and direct the energy produced mentally, the same as in the bio-electric gentle bounce for health (See Fig. 15).

6. As a rule of thumb, to cause healing to take place in a weak spot do the appropriate lymphasizing techniques 15 seconds, every 15 minutes. (Remember the story of Malin Lewis and his 98-year-old mother.)

7. During Step One and Two, to help speed up the healing process, add the pressure, massage, and light fast stroke techniques described in Session Two.

DIRECTIONS FOR STEP TWO

1. Begin to do *The Soft Walk* anytime you feel like it. You may even want to begin with Step Two. This is where you will probably spend most of your time. It may take a little while to "get the hang" of it, but once you do you will enjoy *The Soft Walk*. Keep your toes on the mat and raise one heel, and then the other; this will cause you to bend your knees slightly. As you get the feel of it you will be able to shift your weight from one foot to the other and sort of rock back and forth.

2. As you build endurance with step two, do the Walker-West-Walk and the other lymphasizing techniques described in Session Two. Also, if you have a radio or record player, lymphasize to a special rhythm. Better still, sing some songs. Your mental attitude is important. The deep breathing while you sing will increase the lymph movement in your body just like doing the Walker-West-Walk. Learn the poem "Bouncy Bouncy Baby" and others and say them while you do Step Two.

3. If you have little children when they see you on a lymphasizer, they will say by their actions, *"If you love me, lymphasize me."* They will be right up there with you.

4. As you gain strength, you will be able to lymphasize until you begin to breathe deeply.

5. As it says in Step Seven, whenever you decide to stop,

slow down gradually. Always end up by doing Step One. If you slow down too fast you will cause trapped proteins, and you will lose your energy. If you follow the laws of lymphasizing, you should always be breathing normally, with no fatigue in your body when you step off the lymphasizer.

DIRECTIONS FOR STEP THREE

1. Do not attempt the Low Jog until you can do the Soft Walk for at least thirty minutes. After that you can get into Step Three and do it as you feel like it. To do the Low Jog, begin to raise your toes just off the mat as you bend your knees in a regular jogging motion, or you may still be shifting your weight from one foot to the other and bouncing back and forth. To increase your activity you may want to swing your arms back and forth or up and down. Let your body decide what to do. It may take several months for many people to reach this point. To help increase your endurance, talk or sing as in Step Two.

2. Before you decide to step off, slow down gradually, go back to the Soft Walk and the Gentle Bounce. When you step off, there should be no fatigue in your body.

DIRECTIONS FOR STEP FOUR.

1. This is where all the fun begins. You can begin to do *the lymphasizer variations* anytime you feel like it after you get to the Low Jog. The purpose of the variations are to begin to tone the muscles throughout the body and to cause you to breathe deeper.

(a) The Front Kick and (b) The Side Kick

2. You will find that it will not be too hard to transition from the Soft Jog to the Front Kick. However, as you kick forward, keep your body feeling like you're sitting in a chair. The second your legs start to feel tired with the Front Kick, do the Side Kick which uses another set of muscles. It is interesting how it is possible to kick higher and higher and increase your endurance by rotating back and forth between (a) and (b). While doing the Low Jog and the variations, you will feel the miracle of lymphasizing take place in your body. On a hard surface you would be tired, but if you OBEY THE LAWS OF

LYMPHASIZING you will not cause any stress and you will have no fatigue in your body when you finish.

3. Feel free to rotate from one variation to another or from one step to the other. Remember, we are after endurance, not speed. The statement by Dr. Van Aaken, "From maximum endurance comes maximum performance," is a true statement.

(c) The Seat Bounce

4. If your legs begin to feel tired, but you feel like you want to keep going, go to the Seat Bounce. Step off quickly, sit on the mat and put your feet on the floor. With the help of your hands and feet gently bounce up and down. You are still lymphasizing. The Seat Bounce requires as much or more energy than some of the others, but you will be resting your legs while you continue to pull trapped blood proteins out of your body. *How can you tell if healing is taking place?*

5. If you are increasing in energy and endurance, you know that healing is taking place inside your body. Just keep it up: *You are lymphasizing your way back to better health.*

(d) Turning the Other Cheek

6. To make the Seat Bounce fun, try bouncing from hip to hip. This is called, "Turning the Other Cheek." Say, "ho, ho, ho," while you do this. Remember to make lymphasizing fun. Let yourself go and really enjoy it. (As a bonus this variation takes the weight off where you don't want it.)

(e) The Pony Trot

7. As your energy and endurance continue to increase, the normal Seat Bounce will become easy, so try this: Bounce up and down without your hands on the mat. With your feet on the floor and waving your arms up and down you will be able to do it. This is called "the Pony Trot."

(f) The Bronco Buster

8. To make the Seat Bounce even more of a challenge, after you are able to do "the Pony Trot" with ease, try lifting your feet

up off of the floor and with the use of your arm movements only bounce up and down and from side to side. This is called "the Bronco Buster." And when you do this, shout HO, HO, HO, HO, HO, HO; and your endurance will increase. Singing, talking, and laughing while lymphasizing will help speed up the healing process.

9. The second you feel any stress, get up and repeat Steps Two and Three. You will notice that you are now beginning to perspire and breathe hard, but you will not have any fatigue whatsoever in your body. You will be moving your lymph and blood proteins the same as if you were running down the road as hard as you could go but with a lymphasizer you will be doing it with no stress or fatigue in your body.

DIRECTIONS FOR STEP FIVE

1. After doing Step Four, or *whenever you are able to lymphasize by using Steps Two, Three and Six until you are breathing deeply for about five minutes,* you will be into AEROBIC LYMPHASIZING. (Refer to section D-16 on page 150.) In aerobic lymphasizing, you will be turning *glucose* into *glycogen.* Due to the fact that you do not lose energy at the bottom of the bounce, this conversion takes place much *faster* and *easier* on a lymphasizer than it does on a hard surface.

2. *Review the four physical laws of lymphasizing on page 140. Remember: Walk-run; walk-run; but do not get tired!*

You Are Now Beginning To Experience The Miracle Of Lymphasizing

3. You are now beginning to experience the *miracle of lymphasizing.* You are breathing deeply; you are perspiring; but your body still feels like your sitting in a chair. To stay in the aerobic lymphasizing zone, you must keep breathing deeply. With the wisdom and great treasures of knowledge, even the hidden treasures, that come from learning about the blood proteins, we are now able to literally "run and not be weary, and walk and not faint," on a lymphasizer. And the same laws that must be obeyed to do this on a lymphasizer, must be obeyed to do it on a hard surface until like a Tarahumara Indian, you can run from sun-up to sun-up with no fatigue in your body.

DIRECTIONS FOR STEP SIX

1. To prove that this blessing is yours, after you finish Step Five you will be breathing deeply and perspiring. Now, after a total of about twenty minutes, it's time to show what LYMPHASIZING is all about. On a hard surface, you would be dead tired by now, but on a LYMPHASIZER, your body feels like you are sitting in a chair.

2. To prove that you are experiencing *the miracle of lymphasizing,* start doing a low, soft jog and hold it for a while. Stay beneath negative stress and fatigue levels. If you raise your knees too high too fast, you will cause stress; and this will cause trapped proteins and you will lose your energy, so start slowly. The more you do it, the better you feel; and the better you feel, the more you will be able to do it.

3. Now raise your knees a little higher, speed up a little, and hold it for a while. Your body should still feel like you are sitting in a chair. Raise your knees a little higher, speed up a little more, and hold it. Continue this process until you feel the "point" of fatigue. The second you feel it, go back to Step Three.

4. As you practice Step Three you will be able to come up and down on the same foot. That is you will be able to touch the mat twice with the same foot as you bounce back and forth. When you go back to Step Three, you will find that within seconds, your body will feel like you are still sitting in a chair.

5. When you have progressed to this point, you can run again to the point of fatigue and come back to Step Three and the fatigue will disappear. You can repeat this process over and over again and each time when you go back to Step Three, your body will feel like you are sitting in a chair.

> "You Will Feel Like Soaring Through The Skies
> When You Learn To Lymphasize."

6. If you doubted before, there will be no doubt when you get to the point that you are experiencing the feeling that comes from being able to run and not be weary and walk and not faint.

DIRECTIONS FOR STEP SEVEN

1. Now comes a very critical moment. Do not step off too

fast. Your whole circulatory system is moving very fast. You are breathing deep and perspiring, but no fatigue is in your body. If you step off too fast you will cause trapped proteins, and drain the energy right out of you. STAY ON THE LYMPHASIZER.

2. In order to keep your energies high, slow down by bouncing back and forth, shifting your weight from one foot to the other. Your feet will be coming off the mat.

3. *Do not slow down too fast.* You must keep your body feeling like you are sitting in a chair. Continue to slow down keeping your energy high until you are bouncing back and forth with your feet on the mat. You will be breathing easier at this point.

4. End up with *the gentle bounce* as in Step One. When you learn the Bio-Electric Gentle Bounce for Health, (taught in Session Four), you should begin *and end all exercise* on a LYMPHASIZER with the *Bio-Electric Gentle Bounce for Health* to help speed up the healing process.

5. When you stop, you should be able to speak in a normal voice, breathing normally with absolutely no stress or fatigue in your body whatsoever.

6. You have now experienced the miracle of LYMPHASIZING. This is the LYMPHASIZING program that I have been demonstrating in almost twenty cities a month. Few people would ever be able to do this on a hard surface. But on a LYMPHASIZER, this blessing can now be enjoyed by almost everyone.

7. Because of an accident which injured my left leg when I was sixteen years old, I could never have done this on a hard surface. It is only with a knowledge of *the blood protein research* that I know what it is like to be able to "run and not be weary, and walk and not faint."

D-22. How To Raise Up A Posterity Who Will Master The Art Of Lymphasizing, Conquer Disease And Live In Peace.

22.1. As you obey the mental, nutritional and physical laws of health, your *ability* to overcome disease will increase.

22.2. You have learned what you must do mentally, nutritionally, and physically to not only help save your own life, but also the lives of over two hundred forty thousand men, women, and children who are being killed every two months in in the United States alone because they do not know about these *seven* golden discoveries and this *one* basic formula.

D-23. *You Are Now Ready To Graduate From The College Of Cause, The College Of Self-Help Pain Relief, And From The College Of Prevention*

23.1. Let us examine the statement about the doctor of the future made by Thomas A. Edison and see if you qualify to become the doctor of the future that he talked about.

23.2. He said, "The doctor of the future will give no medicine, but will interest (teach) his patients in the *care* of this human frame, in *diet*, and in the *cause* and *prevention* of disease."

23.3. You now understand how to *care* for your human frame. You know mentally, nutritionally, and physically what you can and must do to *heal your body* and *keep it healthy*.

23.4. You now understand *diet! You know more about what foods will cause disease and death and what foods we are going to have to eat to prevent disease and cause healing to take place in the body.*

23.5 Also, you now know that trapped *blood proteins* are the *cause* of pain, loss of energy, disease and death, and what we are going to have to do mentally, nutritionally, and physically to untrap the blood proteins and keep them circulating in the body via the lymphatic system to *prevent* and if possible *reverse* disease.

23.6. You now know that it is the formula and the seven golden discoveries that gives men the ability to teach these principles, and you know that it has taken the most modern scientific discoveries to write them, yet no man can take the credit for them. For these discoveries were not originally made by man. They were made by The One who made the body. And you now know that those who have a complete understanding of these *seven* golden discoveries and this *one* basic formula can be qualified to become the doctor of the future that Thomas A. Edison talked about.

23.7. With the knowledge that is in this book, you can now become qualified as a registered Lymphologist and teach people what they must do to conquer disease and live in peace. To learn about the teaching opportunities in The World-Wide Family

Health Education Program, write to The International Academy of Lymphology, P.O. Box 351, Orem, Utah 84057.

D-24. The Powers Of Hate To Be Replaced By Love. Golden Families Who Are Willing To Conquer Disease And Live In Peace And Harmony Will Be Established

24.1. How fast will we be able to conquer disease and establish peace? Just as fast as we can get a knowledge of these seven golden discoveries and the one basic formula to the nations of the earth! As this takes place, the kingdoms of the adversary will fall and they will be replaced with a kingdom where love, inner beauty, and peace abound.

24.2. A people will come forth who will be willing to establish such a kingdom. This people will be willing to combat with and contend against the evils that everywhere exist. They will govern their homes in righteousness and bind the adversary. They will bring up their children with a desire in their hearts to let love rule the emotions, and wisdom the appetite. These will be people who will be able to "run and not be weary, and walk and not faint." The mental, nutritional, and physical forces that are now causing destruction on the earth will pass them by as the destroying angel did the children of Israel, and not slay them.

24.3. As we said in the beginning, the Blood Protein Research and the Art of Lymphasizing will have such a dramatic effect on the lives of those who learn the concepts, and apply the principles, that they will have a desire to help get this message to the nations of the earth.

D-25. You Can Now Defend Yourselves In The Battle Of Life And Death

25.1. With the knowledge that is in this book we are now ready to defend ourselves and our loved ones in the toughest battle we have ever faced. This is not a make-believe battle; it is a real battle. It has been stated over and over that more than two hundred forty thousand men, women and children are being killed every two months in this country alone, *because they do not know about this research*. This is like *three* atomic bombs hitting the United States every *two* months, eighteen per year.

There has never been such destruction of human life since the beginning of this nation. As revealed by The Dietary Goals for the United States, our *destroyers* are the greatest financial industries and interests in the world. For gold, silver, and material possessions, they are now *slaying* people throughout the world with killer diseases, *torturing* them with crippling diseases, and *binding* them down *and keeping them in darkness* as to how they are doing it.

25.2. With the additional light and knowledge that has come from the Blood Protein Research, we are able to not only escape them, but we will eventually be able to stop them. For them to continue to slay us for power and money, they must keep us in darkness as to how they are doing it. The Blood Protein Research and The Art of Lymphasizing is the most important message for health and world peace on the face of this earth. It will enable us to bind the adversary and literally help save the lives of millions of people.

25.3. As we said earlier, as people gain a knowledge of *The Dietary Goals for the United States,* the door to safety will be opened, and these *seven* golden discoveries and this *one basic formula will give them the additional knowledge that is needed to bring them through it.*

25.4. *May we have the love and the courage to help get this knowledge to the nations of the earth as fast as possible, that we may help develop a golden civilization where love* will rule the emotions, and *wisdom* will rule the appetite. This civilization will be composed of people who will conquer disease and live in peace.

SESSION IV

THIS SESSION CONTAINS:

A
The new medical research by Dr. Fuller Royal, M.D., Dr. Daniel Graupe; Dr. Joseph Waltz, M.D.; and others who are using electricity to diagnose, prescribe and treat disease with great success.

B and C
How to do the Bio-Electric Gentle Bounce for Health and the other advanced self-help bio-electric lymphasizing techniques. (Pictures and testimonials included)

D
Testimonials of a few more (approximately 50) people who have applied these techniques.

E
Additional scientific evidence with testimonials gives validity to the transition program taught in Session Three.

F
Special acknowledgments to those who helped to make *The Golden Seven Plus One* possible.

G
Special recognition to individuals and manufacturers who helped finance the first edition of this book.

H
My story behind this book.

A. NEW MEDICAL DISCOVERIES GIVE CREDIBILITY TO THE ADVANCED BIO-ELECTRIC LYMPHASIZING TECHNIQUES

1. To help you understand these advanced lymphasizing

171

concepts it is necessary for you to know more about the new medical research that has been done and is being done in this area.

A-1. Electricity Used By Medical Doctors To Diagnose And Prescribe

1.1. In an article, "Body Electricity Offers New Hope," by Paul Harvey, published in the Phoenix Republic and Gazette on April 9, 1976, he states, "The fastest growing medical specialty today is called Electro-Medicine or Electrical Physiology.... Only now are responsible researchers considering *electricity for treatment* as well as for diagnosis. Broken bones which might have required six months in a cast to heal, now—with properly applied electricity—can heal completely within six weeks." In Session Two, I gave you the report published in the January 1973 issue of *Science World Magazine* entitled, "When Bones Heal, is Electricity the Key?"

1.2. Within the last five years a new medical science has been started, called "Dolorology" or the science of pain. Medical researchers in "pain clinics" are now using electrical devices to help relieve pain and help speed up the healing process.

1.3. The nation's first pain clinic to use electricity was at the University of Washington in Seattle. I called this university in February 1977 to confirm the report given in the Chicago Tribune Tuesday, February 22, 1977. Dr. Bonica, the director of the clinic, was reported to say, "The field of pain research which has stagnated for almost a century has been reborn." What has happened in this area since that time has proven him right. There is another pain clinic in the College of Medicine in Tucson, Arizona. Dr's. Charles and Marlys Witte, two of the world's leading lymphologists, are at this college. They have one of the few lymphology laboratories in the world.

1.4. Let me say that the use of electricity to relieve pain is not entirely new. In 43 A.D., a Roman physician named Scribonius Largus used an electric fish to cure the pain of gout and migraine headaches. Unfortunately, the natural batteries of the fish were often so powerful that it killed some of the patients, so it was not practiced very much.

1.5. The pain researchers, who are working with electrical devices that are held on or even near whatever part of the body is in pain, state that "no one is exactly sure of why these devices work: but the one undisputed fact is--THEY DO WORK!"

1.6. At the Nevada Clinic of Preventive Medicine, in Las Vegas, Dr. Royal, M.D., and Floyd Weston are now having great success with a Bio-Pulse machine from Germany and the Dermatron machine which they are using to diagnose, treat and prescribe electrically. I would like to see clinics like this in every city in the United States.

1.7. Pete Peterson in Orem, Utah, is building machines to be used in medical clinics. He is working with the Nevada Clinic and has spent time with Dr. Joseph Waltz in New York. When I spoke to him he said that he is able to confirm the work we are doing with the bio-electric lymphasizing techniques, and that he is willing to help us in this research. There is also a lymphologist in Israel and another in Poland who may be able to document what is happening in the body with these techniques.

A-2. Eyes, Thoughts And Muscles Work Electrically

2.1. In the February 1973 issue of *The Family Circle* article entitled, *"Electrical-Medicine,"* it says "We seldom stop to think that our bodies run on electricity—but they do. And now electricity is being put to use to speed healing, and to ease pain...."

2.2. In 1976, during my seventh year of teaching chemistry, I saw several new scientific films dealing with body electricity. One of them showed a man paralyzed from the neck down, turning a wheelchair by using the electrical energy coming from his eyes. They wired him up with a shield located on each side of his face. After he pressed a button to make his electric wheelchair go, he would look at the shield to the left, and the wheelchair would turn to the left. He would look at the shield to the right, and the wheelchair would turn to the right. Another film, *The Incredible Machine*, showed a man wired up with electrodes going from his brain to an electric train. He could start, stop, slow down, and speed up the train just by thinking about it. They are now able to do this with children. However, in order to make it work, they have to magnify the electrical thought-wave. Keep this in mind because we use this principle in some of the Bio-Electric Lymphasizing techniques.

2.3. Also, in 1977, I talked to Larry Upjohn and confirmed

the fact that he had developed a device at the University of the Pacific in Stockton, California, which enables a person to activate a typewriter using the electrical energy in the forehead muscles. This proves that electrical impulses from the brain can be used to do useful work through the nerve endings in the muscles, etc.

A-3. *The Work of Dr. Graupe:* *"Bionic Arm" Controlled By Thoughts*

3.1. Using these concepts, it was reported in the news that Dr. Daniel Graupe, professor of electrical engineering at the Illinois Institute of Technology in Chicago, has developed a thought-activated artificial limb.

3.2 I called Dr. Graupe on January 5, 1981, and he confirmed this report. He said that he was also working on research to help paralyzed patients. He said that the "bionic arm" is not yet on the market because of the limited number who require it. However, after talking with him, I know that he is anxious that more people know what is going on in this area. He is sending me more detailed information on the work he is doing with his permission to reproduce it.

3.3 The "bionic arm" is unique in that is can be used by above-elbow amputees and performs seven functions--lifting and lowering the arm, grasping and unfolding the hand, turning the wrist clockwise and counter-clockwise, and maintaining a position. Electrical impulses from the brain, which control movements of healthy limbs, are picked up by an electrode placed on the amputee's surface skin. A micro-computer inside the artificial arm receives the impulses and translates them into the desired limb motions.

A-4. *Dr. Joseph Waltz Uses Electrical Stimulation To Help* *Previously Helpless Cerebral Palsy, M.S. And Polio Patients*

4.1. In Session Two, I told you about the marvelous work that is being done by Dr. Joseph M. Waltz, Director of the Department of Neurological Survey at the St. Barnabas Hospital in New York.

4.2. I have now received a letter from him giving me permission to use an abstract called, "Multi-Lead Spinal Cord

Stimulation For Control of Motor Disorders," which he sent me. This is a report on "160 patients undergoing chronic spinal cord stimulation for various disorders of the motor system and comparing the results obtained using older conventional two electrode bipolar stimulation with a newly developed four electrode multiple level system." Improvement was noted in 84% of the 75 patients with cerebral palsy, 67% of the 42 patients with dystonia, 62% of the 21 patients with torticollis and 73% of the 22 patients with post-traumatic neurologic loss.

4.3. When the four electrode system was used, the "marked to moderately improved patients increased from 57% to 84% in cerebral palsy, from 44% to 82% in dystonia, from 53% to 75% in torticollis and from 53% to 80% in post-traumatic neurologic conditions. There was a corresponding marked drop in unimproved patients in each condition."

4.4. It is interesting that "spinal cord stimulation had its inception in 1967 with initial trials designed to close the gate on pain transmission," and led the concept of neuro-augmentation and modulation. The role of spinal cord stimulation was expanded in 1973 by Cook and Weinstein, with their report of *improved motor function* in an M.S. patient *being treated for pain* . . . ." "The possibility of altering other motor disorders with stimulation prompted us to apply minute electrical impulses to the surface of the spinal cord to improve motor function. Our investigation in this area began in 1975 and we have now carried out spinal cord stimulation in over 200 patients with motor disorders, including cerebral palsy, dystonia, torticollis, post-stroke and post-traumatic spasticity. . . ." (See Figures 1-4).

4.5. "Spasticity was decreased, both objectively and subjectively in 95%, with many of the patients commenting on feeling more relaxed and less nervous. . . ." "Hand function was improved in 81% with patients carrying out activities which were impossible prior to stimulation, including feeding, holding a knife, fork, spoon and cup, brushing teeth and turning electrical appliances on and off. *Painful* spasms and abductor spasms have been abolished or markedly *decreased* in *all the patients* with this problem . . . ." "Bladder control was improved in 80% of the patients who had demonstrated dysfunction prior to stimulation. Sitting posture and balance improved in 83% in many instances allowing patients to sit unsupported without restraining straps or side supports. Head and neck stability was improved in 72% with many patients able to hold the head erect. Many patients showed increased ability to control their wheelchairs; and in several instances, arrangements were made for the patient to obtain electrical wheelchairs because of the increased hand function. . . . " "Walking was improved in 39% of the cases, characterized by a decrease in spasticity in the lower extremities, feet more flexible and flat on the floor; and speed and smoothness of ambulation increased."

4.6. "Speech was improved in 81% . . . ." "Swallowing was improved in 68% and drooling was decreased or abolished in 75%."

4.7 The knowledge that electricity dissipates the blood proteins helps us to understand why those who are using electricity are getting such good results.

4.8 Three out of four are receiving dramatic results. Dr. Waltz confirmed the following on the telephone:

4.9 An eighteen-year-old girl confined in a wheelchair was able to walk unassisted and feed herself after this treatment.

4.10 A seventeen-year-old palsy victim was suddenly able to control her bladder, speak clearly and use her hands again.

4.11 A young woman, once paralyzed, is now getting around on crutches and may soon be walking without crutches.

4.12 A 33-year-old woman is now able to move her head again and is free of pain.

4.13 A 14-year-old boy is now able to use his right hand for the first time in six years.

4.14 The four-electrode system is presently available only at the St. Barnabas Hospital. However, Dr. Waltz hopes that it will soon be available through other neurosurgeons throughout the world.

(a) *Complications.* "There were no deaths or serious complications...." "Three patients (1.8%) complained of pain at the stimulation site and required removal of the system. There were fourteen instances (8.7%) in which electrode displacement occurred and required repositioning. Broken electrodes occurred in 17 patients (10.6%) which were replaced without difficulty. Infections were encountered in 10 patients (6%) which necessitated removal of the system. However, there were no residual symptoms in these instances."

(b) Discussion

(1) "Chronic epidural spinal stimulation is capable of altering seemingly widely separated neurologic symptoms. We have observed reversal of the torticollic neck, the dystonic spine and foot, the spastic extremity, and the abolition of intractable seizures. This neuro-augmentation of modulation may result from direct electrical influence on nervous tissue, indirectly via chemical neuro-transmitter substances, or perhaps both. However, to effect symptoms as we have observed, the mechanism must be via some diffuse system which is accessible to our stimulating electrodes. The most likely system would be the ascending and/or descending raticular formation. In any case, the level at which these systems are stimulated, the polarity of the electrical field, and the frequency of the stimulation are critical in achieving a satisfactory result and these parameters must be individualized. The four electrode multi-level system which we have developed allows this individualization, and the improved results in this series confirm this theory.

(2) To further improve the therapeutic response, we are continuing to analyze and correlate our clinical results with the various stimulation parameters, including frequency, polarity, pulse width, impedence, site of stimulation, and evoked potentials.

(3) We are also investigating the possible neuro-physiologic neurotransmitter mechanisms which may lead to further understanding of the type of brain and spinal activity initiated or altered through spinal cord stimulation and which may further elucidate the mechanism of stimulation in the treatment of the motor disorders and the underlying neurologic abnormality.

A-5 Pictures and Letter Sent By Dr. Waltz

5.1 To help you understand the types of patients that were treated, I am including some pictures and a letter Dr. Waltz sent with this report.

5.2 The whole world should thank Dr. Waltz and others who are doing research in this area, for they are going to help bring to pass an age of healing that has never been known before.

5.3 The letter from Dr. Waltz shows how open he is to new ideas and how anxious he is to get his knowledge to others.

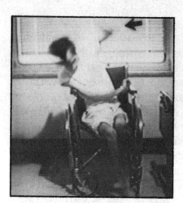

A

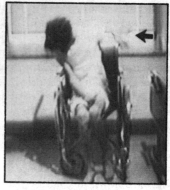

B

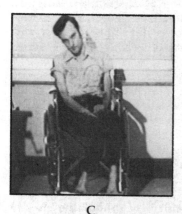

C

Figure 1   (ABC) Cerebral Palsy

The marked uncontrolled athetosis is shown preoperatively (A,B) in this 24 year old Cerebral Palsy patient with spastic quadriparesis and athetosis. The constant athetotic movement precluded any useful function in the upper extremities.

Following spinal cord stimulation (C) he is now able to sit straight and the athetosis has been eliminated with improved function in the upper extremities.

Figure 2   (ABCDE) Cerebral Palsy

18 year old quadriparetic Cerbral Palsy patient preoperatively (A,B) was unable to take a few steps (only if assisted) and unable to use her hands in everyday activities.
Essentially wheelchair bound.

Following spinal cord stimulation (C,D,E) she is able to ambulate unassisted, drink from a straw and feed herself. She is also free from drooling.

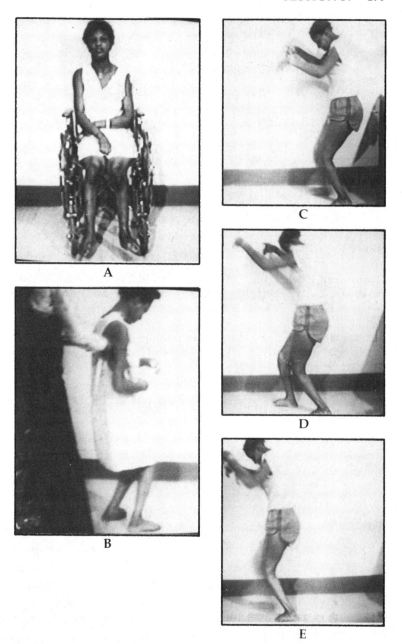

A

B

C

D

E

Figure 3   (ABCD) Dystonia

Dystonia of 5 years duration in a 9 year old boy was manifested by severe axial retrocollis, walking difficulty and poor hand function (A,B)

Postoperatively (C,D), the patient demonstrated improvement in the axial deformity, walking and hand function.

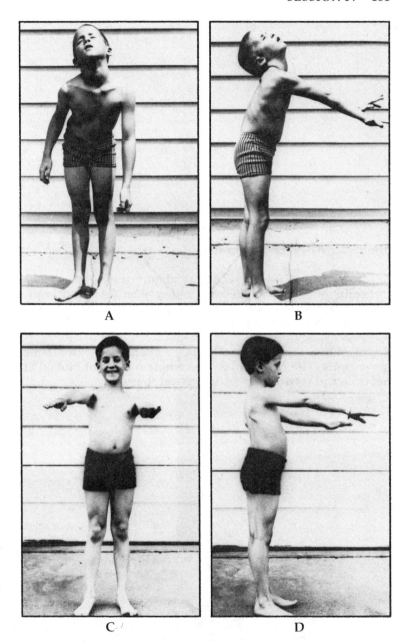

A   B

C   D

Figure 4   (ABCDEF) Torticollis

Severe spasm of the cervical musculature due to spasmodic torticollis burdened this 33 year old woman for seven years. Preoperative photos (A,B,C) show the patient attempting to turn her head to the right, in mid-position and to the left.

Postoperative sequence (D,E,F) demonstrate the same movements. The patient now has complete range of motion of her neck and is without painful cervical spasms.

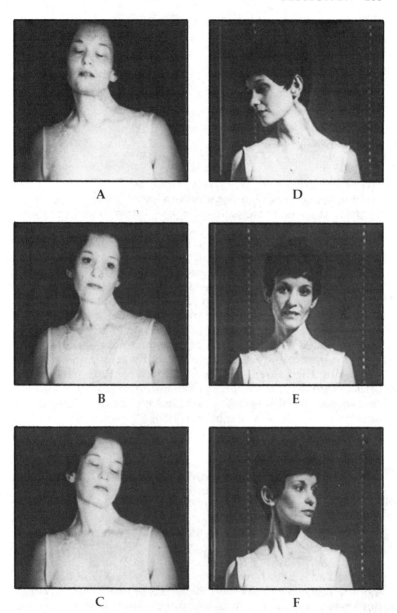

A   D

B   E

C   F

ST. BARNABAS HOSPITAL
4422 Third Avenue
New York, New York 10457

December 18, 1980

Dr. Corwin Samuel West
244 So. Englewood
Orem, Utah 84057

Dear Dr. West:

I had the pleasure of talking with you yesterday and learning of your interest in my work. I would be most interested in follow-up as to our discussion and the possible neuro-stimulating effect on proteins. I have enclosed with this letter reprints which are presently in press. One paper discusses spinal cord stimulation in general and was an earlier paper in 1979. The second paper compares the use of the two-electrode system with the four-electrode system, which I originated showing the improved results. I have also included with this letter a reprint from Patient Care Magazine, which came out in the later part of 1978, some updated statistics regarding the material presented there and also an outline which I am presently sending to patients discussing the present results and the technique which I am using. If you have any questions regarding this do not hesitate to contact me. By all means, if you find any of this information useful to you, please use it in your book.

Sincerely yours,

Joseph M. Waltz, M.D.
Director
Department of Neurologic Surgery

A-6. Thanks To Doctors Who Are Willing To Share

6.1. Dr. Royal, Floyd Weston, Dr. Waltz, Dr. Daniel Graupe and others have proven that they have the heart of a Lymphologist. The International Society of Lymphology is *not* a pure medical society. They are willing to share any information they have to help bless the lives of others.

6.2. I have never seen a more gracious and considerate group of people in my whole life than the doctors who attended The Seventh Congress of Lymphology in Florence, Italy, in October-November, 1979, and The Eighth International Congress in Montreal, Canada, in September, 1981. Lymphologists have come close, in my opinion, to mastering the mental art of lymphasizing which is to love, bless and to do good.

B. A LIST OF THE ADVANCED BIO-ELECTRIC LYMPHASIZING TECHNIQUES WHICH CAN BE DEMONSTRATED BY A QUALIFIED INSTRUCTOR

1. The Bio-Electric Gentle Bounce for Health. (C-2)
2. The special Bio-Electric Eye Exercise. (C-8)
3. The Bio-Electric Breathing and Directed Thinking Techniques. (C-9)
4. The Bio-Electric Wheelchair Technique. (C-10)
5. The Bio-Electric Pin-Point Technique. C-11)
6. The Bio-Electric Energy Field Technique. (C-13)

B-1. Definition Of Bio-Electric Energy:

1.1. Bio-electric energy is energy produced by the body, directly or indirectly, that can be used to dissipate "trapped" clustered proteins out of damaged areas of the body.

1.2. Note: This information is not given to diagnose or prescribe. It is offered only as an explanation of how these techniques work and why they work. If you decide to apply these techniques, you do so by virtue of your free agency.

1.3. As a result of the blood protein research, we can now explain how and why these bio-electric lymphasizing techniques work. Whether you completely understand the explanations or not--the one undisputed fact is: if used properly --THEY WORK! I have seen people use these techniques with success about 98% of the time.

C. EXPLANATIONS WITH PICTURES, AND STORIES ILLUSTRATING THE ADVANCED BIO-ELECTRIC LYMPHASIZING TECHNIQUES

C-1.   The Story Behind The Bio-Electric Gentle Bounce For Health,
       And The Special Bio-Electric Eye Exercise

1.1. The following story behind the *Bio-Electric Gentle Bounce for Health* will explain how and why it works.

1.2. This lymphasizing technique became a part of this program in 1976 as a result of my seeing the two films mentioned in A-2 , Page 173.

1.3. The first time I saw a *lymphasizer* was at an N.H.F. Convention in Phoenix, Arizona. When I observed people jumping up and down on them, the theory of how a *lymphasizer* could be used to convert mechanical energy into electrical energy flashed through my mind.

1.4. I had just recently seen the film showing how they could put electrodes from a person's brain to an electric train, and magnify the thought wave and start, stop, and speed up the train just by thinking about it.

1.5. I said to myself at that time, "I believe a person can create an electrical field by moving up and down on that unit." As a compass will tell you, the magnetic fields go around the earth from North to South. When you put an armature in a magnetic field, you convert mechanical energy into electrical energy. This is how they make electrical generators. As the body moves up and down through this magnetic field, it acts as an armature and it generates electricity going up and down. Howard Mott of Everett, Washington, and other electrical engineers have confirmed this fact. I thought to myself, "If the body could generate enough electricity by moving up and down on this unit, the electrical energy produced could magnify the thought wave, and a person could then mentally direct that energy into any area of the body he wanted to; and if this works, this discovery would increase the circulation and help relieve pain, and cause healing to take place."

1.6. I went up to the group at the convention who were demonstrating these units and said, "I believe I know how those units work better than you do." When they asked me how, I tried to explain it to them. They believed me enough that Karol Truman and two others traveled from St. George, Utah, to attend two of my complete seminars in Arizona, which at that time lasted two days each.

1.7. After the second seminar they let me take what I now

call a *lymphasizer* to my office in Mesa, Arizona, to experiment with it. I had a patient who had pain in her arms and legs and they were very tender to the touch. I said to her, "Let's go into the other room, I have an experiment that I want you to try." I told her to stand on the *lymphasizer* and to put her hands on her chest to prevent the energy from going out of the fingers. I had seen a scientific film showing energy as it comes out of the hands and feet. (I have since found that this Lymphasizing Technique works whether you put your hands on the chest or not, but it works better if you capture this energy.) I asked her to gently move up and down, keeping her feet on the mat and to think of her leg which was very sore to the touch. She did what I now call *The Bio-Electric Gentle Bounce for Health* and most of the pain disappeared in seconds. I could hardly believe it! We got excited. My theory was right; it worked exactly the way I thought it would, only a lot faster.

1.8. I called the manufacturers and made an appointment for them to come to my office. When I showed them *The Bio-Electric Gentle Bounce for Health,* they became excited. Karol Truman was able to take pain out of a scar in the arch of her foot in about five minutes. She had experienced this pain for approximately 25 years. After this excitement wore down a little, they said to me, "How would you like to teach the blood protein research all over the United States?"

1.9. I will never forget that occasion. I had been asking the Lord since 1974 to help me get The Blood Protein Research to the world, and the door opened just in time. When you read *my story behind this book* at the end of this session, you will understand what I mean.

C-2. *How To Do The Bio-Electric Gentle Bounce For Health*

2.1. I stand as shown in the illustrations with my hands on my chest.

2.2. To *"generate"* I move gently but rapidly up and down *WITHOUT HAVING MY FEET LEAVE THE MAT.*

2.3. Using the BODY CHART below, I generate up and down 2-4 times for each part and just think of each part as I do it. (I may want to say each part out loud. I can also add, "Old toxins out; new fluids in," every now and again to make it fun. Also, if my legs are feeling "tight" in the calf while I am generating, I just shift my weight gently from one foot to the other by raising one heel up and then the other.)

2.4. For those who decide to do this, do not go too long at first. Listen to your body. As we said in Session Three, if your body is very toxic, you may get sick in just three gentle bounces. If you do, *stop* and *come back a little later* and do it again until you can keep it up for one or two minutes. Many have to allow about *two weeks* or more to build up to *five minutes* at a time. Remember, the key to healing in the body starts with an "E." The word is *"endurance." Listen to your body;* it will tell you how long you can do it without causing stress or fatigue. (See the *note* on the bottom of the BODY CHART.)

C-3. Dr. West's Body Chart

3.1. This is the bio-electric lymphasizing exercise sequence for Step One of the lymphasizing program taught in Session Three. I put this chart on the wall, and bio-electrically generate and direct the energy into these and other areas of my body by just thinking of the body part as I generate. (Taken from The Lymphatic Exercise Home Study Program by C. Samuel West, N.D.)

3.2. To keep the blood proteins circulating after doing The Bio-Electric Gentle Bounce for Health, it is necessary to do the *breathing, stroking, brushing, and massaging* techniques for the areas of the body that need help as often as possible; fifteen seconds every fifteen minutes, if necessary. <u>For additional benefits</u>, I do the other LYMPHASIZING Techniques in Session Two while I do The Bio-Electric Gentle Bounce for Health.

3.3. To know how to use a lymphasizer bio-electrically to dissipate blood proteins makes this book priceless, and it turns a LYMPHASIZER into one of the most valuable pieces of equipment ever devised by man!

3.4. Because of this discovery I was invited to go all over the United States to teach the blood protein research and how to use the *lymphasizer* and *the other bio-electric self-help pain relief techniques* to help relieve pain and speed up the healing process. Jerry Hinkle traveled with me a lot and Maple, his wonderful wife, spent literally hundreds of hours on the phone setting up appointments. She says that her ear would get so sore that she could not lie on it at night.

3.5. Without their help and the help of many others, it

DR. WEST'S BODY CHART

Exercise Sequence For
"The Bio-Electric Gentle-Bounce-For Health"

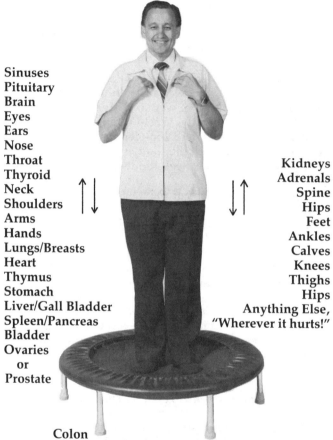

Sinuses
Pituitary
Brain
Eyes
Ears
Nose
Throat
Thyroid
Neck
Shoulders
Arms
Hands
Lungs/Breasts
Heart
Thymus
Stomach
Liver/Gall Bladder
Spleen/Pancreas
Bladder
Ovaries
  or
Prostate

Kidneys
Adrenals
Spine
Hips
Feet
Ankles
Calves
Knees
Thighs
Hips
Anything Else,
"Wherever it hurts!"

Colon
a. Descending (down L. side)
b. Transverse (across middle, R. to L.)
c. Ascending (up R. side)
d. Transverse (again)
e. Descending (again)
f. Repeat several times

Note: To speed up the healing process I add the
lymphasizing techniques in Sessions One and Two.

Figure 5

would have been impossible to write this book. Little did I realize then that the blood protein research would develop into a message that would teach people how to "run and not be weary, walk and not faint," and conquer disease and live in peace.

C-4. Dorothy Howard Reversed Her Sixty-Five Year Old Crippling Condition Due To Polio, In Four Months By Using The Bio-Electric Gentle Bounce For Health

4.1. Many who will read this book have heard me talk about Dorothy Howard. She was stricken with polio when she was about 10 months old. She was sixty-five when she came to one of my seminars in Seattle, Washington, and learned about the blood protein research and bio-electric lymphasizing. She was all bent out of shape and her body was in pain. Her left leg was paralyzed, leaving her heel about three inches off of the floor when she walked.

4.2. She got the concept of the basic formula and how the bio-electric gentle bounce which moves lymphatics could also dissipate the "trapped" clustered proteins out of her leg and would cause healing to take place. She decided to try it. Within one month she told me her leg was getting stronger, and that the doctors could hardly believe what was happening to her. In four months, her heel was on the floor for the first time in her life, the pain was out of her back, she was moving her toes and some of the feeling was coming back into her paralyzed leg.

4.3. Dorthy Howard is a woman everyone will remember. Everyone loved her, and before she passed away, she was able to direct hundreds of people into the path of health and peace. (Read the testimonial letters in this session.)

C-5. Doors Opened To Other Discoveries

5.1. I will never forget the step-by-step process that it took to find The Seven Golden Discoveries which made it possible to write The Formula giving the cause of death at the cell level and revealing what must take place to relieve pain and heal the body.

5.2. With this knowledge, it is now possible to explain how and why the following types of therapy work to help cause healing in the body: zone therapy, reflexology, iridology, color therapy, the herbal remedies, the naturopathic remedies, the homeopathic remedies, the electrical devices used in pain clinics and every other healing art known to man.

C-6. *This New Blood Protein Research Teaches The Cause Of Disease Which Enables Many People To Know What To Do To Take Care Of Their Own Problems.*

6.1. With the complete understanding of this basic formula, people will learn how to teach why the healing arts work. Then people will be able to know how and why to use these services to help relieve pain and cause healing to take place in their body.

6.2. As one man said, "There is a difference between giving a person a fish and teaching him how to fish. If you give him a fish, you feed him for a day. If you teach him how to fish, you feed him for a lifetime."

6.3. With this book, and in The Golden Family Self-H.E.L.P. Centers, we can teach people that the cause of pain, loss of energy, and disease *is* breaking the laws that cause trapped blood proteins; and what they must do to help untrap the blood proteins to keep them circulating in the body via the lymphatic system. If they go out and start to master *the art of lymphasizing,* and if they get a *lymphasizer* and start to do The Bio-Electric Gentle Bounce For Health and the other bio-electric lymphasizing techniques to dissipate their own blood proteins, they can help increase circulation which will relieve pain and cause healing to take place in their own bodies. They can raise up a golden generation of people who will conquer disease and live in peace, which is not only their prerogative, but also their solemn duty. Everyone has the responsibility to do all they can mentally, nutritionally and physically to relieve pain and cause healing to take place in their body.

6.4. I have seen aloe vera take pain out of burns and cayenne pepper stop bleeding outside and inside. Being high in potassium and other nutrients, these and other foods like bee pollen, barley green juice, wheat grass juice, Wachter's Sea Products, the herbal remedies, the naturopathic remedies, Research Formula #2, Blue-Green Manna, Spirolina and GH3 have a special ability to re-establish the delicate chemical balance in the cell which will increase the energy fields, and dissipate the blood proteins. If there are no trapped blood proteins, the body is in a negative sub-atmospheric pressure with no excess fluid or excess sodium around the cells. The chemical balance in the cells is right, the cells have oxygen, and the generators (the sodium-potassium pumps) are working properly. Therefore, there is no pain, loss of energy or disease. *To find out why something works, all you have to do is find out what it does in the body--then with the seven golden discoveries and the basic formula you will be able to figure out why and how it works.* This is exciting because everything begins to make logic and common sense. Remember, I found this formula, but no human being can take credit for it because it was made by The One who made the body. This is why its validity has never been questioned. To try to prove this formula wrong would be like trying to prove that the cells and the blood proteins in the body do not exist.

6.5. When I went to school thirty hours per month for a year- and-a-half to become a Naturopath, every time they would explain why a herbal remedy or other natural remedies worked, I would just sit there and say out loud, "It's moving out the trapped blood proteins." At the beginning of the year some of the Naturopaths would jokingly say, "Shut-up about the trapped proteins." Finally, because this research was so important, they asked me to teach a ten-hour course to the Naturopaths on the blood protein research. *At the end of the year and one-half, almost all of them knew that herbs, naturopathic remedies, the homeopathic remedies, and all the other energy producing therapies work at the cell level because they have the ability to dissipate the trapped proteins.* Through iridology you can learn where the trapped proteins are. Then as you use the natural energy producing therapies to dissipate the trapped clustered proteins, you can watch the healing lines appear in the eye. Isn't that exciting!

6.6. This research explains why things work at the cell level, and this is why it is so important. This is the only book in the world that contains The Seven Golden Discoveries and The One Basic Formula which reveals that "trapped" blood proteins produce the conditions that cause pain, loss of energy, disease and death at the cell level.

6.7. Now you know what the first law of lymphasizing is: LYMPHASIZE ON A LYMPHASIZER BIO-ELECTRICALLY ONCE OR TWICE A DAY, THEN BREATHE DEEPLY BY DOING THE WALKER-WEST-WALK EVERYWHERE YOU GO, OR AS OFTEN AS POSSIBLE.

6.8. As you do this Bio-Electric Gentle Bounce For Health once or twice a day, you will help dissipate the blood proteins out of every organ in your body. (See the BODY CHART.)

6.9.. Then to keep the blood proteins circulating so healing can take place, *it is necessary* to breathe deeply everywhere you go, or as often as possible. If you are not willing to do this or if you don't have the time or whatever your reason you do not do it, you will not receive the health that is possible for you to receive. In order for the body to heal, the blood proteins must be continually removed from the spaces around the cells by the lymphatic system.

6.10. Now you will understand the poem that my "angel" wife wrote more than ever. Let's look at it again.

C-7. *Poem, "Bouncy, Bouncy Baby" by Johna May West.*

> Bouncy, Bouncy Baby,
>   We don't rock anymore.
> We just get on a *LYMPHASIZER,*
>   And bounce from shore to shore.
>
> Bouncy, Bouncy Baby,
>   We don't rock anymore,
> We just get on a *LYMPHASIZER,*
>   And bounce forever more.
>
> Lymphasizers are magic,
>   Lymphasizers are grand,
> *When you learn how to use one,*
>   You will understand.
>
> Rocking chairs are super,
>   Rocking chairs are great,
> But when you get on a *LYMPHASIZER,*
>   Old age will have to wait.
>
> Now you can jump on the bed,
>   And you can jump on the couch,
> But when you buy new furniture,
>   Your husband will say "OUCH"!

So if you love your family,
You know what you can do,
Go out and get a *LYMPHASIZER*,
And tell them, "I love you!"

7.1. Now, keep on *LYMPHASIZING!* Read the testimonials in this session. If you haven't done so yet, get a lymphasizer and start doing the *run and not be weary, walk and not faint lymphasizing program* that we gave you in Session Three.

7.2. Remember, the key to healing in the body starts with an "E." The word is "endurance." The secret is to know how to obtain endurance without causing negative stress or fatigue in the body.

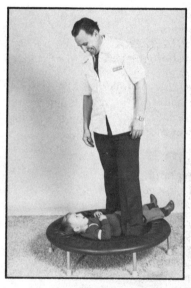

Figure 6
Bouncy, Bouncy Baby

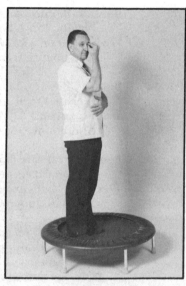

Figure 7
Bio-Electric Eye Exercise

C-8. The Special Bio-Electric Eye Exercise

8.1. Using the Bio-Electric Gentle Bounce for Health technique, I put my *left* hand on my abdomen and my coned fingers of my right hand on the *left* eye. Then I reverse the hands for the right eye. I can also put the coned fingers of both hands on both eyes.

8.2 On October 22, 1981 Bernardine R. Schramm in Ohio wrote:

Dear Dr. West,

I do the special Bio-Electric Eye Exercise morning and evening.

I make a cone shape with one hand and put the other hand over my navel--crossing over I put the coned hand on the other eye and say, "Thank you Lord for perfect sight." I do it to my ears also. It has helped both.

I now have 20/20 vision in my left eye with my glasses which I never before had. My eye doctor says my eyes are improving each time he sees me.

Sincerely

Bernadine B. Schramm

C-9. The Breathing and Directed Thinking Technique

9.1. (See Figs. 8-13) When I am not on a lymphasizer, if I want to direct energy mentally into any area of my body, I generate energy by breathing deeply in through the nose and out through the mouth three times and hold the third breath. This takes the pressure off of the Thoracic duct in the chest and the lymph shoots into the blood stream like a geyser. As I hold the third breath, I mentally direct the energy I have accumulated into the desired area, to help dissipate the blood proteins. It is not as easy as doing it on a LYMPHASIZER, but IT WORKS! The following pictures will show where I put my hands to increase the energy flow as I mentally direct energy into my body.

9.2. Fig. #8 is referred to as a master position and can be used while I mentally direct energy into any part of my body. It is specifically for the lungs.

9.3. Fig. #9 is for the heart.

9.4. Fig. # 10 is for the thyroid and throat area.

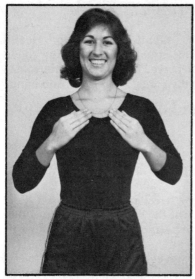

Figure 8 Master Position (All Body Parts)

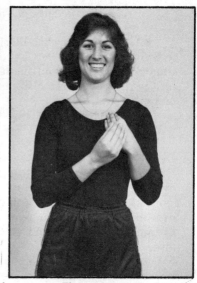

Figure 9 Heart

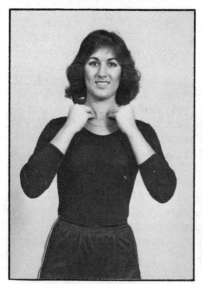

Figure 10 Thyroid

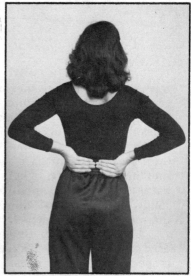

Figure 11 Kidneys/Adrenals

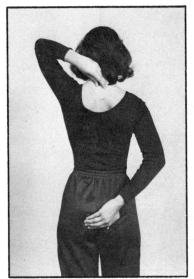

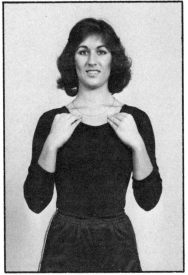

Figure 12 The Whole Spine   **Figure 13** Lungs, Sinuses (Same as Fig. 8)

9.5. Fig. # 11 is for the kidneys and adrenals,

9.6. Fig. # 12 is for the whole spine.

9.7. Fig. # 13 is for the lungs, sinuses, pituitary gland, etc.

9.8. I combine these with the basic self-help techniques in Session Two and the other advanced techniques in this session. Also, to obtain the maximum benefits the mental and nutritional laws must be obeyed.

9.9. Mr. Crowley of Everett, Washington, told me of a woman who came to one of my lectures in Seattle with a very bad curvature of the spine. She sat in front of him and when I talked about this technique she turned to him and said, "Do you think I could do that?" He said, "I know you can." Six months later, when I went back he said he saw her again and her back was straight. He said she told him that she did the Breathing Directed Thinking Technique eleven times a day for the whole six months to dissipate the blood proteins. That is what I call, "moving mountains." (See Fig. 12.)

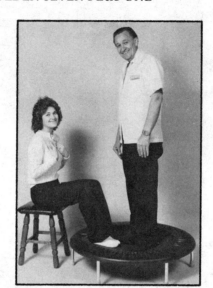

Figure 14

(Demonstrated by Dr. West and his daughter, Debbie)

C-10. The Bio-Electric Wheelchair Technique.

10.1. (See Fig. 14) I once had a whole room full of M.S. patients at one of my lectures in the home of Malin Lewis in Phoenix, Arizona. It was exciting as they began to understand the seven golden discoveries and the basic formula. But it was more exciting when I had them put their feet on the *lymphasizer* and as I would jump up and down, the magnetic electrical energy that was generated from their legs moving up and down magnified their thought waves enough that when they mentally directed this energy into their arms and legs, the tenderness and the pain started to come out of their arms and legs. They got so excited they literally began to crawl out of their wheelchairs to get onto a *lymphasizer.*

10.2. One beautiful young woman who had M.S. has now helped 60 other M.S. patients with this, along with other advanced techniques which we cannot teach unless we are teaching licensed physicians.

10.2. Following are some pictures and the testimony of a

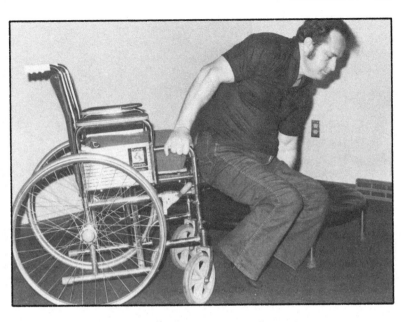

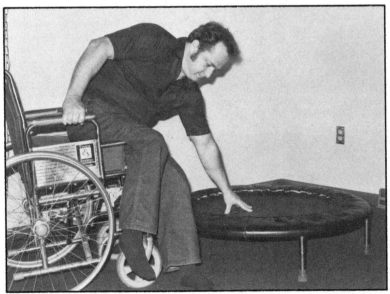

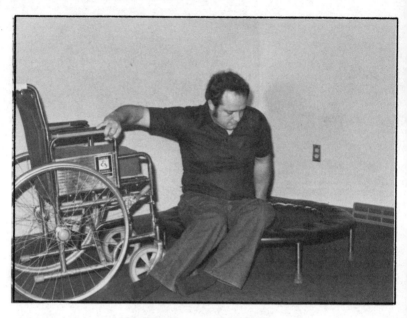

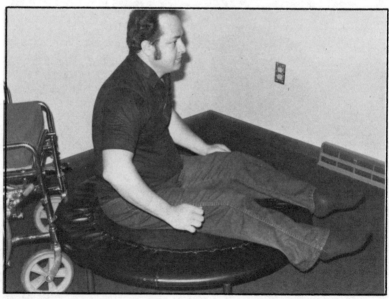

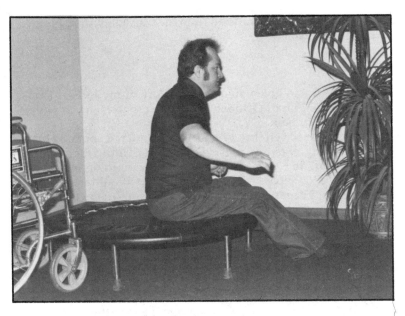

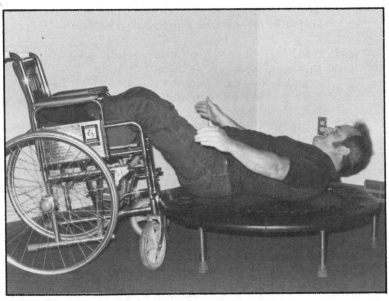

young man who was paralyzed from the waist down and how he used a lymphasizer.

Dear Dr. West,

I would like to give you a short history of my injury. I was paralyzed the 29th of October, 1969, in a car accident, in which my back was broken.

Damage was to vertebra T7 and T8. I do not feel, nor do I have control of any organ or muscle below T6. Until I bought my lymphasizer 7 to 8 months ago, I had done nothing in the last eleven years to exercise my body. Right away I could see and feel a difference, I began to feel burning sensations in my toes, feet, legs and in my buttocks. Using the lymphasizer every day for the past few months I have seen the muscles in my legs and arms rebuild and become stronger. I know with all my heart that the lymphasizer is the best way to exercise and to stay healthy.

Sincerely yours,

Raymond E. Modlin

C-11. *The Bio-Electric Pin-Point Technique.*

11.1. (See Fig. 15) I have been able to relieve pain with this technique that I could not relieve in any other way.

11.2. I can use this technique by myself or with someone helping me. By myself I only have half of the energy as I do with someone else.

11.3. I will never forget when my luggage strap slipped off my luggage carrier in the airport one day, and the metal end hit me in the mouth and broke my lip. I was in trouble; I had to give a seminar that night. A Sky-Cap was standing there, and he saw it happen. I went over to him and said, "I don't care if you believe this or not--do it." I curved my fingers on my left hand as if I were holding a bottle. I asked him to put his left finger tips on my left finger tips. Then I coned my right hand and put my finger tips on my lip and asked him to put his right hand on top of my right hand. He did so. He knew I was in trouble and he didn't argue. In about two minutes, the energy dissipated the blood proteins, and most of the pain was gone. I said, "Thank you," and he looked at me as if I was crazy. When I got on the plane, my lip started to swell up again, so I put my left hand on my abdomen to tap into the energy field around that part of the body, and then I put my right coned fingers on my lip. The swelling would go down. I would turn loose and after a while it would start to swell. I kept doing this all the way up until the time of my lecture. When that time came, I could not even feel a scar and no one knew that I had been hurt. If I had not known these techniques, I would have had a very sore lip and a difficult time lecturing that night.

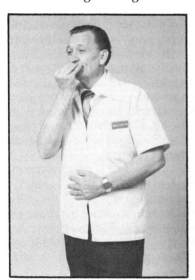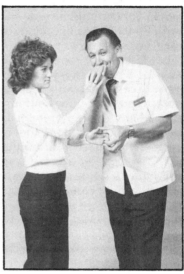

Figure 15

C-12. Details Concerning Energy Flow While Doing The Basic Bio-Electric Self-Help Techniques Described In Session Two.

12.1. By the way, this is why the hands are on the body in various places while doing the basic Bio-Electric Self-Help Techniques. In the case of migraine headaches, if a person puts his hand on the leg instead of the abdomen, it does not work. I have proven hundreds of times that there is not enough energy transfer from the leg. Put your hand on the abdomen and the energy transfer works.

12.2.   In the techniques where you put your hand upon the shoulder and stroke the liver and gall bladder with the other hand, the energy going out of the hand on the shoulder goes down the arm and increases the energy going out of the other hand that is doing the Light Fast Stroke.

C-13.   *The Bio-Electric Energy Field.*

13.1.   I learned this technique from Dr. Decker, a chiropractor, whom I studied under before he died.

13.2.   (It would be unkind if I did not show appreciation to Lynn Radcliff, Ina Bryant and Stanley Burroughs for helping to open my mind to energy currents in the body. Also Dr. Roy, D.N., N.D., and Dr. Harold C. Swanstrom, D.N., N.D.,have played a big part in my life. Both doctors taught me a great deal. What I learned about physiology, nutrition, and how muscles work to pull the bones out of place is priceless. Knowing that trapped or clustered proteins in the muscles is what causes the muscles to pull the bones out of place helps me to know how to use these bio-electric techniques properly.)

13.3.   *The bio-electric energy field* is a very powerful technique. It works. To create this energy field, I curve all of my fingers on both hands like I am holding a big soft ball. Now I put my hands in front of me with the fingertips of one hand about one-half inch away from the finger tips of the other. I begin to rotate my hands clockwise, keeping my fingers no farther than 1-2 inches away from each other. Energy is dispersed from the finger tips. Most people can feel the energy field that is created as they rotate their hands through the magnetic field going around the earth (See Figures 16-16C).

13.4.   To make the energy field big enough to dissipate clustered proteins, I continue by making a heart shape with my hands for three-five minutes. I start with my hands in front of me, then I bring both hands up and around and down. Without breaking the motion, I throw the energy in at the bottom because that is where the smashed finger, burn or whatever, may be.

C-14.   *Bio-Electric Energy Field Reverses Injuries.*

14.1.   My little boy, Benjamin Alexander, smashed his

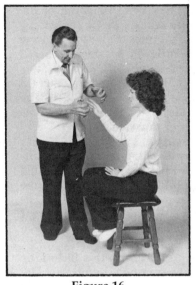

Figure 16

Figure 16A

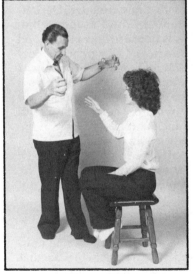

Figure 16B

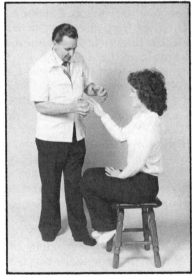

Figure 16C

fingers in the back of the door. They were bleeding at the knuckles. My wife held his hand up while I threw the energy into his fingers. Within two or three minutes, he stopped crying and was looking around with a smile on his face. When I stopped, he got on his little tricycle and took off. The next day the fingers were black and blue. As I began to examine them, I found that there was absolutely no pain in the fingers at all. The energy produced by this technique dissipated the blood proteins and reversed that injury in about three minutes.

14.2. Another son, Joseph Anderson, got hit in the mouth with a little play truck. His lip was bleeding all over his shirt. My older son, David Samuel, stood behind him and held his face up so I could throw energy into his lip. In about five minutes, he was not crying. I told him to lay down and do *The Bio-Electric Pin-Point Technique* on it. He did. In the morning, I asked him if his lip was sore. As he pushed in hard, he said, "No Daddy, it doesn't hurt."

14.3. I have seen the energy produced by this technique relieve pain of a burned arm, my own smashed thumb, etc. The first time I used this technique was when a young lady came to me with a turned ankle, walking with crutches. She had been here one time before I learned this technique from Dr. Decker. The next time she came in was the first time I used the Bio-Electric Energy Field Technique. I was not sure how much good it would do, but I asked her to lie down, and I propped her foot up so I could put the energy field around her ankle. I told her I did not know if this would work or not, but that I would give it the "good old college try." I threw the energy into her ankle until I was so tired that I could not do it anymore. I stopped and said, "OK, get up and try it." She sat up and stepped down off of the table slowly. She stood up and slowly began to take a few steps, and the steps got bigger and bigger; all at once she began to yell, "It's gone, it's gone, it's gone!" and she went running around the room. Well, that was my first experience, and after that I did not doubt anymore.

14.4. But the most wonderful thing I have seen with this technique was with Scott Nydegger. He was sent to me at my clinic in Mesa by a precious M.S. patient. When he came in to see me with a friend, he was in so much pain from a steel bar that had been put in his back when he was smaller to hold his back straight, that he could not get out of pain no matter what he did.

I asked him if he could lie down and he said, "Yes." When I saw the tears roll down his face, I said, "I thought you could lie down." He said, "I can, but it hurts." I asked him to stand up. I found that I could not touch his back anywhere without causing pain. I did not know what else to do, so I told his friend to make the energy field and throw it into his chest with one hand and into his back with the other. Scott had to stand sideways for him to do that. One week later, they came bouncing into my office. Scott's friends arms were "shot" but the pain was out of Scott Nydegger's back for the first time in years. His problem was reversed in one week. That was about four years ago. I called him in December, 1980, and asked how he was doing. He said he was just doing great, no problems; he is getting married soon.

D. WRITTEN TESTIMONIALS OF A FEW OTHERS WHO HAVE RECEIVED HELP AS A RESULT OF APPLYING THE SELF-HELP LYMPHASIZING CONCEPTS

1. We are here including some of the written testimonials that we have received from those who have obtained help as a result of applying the Bio-Electric Lymphasizing Self-Help Pain Relief Techniques and the other principles and concepts that are being taught in this book.

2. There are thousands of people all over the United States and many in Canada who are enjoying the blessings of being able to reverse their injuries and help relieve their own pain.

3. The following are a few of the testimonials that we have received. We give them here because of the joy that comes from having someone tell about the blessings they are receiving from following the principles and concepts which have brought relief to them and have caused healing to take place in their body.

4. If you knew some of these people personally, it would cause even greater joy, because as you will learn by reading their testimonials, some of them, with the understanding of the principles and concepts, decided to use these *bio-electric and other self-help pain relief techniques* and obtain relief from pain when nothing else worked.

5. These testimonials are printed as they were written by their authors. Italics are used for underlining.

Letter 1   March 2, 1981

To Whom It May Concern:

It it were not for Dr. C. Samuel West, I could not be serving my third term, in thirty years, as Mayor of Pleasant View City. It is now 3 1/2 years since I first attended a lecture, September 7 & 8, 1977, of Dr. West. Since that time, I have never had any of the pains that were plaguing me at that time.

When my chiropractor had given up trying to relieve my pain, January 7, 1975, I went to Dr. Marian J. Haslam, an orthopedic surgeon. He took x-rays and told me that I have had "Spinal Stnosis" all of my life; a structural condition that tends to shut off the spinal canal ventilation to my legs; that the condition could only be helped by chiseling the opening larger around the spinal canal where the vertebras are offset in my lower back. He said he wouldn't advise the operation, that he didn't think it would get worse, and would not shorten my life.

A few months later it had gotten worse and limited me to just 2 or 3 minutes on my feet without excruciating pain in my back and legs. I decided I should have an evaluation from another doctor. Orthopedic Surgeon, Billy A. Allison, took more x-rays and had nerve sensitivity tests in the hospital. He gave me the same information and advice. He said they don't operate on many with my condition, because less than 2% of the people have this structural condition; but he would like me to come back every six months for a check on my condition.

I took Dr. Allison's x-rays to another Chiropractor and had 8 adjustments, without any relief. Then I went to a nature doctor who had many degrees besides that of chiropractor. He really worked me over in his office at the Crystle Springs a number of times. I felt good, as long as I would swim in the pool, but had excruciating pain just getting back in my car to drive home.

I was also plagued with constant pain in my right upper arm. About two years before my attendance at Dr. West's lecture, in October 1975, I took my wife and our daughter, Cherie, Mrs. Dr. Keith M. Wayment, of Akron, Ohio, to a 5 day Advisory Council Seminar at the beautiful Wentworth By-The-Sea, in Portsmouth, New Hampshire. The second day there, I got an unbearable pain in my elbow. We went to the Portsmouth Hospital. The doctor said I had Calcific-Tendinitus in my elbow. He put my arm in a sling and gave me pills to take. He said the pills would relieve the pain in about 24 hours. The pain was not relieved, but got worse.

After the seminar, we drove to the home of Dr. Robert Dowst in Malden, Mass. Dr. Dowst and family were our son, LaMonte Barker's first family converts while serving in the New England Mission, under President Paul Dunn. Dr. Dowst took me to St. Elizabeth Hospital in Boston and had a doctor inject cortisone into the elbow. The doctor said that would force the pain out of the joint within one hour, but it might settle in the muscle.

The doctor was right. From that date, for nearly two years, to September 8, 1977, I was up most nights, bathing my arm and shoulder in hot water and applying Icy-Hot or some other liniment to relieve the pain.

My sisters, Grace Judy and Louise Thompson, told me about the coming of Dr. West, September 7, 1977. They had attended his Self-Help Clinic when he was in Ogden 15 months before. I was convinced, by the doctors, that nothing could help my condition, but attended Dr. West's Clinic in respect to my gracious sisters.

Needless to say, I received hidden treasures of knowledge, and immediate relief from all my pains and a new way of life that relieved me of 37 pounds of overweight in the form of toxins and poisons, during the next two months. I have enjoyed every moment; have never felt hungry or thirsty. I weigh less and feel better than at any time since leaving Weber College, 50 years ago.

I served as Town President of Pleasant View, after being elected to the Town Board, in Pleasant View's first election, held November 1949; being elected by a majority of one vote, not knowing that my name was on the ballot until 8:00 o'clock the day of the election.

In 1965 I was elected to another four year term as Mayor of Pleasant View City.

November 8, 1977, I was elected to my third term by 54% of the vote, with four other wonderful men running for office. This was an answer to my prayer, "If the Lord wanted me to help lead my people again, I desired a clear mandate from the electoral."

If it had not been for Dr. C. Samuel West's Self-Help Clinic, I could not have served this term as Mayor.

Sincerely,
Peary B. Barker, Mayor

Letter 2

Dear Frank and Dr. West,

Here is a letter I am hoping will *help* and *encourage many people*. I am a young woman of 28 years old and have been married for 8 years now. In those 8 years I have been in and out of the hospital so very, very often. I had one operation after another. The first year we were married I had my first operation for an ovary that had ruptured. After the operation the Dr. told me that I am to thank the dear Lord every day to be alive. Because I had hemorrhaged and the Dr. said in *1 more minute the blood would have gone over my heart*. The Dr. took half the ovary and the other half he patched up, but in less than a year the same thing happened to the other half, so I went through it all again. With each time growing *bigger tumors* and *cysts*. In a little over half of another year my other ovary did the same thing and this time my heart *stopped* when I was in the recovery room. The Dr. really *worked* at me and had my heart going again in a short time. After I had this operation I was still *sick* and full of *pain* as I was before I had the operation.

Here I was sick as could be again and just had undergone an operation. So, the Dr. put me under some more tests again and they found something else wrong again! It was not a week since I had the last operation and the Dr. said to me. He is so very sorry, but I must go right to the operation room again for another operation. I said, "Oh no," it just cannot be (me again), (but it sure was me again!) I had all these operations and my body just couldn't *even begin to get built up.* "It was all, just way too much for me!" In a short time after this last operation my body gave out and that means *my muscles* and *nerves* went *completely.* I then went into this *muscle condition.* I couldn't talk for over 2 months and to eat was the same thing. I also had *no strength at all.* That means I couldn't put my arms up and down and walking was out for some time. After a while someone would help me to walk. (Also with all these operations they messed my *back completely* too.) After I did get out of the hospital I still had so much pain, because of a *very, very bad back.* This is when I started chiropractor help and really did get a lot of help too. But my back was soon out of place again and my muscle would be hurt too from my back. I was still looking for something else to help me further. So, this is when *Dr. West was an answer to prayer.* My husband and I went to one of his Self-Help Clinics and we knew we just had to go back to the next one to find and get more help. This was when I first met Dr. West and knew that he was the *one to help me even more! (And he sure did!)* Dr. West had said I was the 2nd worst person he ever worked with. At first I had to sit on a chair and my husband would get on the rebound exerciser and we together would work for a few minutes. We did this quite often each day. In a few weeks I was on it myself, and in a few months I was feeling so much *Strength* coming to my body. My insides, I could feel getting stronger. And the *Chiropractor* and my *family Dr. even saw a big change in me.* My *family Dr. said, if he wouldn't have seen me with his own eyes* he wouldn't believe that I was the *same person.* We will have our rebound exerciser 1 year the end of May. And we wouldn't give it up for *all the world.* Now, I am up to 15 minutes of running and jumping on our rebound exerciser at a time. (Just Wonderful) We also have the most *wonderful news* that could have ever happened for us! I now am pregnant and our first baby is to come the end of Aug. or the beginning of Sept. The Dr. said that if I wouldn't have gotten so much strength in my insides I could never be carrying this baby. *I also want everyone to know this rebound exerciser is the best thing I ever found for my pain without taking pills.* We thank our Dear Lord each day for his many blessings and for letting us come to know *Dr. West and Frank & Kathy Angelo.*

> Our love & Prayers
> Go to You All,
>
> Laverne & Paul Groff

P.S. By the way, you see it is all due to the Dear Lord and Dr. West for my carrying this baby with *only 1/2 of an ovary!* I just had to add this yet. "Thanking you all again."

Letter 3

TESTIMONIAL OF
Mrs. Florence M. Franet

(Teacher of Aphasic Students, Mt. Diablo Unified School District, Concord, CA)

After attending a lecture and workshop by Dr. C. S. West, I purchased a (MT) mini-trampoline for my own use and that of my family. I felt so good as a result of using it, I knew I had to share it with my students too. Transporting it back and forth to school daily became a real chore, so I purchased a second one for the specific use to be for the students in the handicapped program. This mini-trampoline was used as a source of daily activites and exercises in my classroom with Special Education Students during the 1976-77 school year. There were six students, ranging in age from 8-9 to 11-7 in September 1976.

The students began using the MT by just trying to stand and balance themselves on it, then bouncing with two feet together and/or running or jogging easily. Three of the students were able to balance themselves from the start, but the other three had to be assisted. Gradually, all could balance alone and begin the exercises, although the most severe student took nine days before she could stand alone. Let us take time here to follow her development.

At the beginning of this '76-77 school year, she could not coordinate her small motor development enough to draw a circle or copy a single letter. She did attempt to write her first name, but one had to know what it was in order to read it. Her eye-hand coordination was nil. Her speech was unintelligible. She used only words and sometimes short phrases. After one month on the MT she was bouncing with two feet together by herself. Following this she developed enough coordination to turn slowly on the MT and in four months time she was running fast, jogging, and dancing. Her language developed along with this. In four months time, one could read her written name and she could draw a circle. In six months time, she was able to trace the letter of her last name, in eight months she could COPY her last name, and after nine months, she could write it herself. She was able to write some other letters by this time too. Needless to say, she was a very happy little girl, her parents were pleased too. Her verbal expression developed along with this written and motor expression. She was using simple sentences, gradually extending them into paragraphs by the end of these nine months. Her receptive language improved too.

Another student, (A.S.), whose large motor development was fairly well coordinated, could bounce and jog on the MT but could not hop on either foot alone without losing his balance. His verbal expressive language consisted of phrases and sentences without verbs. His comprehension (receptive language) was impaired. After five months he could hop on either foot for 300 or 400 counts, and after six months he could jump rope while on the MT, and after another month he was SKIPPING rope on the MT. His expressive verbal language had developed considerably during the first three or four months, and the receptive language improved by about 2 1/2 to 3 years.

All of these students showed growth in their coordination, language skills, health, and attitudes. I had expected to see growth for each student during the school year and had worked with the Aphasic students for five years previous to working with the group, but this growth far exceeded expectations and I attribute this additional gain to their developments and total stimulation by use of the MT, (mini-trampoline).

This 1977/'78 school year, I am using the MT with high school age Aphasic students, and again I am seeing beautiful developments in physical coordination, muscle development, self-concepts, and language skills. We coordinate the MT's use into math and social studies programs. A 3" to 4" cross is on each wall (for N, S, E, & W directions) at eye-level. The assignment may be to bounce 360 times total but to divided it equally while facing each of the four directions.

Some of the better coordinated boys decided to challenge one another to see who could hop on one foot the most number of times. They started out with a 100, then 300, 700, and 1000 (one thousand!) It was getting to be too difficult trying to count the number of times accurately (taking longer to say a number than to take a hop) so we began to use a stopwatch, and they set five minute periods of time for themselves. Each of the three boys could do this on one foot but not the other, so each was challenging himself to develop his weaker side. One boy did it in three weeks time, a second did it in seven weeks time, and the third is still trying to master that second side. After six months time now, he is very close to mastering it.

I would like to see all of our handicapped students have the opportunity to use a MT on a daily basis in order to minimize their handicaps more rapidly.

Aphasic is a severe language handicap attributed to neurological brain damage. The student' handicaps vary greatly, the problem being expressive, receptive, or both, and auditory or visual or both. The motor coordination usually is poorly developed also.

MSS refers to Most Severe Student in this particular class.

Letter 4

Dear Friends, Dr. West and Family,

Greetings to you in the Name of our Lord. Hope this finds you in good health. We are all busy and feeling well. A blessing indeed that I will not take time and write you as I promised to do long already. I knew you would like to hear some interesting facts about results of using the Rebounder. Our first experience you know but will write it down how it was.

Our granddaughter 8 years of age, Mary Lu Fisher, got sick one morning at 4 o'clock. She was breathing so hard that our daughter, Miriam, heard her from the other room. She needed oxygen very bad. Miriam gave her catnip and peppermint tea. She only drank a little at a time and soon was semi-conscious. Being alone and not knowing what else to do Miriam put a comforter on the Rebounder and layed her down and bounced her slowly for 3-4 hours. Mary started to get oxygen and started to talk and went through 3 sweats. Miriam had to change her clothes 3 times. Her breathing soon became normal and mucous was broken and by about 8 o'clock she asked if she may go to school. That afternoon she really coughed up lots of mucous. This was our first experience with the Rebounder. This I believed saved Mary's life. We feel grateful to God to give us something so simple to use to help our sick ones and we can have it to use in our homes.

Another experience with a friend of ours a mother who fell from the sink top and lumped her head against a refrigerator. She had a concussion and a very bad neck problem. She went to a chiropractor for treatments for 2 or 3 months and got good results for her neck but her pressure in her head was still severe. We started her slowly on the Rebounder. She could hardly take it for a few bounces as it caused so much pressure in her head.

gave her a Rebounder to take home and to use slowly every 15 minutes. This was Monday she started, till Friday she could bounce 5 minutes at a time and did some of her housework. She was going on the Rebounder every 15 minutes from Monday to Friday. Her husband bought the Rebounder and they were both happy.

Another wonderful experience in our family again. Our grandson, David Fisher, 11 months old, fell into a septic tank as the ground caved in at the time he crawled over it in the backyard. We believe it went 8 or 10 minutes until they had him out of the water. They could not find a pulse or feel any life but they were working on his body. After awhile life seemed to be coming back. He was in the hospital in serious condition for 3 to 4 weeks and the Doctors said he had definite brain damage and irrepairable brain cells. They took him home from the hospital helpless and also blind. The mother and father could hardly wait to get him on the Rebounder plus giving him good food supplements and also stopped giving his drugs which he was supposed to have for a year. The Doctors were afraid he would get convulsions. The first week he was restless but they didn't give up. After the 3rd week the little boy seemed just about normal. His eyesight and everything else seems normal. At six weeks the Doctors wanted to see him again at the hospital. They said this can't be the same little boy, but it was. The nurses flocked around him too. I could hardly believe the change. We want to give all the honor and praise to our Heavenly Father for healing him. He is the Great Healer. Also for the sending of good friends and Doctors like Dr. West to teach us these simple ways of helping our loved ones.

We could tell you many more Asthma and Pneumonia cases where people helped themselves and also many back problems, headaches, constipation, mental problems, if I had time. I would write a book but want to share these with others hoping it will help them.

Now we are wondering when we could get you into the vicinity again. I know many people would like to meet you and learn more. Many have never heard you yet. Just drop us a few lines and we'll try and get a place for you.

Wishing you God's blessings and His guidance in your work. He never fails us does he?

Best wishes to you and your family

David and Sarah Glick and Family
Lancaster, PA

Letter 5

Dr. West;
Last summer I attended your lecture and clinic. I previously had cysts in both breasts. My doctor, a naturopath, told me it was a lymphatic condition. After 3 months of your program-- suddenly no more cysts were in my breasts.

Many thanks to you.

God bless you.

Deb Shepardson
Morgantown, PA

Letter 6

April 20, 1977

Dear Dr. West:
I would like to relate an experience in connection with the use of the Vitalizer.
I am 56 years of age and have had an eye problem since I had the measles when I was seven years old. In the early forties I was told I had corneal dystrophy and that nothing could be done to stop the deterioration since it was hereditary. Then in 1972 I began to have corneal ulcers and spasms of the eyes. In using the ophthmalic medication to cure the ulcers my eyes reacted to the medicine which caused severe iritis. Then all medication was stopped. I went from one eye specialist to another only to be told that my condition was systemic and hereditary and no treatment would be effective. Finally, I went to see Dr. Carey Reams in Roanoke, Virginia, and he told me I was not assimilating Vitamin A and was not getting sufficient oxygen. While there I heard you speak on the lymphatic system. About three months later I attended your workshop in my hometown in Texas and decided to purchase a Vitalizer. After five or six weeks of doing

the exercises I noticed I did not have as many spasms. I haven't had any ulcers recently and my eyes continue to improve. I am therefore elated at the progress my eyes have made in such a short time, and I owe it all to the Vitalizer.

Thank you, Dr. West, for teaching me about the lymphatic system and the importance of proper diet and exercise to rid the body of toxins. This is so vital in restoring our health. Keep up the good work!

Sincerely,

Mrs. Jim H. Owens
Texas

Letter 7

9/9/78

To Dr. West,

I attended the convention at Bucknell in Lewisburg the first week of Aug. of 1978. At the time I was a diagnosed Hypoglycemic. Had high triglycerides & hypertension. I was taking between 8 to 12 pills a day: Diurel for Hypertension; Benedryl for allergies; Fiornal for headaches. Blood pressure 180/100.

I had the feeling of exhaustion and just wasn't interested in life, but went throught the motions out of necessity. I left the Self-Help Class with a sincere desire to do what I had learned from Dr. West. Exactly 1 month later I have a new desire to live & help others, my energy is almost frightening at times. My blood pressure at this time is 120/85. I feel great, have no allergy problems and do not suffer from any symptoms of hypoglycemia. I am anxious to see Dr. West again to report on further progress. I am losing inches very fast & to date have lost 11 lbs. The pain in my back is gone. Also I could not cross my leg before.

Sincerely,

Marie Nave

Letter 8

11/28/78

Dear Dr. West.

I had severe back problems last summer. It was so bad I was limping around for a day or two dragging my left leg. We applied your method. I walked away and I was well. I could not believe it. It really works. Have nice holidays and best wishes for a wonderful New Year.

Sincerely,

Karola Parkin

Letter 9

January 31, 1977

Dear Dr. West:

It is with sincere gratitude that I write this letter of thank you to you. You have no conception of the hours I have spent in prayer asking for someone to come into my life to teach me the techniques I have long studied; to enable me to heal my own body with the forces within.

I have lived through a series of accidents, beginning with a severe back injury at the age of eleven, coupled with a congenital curvature of the spine, that spiraled into one back and head injury after another, which left me a partial cripple, with my left leg nearly three inches shorter than my right leg.

Over the years I have slowly been able to regain my physical well-being, overcoming insuperable odds.

For a long time I lay a helpless invalid, unable even to "crawl like a seal" across the floor. X-rays showed unrepairable deterioration and damage to the discs in my spine and to the cartilage in the toes, elbows and knees, and portions of the bones in my knees.

By charging my body through prayer and meditation (not to take lightly the efforts of a Chiropractor) I began slowly to properly right my condition, and within the past five years have made fantastic strides in this area. May I add here that all of my "right eating" could not stop the failing of my body chemistry, which I am presently fighting so hard to reverse. For the past four years it has been an up and down thing with me. Some days

I can walk and some days I cannot even rise out of the bed. It is only just recently that I have been able to walk with some degree of confidence without the aid of crutches, or with a very noticeable limp. Until my recent meeting with you in Gainesville, Florida, I thought perhaps that my above condition was as far as I was destined to progress. And I do mean ABOVE condition, for I cannot bless my Father in Heaven nor thank you enough for what you have given me. I shall shout it from the mountain tops! You have given me my one "missing link". The link I knew I MUST have to go on.

I am not quick to accept the theories or ideas of those who have "a message". I am guided by the Light of my Innermost Consciousness, and if it is "Rubbish", I cast it aside, quickly. Your teachings have not been cast aside.

Please continue to learn, and grow strong and attain wisdom, always remembering that you are only the teacher and not the Doer. I wish you God Speed in spreading your message of healing. Perhaps you have not yet come to know just how great your work is, and how much greater it is to become. You must realize, however, that by and large, you are speaking to the "Mass", who largely have no conception of your message, thus you must not feel saddened, for you can only sow the seed. If the ground is fertile, the seed will fruit and multiply.

May God go with you, always; and, again, thank you for being.

In His Name, I remain, Truthfully Yours,

Penny C. Condrey

Letter 10

April 2, 1977

To Dr. West:

A year ago this last November and December I was in so much pain I truly thought I was going to die. The doctors couldn't figure out why I had so much pain. After lots of x-rays it showed I had a hiatal hernia and lots of spinal trouble. From January to November 1976 I went to a stomach specialist to try and get my hernia under control and an Osteopath for the back. I went 2-3 times a week. I continued to have lots of pain. I had so much pain in the hip joints and low back I couldn't turn over in bed without physically using both hands to turn my hips. The adjustments just wouldn't hold. I was lucky if they held one night and I could have one night's sleep without pain.

On November 8, I got a Lymphatic Exercise Unit. I started "bouncing" on it with my palms and hands on the collar directing energy like Dr. West said. I would try anything no matter how goofy it sounded. I did this every time I had pain, every half hour or so and just for ten times at first. That was all I could do. After three days I was sleeping at nights without pain. I couldn't believe it. I gradually worked from 10 to 15 to 20 to 50 to 75 to 100 bounces each time I had pain. I told the Osteopath what I was doing and even let him try an Exercise unit. He didn't and doesn't believe that's why I improved. I did not blame him for I couldn't believe it either, but don't see him for adjustments anymore.

N.I.E.
Seattle, Washington

Letter 11

Jan. 9, 1977

Dear Dr. West,

My wife and I are so excited about what you have taught us in your Self-Help Clinic we want the whole world to know about it. We heard your lecture and workshop in Seattle, Wash. the last weekend in October of 1976. Since that time many wonderful things have happened.

My wife has suffered for the past 15 years from migraine headaches, sore joints, and stomach disorders. She visited a Chiropractor on the average of twice a month. She has gone through all of the major health clinics available in Seattle. Among those were the Mason Clinic and the University Hospital Pain Clinic. We were fed up with doctors telling us to go home and learn to live with it or it's all in your head.

The fantastic thing about it is the fact that after your workshop in October we have not seen a chiropractor or a doctor for any illness or any problem. Yes, she still has her migraine headaches but we are able to control them thru your Accu-lymphatic Exercises.

We are believers and wish to promote your program with all the vitality that is within us. We'll see you in Seattle, with as many guests as we can bring, the next time you are here.

Sincerely,

William C. and Nina M. Dearinger
Seattle, Washington

Letter 12

April 10, 1977

Dear Dr. West,

Since I have been twelve years old, I have had severe migraine headaches, sometimes twelve to fourteen days at a time, without ever letting up.

When I was between thirty-five and forty years of age, they would get so bad they would never let up. I could not eat and all I could do is to get in a dark room and have everyone leave me alone, as I could not stand the slightest noise. And these continued this way until I was seventy-four when I met you. Until I met you no matter what I tried, or who I would go to, for help, it never worked.

I had a headache for three days when we came to you, for the purpose of helping my wife Mary. After you treated Mary, you worked on me, and told me what to do, to prevent these headaches. Before I got home the headache was gone. Praise the Lord and thanks to you, I have been able to control them ever since. In fact, I don't know what it is to have a bad headache any more--May the Lord bless you, Dr. West and keep up your work. And thanks for making me my own doctor.

With love and appreciation,

Norman C. Favinger
Mesa, Arizona

Letter 13

October 30, 1978

Dr. Corwin West,

I was in an accident in which I ran into a telephone pole. For a couple of months, I was in pain and my right side was tingling and feeling fuzzy.

I went to two different doctors within 3 days and they just wanted to give me some pain pills.

It was frustrating to me that they weren't dealing with the cause of my problem.

So, when I heard about Dr. West being in town, I decided to try out his technique. He showed me in just a few brief minutes some exercises and stroking methods to relieve the pain in my lower back and neck. I felt immediate relief and did the exercises each night and used my sundancer along with the stroking.

Within a week, I was as active as before and experiencing no pain.

Thank you for your help in helping me,

Bev Schurig
Mesa, Arizona

Letter 14

February 26, 1977

Dear Dr. West,

My back hurt me so bad day and night for a week until I could not sleep over and hour or two at a time nor could I sit at lengthy periods. Today, my pain left and what a relief it was.

If I had not experienced these things it would be impossible to believe it. I appreciate all that was accomplished. I intend to put in practice all that I can remember. Surely this was the best 5 hours I have ever spent for I learned how to really live a healthy and satisfied life.

May the Lord keep His hand upon your ministry.

Sincerely,

Betty McNab
Hobe Sound, Florida 33455

Letter 15

February 23, 1977

Dr. West:

I have attended three of your workshops with great interest in what you have had to say. I have had very bad headaches and backaches for over forty years. I have spent untold amounts of dollars and agonizing hours with no real lasting relief. I had come to the point of concern that I was going to have an examination to see if I had a growth in my head causing pressure on the brain. Well, I got an Exercise unit and I did the stroking. I was able to get very temporary relief until I got to ask you some questions and you showed me that my problem was old and deep and needed some special hard rubbing to break it loose. Well, that was done-it was very painful but I have not had a headache or backache to speak of for 6 months. I have to do my exercising regular. I don't dare miss it but I do the low bounce for 5 minutes, going through the exercises you taught me-then I jump rope the Vitilyzer 100 forward and 100 backward, with a good vigorous jump. Then I do 5 minutes of a moderate jogging to saturate my blood with oxygen. Then I jump a little more and wind up with a few fairly strenuous exercises totaling up to 15 to 20 minutes. I do this twice a day. I feel better than I have in many years. I know that exercise has to be done every day. It is wonderful. Until you have the contrast you can not really realize the power of this exercise-it is very powerful. Thanks for your instructions and help. It has made a new life for me.

Sincerely,

Keith P. Brown

Letter 16

October 13, 1977

Dr. West:

I was playing softball and sprained my ankle sliding into home. I went to the hospital and the doctor said use crutches, so I did. The next day I went to Chris Wordens house and she said I can help you. So I let her do it. With this electrical field she created with her hands she stopped the pain. Within 5 minutes I walked out of the house on the ankle that I couldn't even touch before.

Keith McElhaney

Letter 17

Dear Corwin:
   Hope to have you back soon. A man bought a lymphatic exercise unit for his 21 year old retarded daughter who was listless the past 4-5 years, not reading, writing, washing dishes, etc.--just throwing 2-3 seizures a day. After 2 weeks on the thing he called the other day to say she was not only doing all those things and more, but asking to go back to school. Neither did she have another single seizure except two the first day she started on it.
   So your ministry is bearing great fruit. Keep up the good work.

Love,

Ben Andrews
Chattanooga, Tenn.

Letter 18

November 30, 1978

Dear Dr. West:

   Last year I went to see an Optometrist. He said I had small catarcts on my eyes. But when I went back to him Tuesday, he said "I'm surprised at the condition of your eyes! The cataracts have not advanced any in size." I didn't tell him that I have been using my Sundancer twice a day since I got it about six months ago and I have been putting energy to my eyes. As I keep at it, I think he'll find that they are better than that next time.

Roberta Leithan
Mesa, AZ 85204

Letter 19

May 25, 1977

To whom it may concern:

For about three or four months I had been much aware of a nagging pain, at first intermittent, then continuous, in the lower right abdomen in the general area of the ovary. A visit to a trusted chiropractor who is more than just a chiropractor (a homeopathic doctor) afforded me no relief. Then I remembered Dr. West's lymphatic exercises which I had just learned and decided to apply them. To the lymphatic exercise for liver and gall-bladder I added a stroking up through the area of the pain. There was temporary relief immediately. Every time the pain returned I repeated the exercise. Within a week the pain was all gone. To prevent a return, I do the exercise every night. For the past three months there has been no pain.

Ms. Elaine Gleeson
Nottingham, PA

Letter 20

January 8, 1979

To whom it may concern:

The other day I felt as if I should visit the nursery. When I got there a baby was screaming with pain. It's hand had got in a door. I quickly began stroking it the way Dr. West taught me. In about 50 strokes later, the baby suddenly stopped crying and was soon playing with the blocks, apparently oblivious to any former problem.

Bessie Eliver

Letter 21

Dr. West,

A few days after you left here (San Diego) early in the summer, I was walking with a friend who had her dog on a leash. A strange dog ran out and attempted to attack my friend's dog. In the confusion I stepped on a pebble which rolled under my foot. My entire right foot bent under my body. The pain was excruciating to remember. But not too excruciating to remember Dr. West's instructions for this very thing.

To my friend's astonishment, I didn't even move from the street. I just sat on my tracks, clamped down on the pain at the same time I began to manipulate (rubbing one section) the other side of my foot to keep the blood flowing rather than allowing it to swell. After several minutes I got up, walked up to a steep hill with no real problem.

While the pulled ligaments took 3 months to heal completely, I was not incapacitated at any time except for the first few minutes, and walked and continued in the regular business of living with no pain or difficulty. I was so thankful for this knowledge.

> Katie McPherson
> LaMesa, CA 91041

Letter 22

Dear Dr. West:

It has been some time since I have had the pleasure of taking your course in Seattle-last fall in fact. Have wanted to write you sooner, but you know, the road to hell is paved with good intentions.

What I wanted to mention specifically was this: I am the 73 year old retired chiropractor who looks askance at every health method that comes along. My wife wanted to take your workshop after hearing the lecture., and I agreed that it would be fine. Well, she made me do likewise, and I am very glad that I did. She volunteered when you asked for women to come up on the stage for demonstration purposes, and what we saw I know could be done with foot reflexology, only in a more extended period of time. This sold me on the idea of presenting my body when you called for people with a short leg to come up. You know as well as I do that the only people with one real short leg are those who are actually crippled. All other cases of short legs is due to spinal trouble: a tilted pelvis, muscular distortion, etc. With the simple little pressure that you asked me to put on one of the pressure points that you named, and at the same time stroking the neck muscles my "short leg" immediately lengthened out to the point where the others in the class could see it happen, and I could notice it when I went back to my seat. Most remarkable was that the pain in my lumbar region was gone! And to think for years I had worked and twisted on pelvic bones to ease pain in my patients and bring the legs to equal normal length!

This has convinced me that the two classes of people who can't stand to be wrestled around: Senior folks and young ones, can be treated in this natural way without pain and discomfort of a harsh treatment. And that is a real boone, believe me.

Hope to see you again in Seattle sometime.

Yours for better health,

Theodore E. Jodar, D.C.
Edmonds, WA 98020

Letter 23

March 1, 1979

Dear Dr. West

I was folding up a stepladder and it slipped and folded up and caught my pointer finger, cutting a deep gash in it. I grabbed my finger and held it tight till it stopped hurting. When I let go, I had lost only 3 to 4 drops of blood and it never did swell or get sore. I put some tape on it just to keep it clean.

La Mont Bell
Mesa, AZ

Letter 24

Dr. West:

One week after we had attended your seminar, we went on vacation. (8-21-76)

Walking down a step path to the beach I slipped and fell, landing on my right wrist and hip. The pain was so bad I thought the wrist was broken. I told my husband to start stroking. He stroked the wrist about 1 minute and the pain completely released. I could move the wrist freely. I then stood up and he stroked the hip and released the pain. When we got home I used the Sundancer and had no more pain. I had a large bruise on my hip a couple of weeks but no pain.

Elenore Vandermode
Sunnyvale, CA

Letter 25

February 20, 1978

Dear Dr. West:
My name is Casey Vaury, I met you in Toronto on February 17, 1978 where you lectured at the Holiday Inn.

I am a massage therapist, naturopathic physician, and physical culturist. I have given many treatments (approx. 20,000) in my clinic and my recovery rate is about 90%

I have worked on the idea for many years that the answer is in the interstitial fluids and lymphatics. I never knew exactly why! *You have shown me why!* You have given me the missing link in the chain. I thank you from the bottom of my heart! I felt very "touched" when you lectured and I still do because this answered my questions which I had for so many years.

Casey Vaury
Toronto, Canada

Letter 26

December 30, 1978

Dr. Corwin West,
This letter is to express appreciation to you for the tremendous service you are rendering to your fellow men by teaching them correct principles of diet and health care.

My wife and I attended your lecture and workshop during the summer of 1976 at Paul, Idaho. This experience was very inspiring and enlightening, and has had a tremendous influence for the betterment of both us and our children's health since then. Because of the knowledge and inspiration gained at your lecture and workshop, and because of continued study and application of natural health principles, and with the help of the Lord, I have been able to care for the health of myself and my family and eliminate the burden of medical care costs.

I would also like to mention that my wife prior to the time of this lecture and workshop had been bothered by a bad hip for several years and we had much expense at chiropractors because of this. Since you showed us at the workshop how to put the hip back in painlessly with the use of body electricity, we have eliminated those trips to the chiropractor.

Thank you so much Dr. West for all you have done and are doing to help people help themselves.

Sincerely,

Gaylin Patterson
Burley, Idaho

Letter 27

January 9, 1977

Dear Dr. West,

My husband and I attended your lecture in Moses Lake, Washington in September 1976. Before that time my husband had a long history of back trouble at one time even having to lay on a bed for three months. Since learning Dr. West's methods we have been able to get his back in and keep it in.

I also had lower back problems a few times a year and since can take care of myself.

We are so thankful for this information and feel we have saved many times the cost.

Clarence L. Crawford

Letter 28

March 8, 1979

My husband has been a bed patient with rheumatory arthritis for more than five years. He had developed bleeding ulcers from the aspirin. After going to Dr. West's class and learning about stroking to relieve pain, I was able to help my husband. He was in so much pain that he called me home from work today. I stroked his arms and legs and back and encouraged him to breathe more naturally, to take deeper breaths. Pretty soon he relaxed and went to sleep. At first he thought he couldn't straighten out his arm but I kept telling him he could. I kept stroking him and soon he could straighten it out. I stroked him several times today. I got him to bounce on his bed a bit while he sat on the edge, too.

At the clinic last night I used Dr. West's discovery on the Sundancer exercise unit to relieve pain in my arms and legs and to straighten up my hips. My back has felt straight and it hasn't hurt all day. I slept at night, which is unusual for me. When I got up this morning it didn't hurt.

Hazel Van Slyker
Mesa, AZ

Letter 29

January 11, 1979

I had constipation after I had my stroke. But after I went to the first lecture and began doing the colon exercise like Dr. West showed us, my constipation problem has been greatly relieved.

Kim Lindsey
Mesa, AZ

Letter 30

I am really thankful for Dr. West's work.

I have been troubled with a pain in my tailbone and hip for the last year. After I stroked my hip, both tailbone and hip feel better. I even have feeling in my right leg, something I haven't had in 12 months or so. The doctor said it was from pregnancy. I am sold 100% on Dr. West's work. God bless him and thank the Lord I was opened to hear about him. Thanks so much Dr. West!

Sharon Farewell
Milwaukee, Wis.

Letter 31

October 29, 1976

Using Dr. West's discoveries my neck is better now than it has been since 1952 when I had a serious accident. They were planning brain surgery for me.

Thank you,

Fran Farrell

Letter 32

March 15, 1979

While attending Dr. Samuel West's lecture at the Holiday Inn in Albuquerque, New Mexico, on March 15, 1979, I heard him teach a method of relaxation and body alignment, which relieved a problem that I had been plagued with for 6 months. Hip misalignment and numbness in left thigh. While doing the simple motion, described in the exercise book, I noticed vital energy surging in my thigh and increased sensitivity returning. I want to thank Dr. West and celebrate his discovery.

With love,

Erwin Hellman
Albuquerque, NM

Letter 33

March 3, 1977

At first I couldn't stand any more pressure applied to my feet, thighs, and arms. After jumping the way Dr. West told me to, it truly was fantastic in the difference in the pain that was so bad before.

Also, I haven't been able to write this long at one time for the last two years. These notes would have taken me days to write. My muscles would jump and jerk and the pain from the top of my hand and up my arms hurt too badly that I could not continue.

Thank you Dr. West,

Esther R. Roy

Letter 34

Dear Dr. West:
   Praise the Lord--The joint in my left hip has bothered me (at times crucially). I hate to tell you how much suffering I've gone through plus doctors. I could never lay on my left side. It does not hurt since I used your exercises. Praise the Lord and you. I have had this trouble for 50 years.

Helen Pluzynski
Morton Grove, Illinois

Letter 35

Dear Dr. West:
   January 9, 1978, when I stroked the hip, it helped and also took pain out of the knee.
   January 11, on the second night of exercise and stroking I slept all night without my knee hurting once. Also my hip and leg.

Lillie Jensen
Mesa, AZ

Letter 36

March 15, 1979

   After attending Dr. West's lecture I applied the principle of Deep Breathing and mentally directing the energy into my sinus problem. I get severe headaches after eating certain foods. In the past I relieved the headaches with aspirin, A.P.C., Actifed, and Fiormal depending on the severity of the attack. Now I simply breathe deeply until the sinuses clear.

Carl Pister
Apache Junction, AZ

Letter 37

I had pain in my tooth for a very long time and after using Dr. West's pin-point technique I feel just fine. I thank you so very much·

> Aria Compagnone
> Norwood. Mass.

Letter 38

February 15, 1979

After going to Dr. West's lecture and applying the principles, within one month, my blood pressure has gone from as high as 180 over 110 to 144 over 84. I give a lot of the credit to the lymphatic exercises.

> Lillie Jensen
> Mesa, AZ

Letter 39

Dr. West:

It may have been my lack of understanding the effectiveness of the Sundancer that prompted me to prove it's value.

When my husband's blood pressure ran exceedingly high after a day at the office, a minute on the Sundancer lowered the Systolic pressure 15 points.

To further prove my point, Mother and my two sisters were visiting. I took their blood pressure reading before and after using the Sundancer for almost a minute. Mother's Systolic reading was high and the Diastolic pressure was low. It lowered the Systolic and raised (slightly) the Diastolic. (Lowered Systolic 15 points). A sister's high systolic pressure was lowered 18 points. A sister whose blood pressure ran low was raised to a normal reading.

The normalizing effect is of tremendous value to me. I am a Corrective Therapist.

> Mildred Huggins, R.M.T.
> Wichita, Kansas

Letter 40

April 13, 1979

I usually went to the chiropractor every two months to relieve the tension built up in my neck and across the shoulders. I attended one of Dr. West's health lectures in November where I learned of the lymphatic exercises. I immediately began using them and have not been back to the chiropractor since. Thank you Dr. West!

I injured a ligament in my knee skiing at Christmas time. Eight weeks later, I was still trying to heal up my knee. I purchased an exercise unit and I started jumping on it one-footed. After two weeks I noticed that my knee had greatly improved. Now 4 weeks later, it seems to be completely healed.

Beth Harris

Letter 41

September 17, 1977

Dr. West:

After doing your exercises today the sciatic pain that I have had in my back for 30 years has gone. How wonderful!

Thank you,

Fern Merrill
Mesa, AZ

Letter 42

March 10, 1979

Dear Dr. West:

Age of 19, I had arthritis and both legs in casts to keep them straight, and thirty different allergies. After spending hundreds of dollars on allergy shots, allopathic methods, the best specialist, my condition got worse. I now have no allergies, or arthritis. I cured myself using God's natural laws of eating and cleansing and within two years I'm now back competing in running and racketball.

Nutritionist, therapist,

Smokey Santillo

Letter 43

January 29, 1978

Dr. Corwin West,

If we had received no other benefit from your class than the energy field it would have been worth more than what we paid for the class.

We have used it on all of our family--especially grandchildren who are always getting bruised.

A week ago our 4 month old granddaughter rolled over and fell from the bathroom dressing table onto the tile floor when her father turned his back for a moment. She received a severe skull fracture which the x-rays showed went in a horseshoe shape from the back of the ear around the back of the head. The skull wasn't depressed so the doctor let them take her home but cautioned them about blood clotting and had them wake her up every two hours to test reflexes.

Our daughter used the energy field three times before the paramedics arrived at their house. They then brought her to our home for the night and we used it two more times at her head. The accident occured at 10:00 p.m. By two a.m. the swelling was down and she slept. By morning there was no discoloration or swelling.

Just this incident alone would have been worth the knowledge we received in your class.

Sincerely,

Vie Hull
Provo, Ut 84601

Letter 44

March 11, 1982

After hearing Dr. West tell how he overcame a turned ankle, I stepped off the edge of a sidewalk and turned my ankle. I set down right away and pulled my foot to the inside and started rubbing it. Within five minutes the pain was gone and I continued on walking to work. This was a miracle since I have turned my ankle many times before and it had always left me disabled for a couple days, but this time I had no after effects.

T. E. Rose
Hershey, Pa.
Harrisburg, Pa.

Letter 45

October 10, 1981

All my life I was always tired and cried easily and could never keep up with the other children. When I was in High School I couldn't hardly finish my day at school after a Physical Ed. class, my muscles were so stiff I could not exercise without it hurting to the extreme and leaving me too tired to study. I sat at home doing needle work and sewing and had no other exercise until my Senior year. I then started square dancing. Needless to say I was ill all year hardly attending school. My nerves were so on edge and I upset very easily. I know now my system was so tight and clogged with all the Animal Protein I ate 3 times a day. My parents had no money and my Mother had to work to provide us with all that beautiful food. They feed us WELL. When I was 17 I was taken to a Chiropractor which started a life time of Misery. After several years of fighting the painful neck, shoulders, and head pains and going to Medical Doctors, with no success, I finally went to a Medical Dr. in 1967, that gave me a shot of cortizone in the back of the neck, then sent me to the Hospital. Of course nothing functioned right after that. I was there for 3 weeks. I was so weak I couldn't hold a pencil. This is when the Dr. started me on prescribed Drugs. Several different kinds and combinations. I managed to go back to work 3 months later in rather a shakey state. I spent the next 7 years in a state of depression, and with my kidneys not functioning half the time. I would swell up till I thought I was going to burst or die. The Medical Dr. had given me more and more drugs with many, many combinations. When after 7 years I became so weak and over medicated, they then gave me a Hysterectomy of which I could not recover from. I was forced to quit my job and I went to bed for 2 yrs. I had a family that I could no longer care for. The Girls had to do all the work, and care for me. They got tired of my condition. I was so drugged by this time I didn't even realize what was going on. I finally contacted a Dr. that trained me in Bio-Feedback. I lay connected to that machine for 8 hrs. a day for 5 months. I improved enough to get up and get to another Chiropractor of which started things to be worse again. My Husbands Health was also deteriorating and he lost his job. He took a new job in another State. We took our personal belongings and left our newly married Daughter and her Husband in our home and left. After arriving to this new Home, 3 weeks later I found my days to be numbered 1-2-3. I contacted the Ladies at the Health Food Store as I knew if I were to go to the Hospital they would only give me more drugs and I knew one more would be the end for me. The girls sent me to a New Naturepath in another State. There we set up Hospital room in a Motel for 5 weeks. With my Husband and I fighting for my life. I had quit taking all my Medication in one day, which included insulin shots, knowing I couldn't take another pill. I remember I didn't have much to eat - one day - 5 spinich leaves then a Lady made a vegetable juice drink for me and some broth, from Vegetables. We had no cooking facilities in the motel and the restaurant was so far my Husband couldn't leave me long enough to go eat, for most of the time. I also remember more than one day of having 12 enemas in a day. It is hard to believe but I held on to my Husbands hand for 2 days, I received enough strength from his energy to stay alive. I was down to my last breath more than once. My Husband took me to the Hospital and I was refused entrance, which was a good thing.

We then came back to our rental trailer and the fight for life continued for 3 more years. I went to Chiropractors and others and finally found I could receive no help. I had heard a little about Dr. West's program so that is when I put in a S. O. S. call to Arizona. He told me what to do until he could get the information mailed to me. I had already been eating natural foods for the 3 years. I brought myself up from "O" with his Lymphatic exercises. After that I no longer felt that I needed to go to a Chiropractor. Since that date we have been caring for ourselves. The first 2 weeks on this program I did this exercise every hour for 24 hours a day. This brought enough life back into my body that I could gradually cut down on the frequency of the exercise. I also purchased a "Rebounder" and started doing the exercises on it. I could barely bounce for a long time then as time went by I could do more & more on it. I can do most anything on it now & jump for 20 minutes at a time, to a full side of a polka record, without being winded. I went to the Dentist periodicaly for the last 2 years and again found my energy was drained & unable to do so much on the "Rebounded", but now I am able to do all my own work, and go to the office everyday to help my Husband in our own Business. I also have an organic garden and juice alot of vegetables & fruits. I have had to eat frequently and in the night. I am now supplementing Aloe Vera juice along with my exercises. I have not had a grain of sugar, a slice of bread, or meat and not even an aspirin for 5 years now. I eat only fresh vegetables and fruits and grains, and feeling better than I have my whole life. I have tried well known instant proteins and Brewers Yeast only to find them to be very toxic forming. My system, also my Husbands, refused them, as they make our necks and shoulders stiff and with pain. Also, our eyes became weaker, and I couldn't take the Sunlight of which I usually enjoy so much. I developed difficulty in breathing and a dry mouth & throat, and again felt listless, and nerves very on edge, and the loss of energy. Other than during this period, I have been without pain now since I started this program of Dr. West.

My regular weight was, as an adult, nearly always 125 lbs. After prescribed drugs I weighed 185 lbs. I lost down to 116 lbs. at the time I started cleansing. I lost during the drastic 75 cleanse, to 97 lbs. I now weigh a natural 115 lbs. My spine & body feels as though it has been set free. I can move & do things that I could never do even as a child & teen ager. I am just recently able to return to the outside world and Public life to some degree, after 8 years of being confined to my house, and years previous, of being very ill.

With Gods help we have managed somehow to get thru this nightmare and hope to enjoy this beautiful world now for the remainder of our lives. It wasn't easy for my Husband as he wasn't in the best of Health either, but he saw me thru and also is on the program & doing well. To me this is a SPECIAL STORY because thru Dr. West's Research & Program he gave me LIFE and for me LIFE will begin at 50.

I believe 100% in Dr. West's program & believe it to be the answer to the worlds suffering. I also believe it to be a difficult task to teach & convince the people.

Mary L. Cox

Letter 46

11/7/81

After hearing your lecture on how to eliminate pain of injury, I want to tell you the following story.

Several years ago I cut off the end of a finger to the 1st knuckle. As soon as it happened, I grabbed it and held it tight until I got to the hospital which ws 10 to 15 minutes. I was afraid to let go for fear the blood would just squirt out. Although the end of the finger was cut off, there was no bleeding or pain when I released the pressure off the injured finger.

Until now I did not know why I did not have any pain. Even the doctor and nurses were amazed that I had no pain.

Sincerely,
Burley Owen
4720 Mesa
Amarilla, Tex. 79109

E. ADDITIONAL SCIENTIFIC EVIDENCE WITH TESTIMONIES GIVES VALIDITY TO THE NUTRITIONAL CONCEPTS AND THE TRANSITION PROGRAM IN SESSION THREE

1.The following is designed for those who need more evidence to convince them that they must change their nutritional program or be destroyed.

2.   Remember, the atomic bomb only took about 70,000 lives. Cancer is taking over 400,000 lives a year and heart disease, over a million lives a year. That is the equivalent of fifty planes, each filled with eighty people, being shot down every day. This research will help keep those fifty planes in the air.

E-1. What About High Protein For Athletes?

1.1. George Beinhorn, writing in the *Bike World Magazine,* April 1975 edition, gives the following information to the bike riders around the world. "Excess protein saps energy from working muscles." With the knowledge of how the lymphatic system works, we can understand how "trapped" protein not only saps energy from a muscle, it will also sap energy from any organ or area in the body where it accumulates. This is *where* and *how* loss of energy takes place in the body. He goes on to say, "It has also been discovered that too much protein is actually toxic. In layman's terms, it is poisonous.... Protein has enjoyed a wonderful reputation among athletes. Phrases like 'protein power', 'protein for energy', 'protein pills for the training athlete', 'ring-in memory', are all false and misleading. Protein requirements, in all the available research, are known to be 25-30 grams of high-quality protein per day. This is much less than people have been brought to believe."

E-2. A Very Well Documented Article Entitled, "Top Doctors Reveal...Simple Diet Change Can Prevent Breast & Colon Cancer," Appeared In The National Enquirer, September 15, 1979. On Page 20, It States:

2.1. Top doctors say a simple change in eating habits can prevent millions of Americans from getting breast or colon cancer--two of the biggest killers in the U.S.

2.2. To sharply reduce your chances of ever getting these

terrifying diseases, *the medical experts say that all you have to do is adopt an anticancer diet that is super-high in (complex) carbohydrates and low in fats.*

2.3. "There is no doubt that if the American public switched to this diet there would be a dramatic reduction in the number of people getting cancer of the colon and breast -- saving the lives of millions of American men and women in the long run," declared *Dr. Julian Whitaker, the former vice-president of the Orthomolecular Medical Society, a nutrition and preventive medicine group.*

2.4. *Agreed Dr. John Weisburger, who is the vice-president of the American Health Foundation and a former National Cancer Institute (NCI) researcher:*
"The chances are very good indeed that if Americans ate a diet that was higher in unrefined carbohydrates and lower in fat, they would have less colon and breast cancer."

2.5. "It is an amazing diet...a very healthy diet," added *Dr. James Anderson, Professor of Medicine at the University of Kentucky.*

2.6. The human diet consists of 3 basic food groups — proteins, carbohydrates and fats.

2.7. Proteins contain the basic building materials of the body and are found in meats, beans, and other foods.

2.8. Carbohydrates are sources of quick energy and include starches found in potatoes, rice and pasta.

2.9. Fats consist of greases and oils, usually stored in body tissues as long term sources of energy. Fat is present in such foods as meat, peanuts and butter.

2.10. Extensive research has convinced scientists that the standard American diet — 40 percent carbohydrates, 40 percent fat, 20 percent protein — is linked to the nation's high rate of breast and colon cancer, which together kill 77,000 Americans and strike another 183,000 each year.

2.11. To drastically cut your chances of ever getting these dreaded diseases, the experts say all you have to do is go on a simple anticancer diet that's super high in carbohydrates and low in fats. Ideally, the diet should consist of 80 percent carbohydrates, 10 percent fat and 10 percent protein.

2.12. But the experts all agree that even if you don't go that high — for example, a 60-20-20 diet — you can still get substantial health benefits from the anticancer eating plan.

2.13. "Detailed laboratory studies document that when you put animals on high-fat diets, you get more colon and breast cancer," declared *Dr. Weisburger, former head of the NCI's Carcinogen Screening Section.*

2.14 And studies on human populations indicate that low-fat, high-carbohydrate diets result in a lower incidence of colon cancer and breast cancer.

2.15. "The incidence of breast cancer in some countries with a lower fat intake is only a fifth of what it is here," explained Dr. Kenneth Carroll, professor of biochemistry at the University of Western Ontario in Canada.

2.16. "There's other evidence, too, that when migrants move from one country to another and change their diet, the pattern of cancer tends to change to that of the country they migrate to."

2.17. A worldwide study of colon cancer by *Sir Robert Williams, head of Britain's National Public Health Laboratory Service,* produced similar findings.

2.18. "In these population studies, we are talking about the *dietary habits* of millions of people," he told The ENQUIRER.

2.19. "There is a pretty good relation between the reported national intake of fat and the reported national prevalence of (colon) cancer. Certainly a corollary of the studies is that there would be a definite reduction of colon cancer if we switched to a diet that is low in fat."

2.20. Breast cancer is now the most common form of cancer among women and colon cancer is the third most common form of the disease among men, according to the NCI.

2.21. Even if you fall short of the 80-10-10 ideal diet, there is no doubt that the anticancer diet "would save lives" said *Dr. Olaf Mickelsen, distinguished visiting professor of nutrition at the University of Delaware.*

2.22. And another expert pointed out that there is no risk of putting on weight because of the carbohydrate-rich diet.

2.23. "High carbohydrate consumption will not cause people to gain weight," notes *Dr. Kelly West, Clinical Professor of Medicine at the University of Oklahoma Health Sciences Center.* "When they eat all the carbohydrates they want and reduce fat intake, people tend to lose weight."

2.24. To change your eating habits under this anticancer diet plan, the doctors recommend that you follow these simple rules:

2.25. Eat more whole grains cereals, rice, spaghetti and other noodles; all bread except white; plain Graham crackers, rye crackers, whole wheat muffins, oat muffins, corn muffins; all fresh vegetables; potatoes; nonfat dairy items; apples, applesauce, apricots, bananas, blackberries, strawberries, cherries, grapes, muskmelon, grapefruit, oranges, peaches, pears, pineapples, plums and tangerines.

2.26. At dinner, eat only moderate amounts of chicken or fish and limit beef and other red meat servings to no more than three times a week. And make sure you use lean meat such as round steak.

2.27. Eat less: fats and oils, butter and margarine, table sugar and anything made with sugar, including cakes, pies, cookies and ice cream.

2.28. Concluded *R. Emanuel Cheraskin of the University of Alabama Medical Center:*

2.29. "If Americans changed to this diet, there isn't any question in my mind that lives could be saved from cancer. IT'S MY OPINION AND PREDICTION THAT WE'RE GOING TO HAVE TO GO IN THIS DIRECTION, OR DESTROY OURSELVES."

THOMAS NESI
and DAVID WRIGHT

E-3. Millions Live--On Low Protein

3.1. "Research cited in *Foods for Fitness* shows that whole populations, numbering in the millions, have lived in excellent health for centuries on as little as 15-20 grams of protein per day, developing magnificent physiques and doing hard physical labor."

3.2. We can now understand that the hard physical labor has a great deal to do with their health and strength, and this is why: Without sufficient vigorous exercise to activate the lymphatics, protein will accumulate or become "trapped" in our bodies, even if we are eating the best kind of foods. Now this may be something that will surprise you: "The United States Government's own 70-gram recommendation was established on the basis of research that clearly showed 30 grams to be *completely adequate.* The extra 40 grams were labeled a 'margin of safety' though one Food and Nutrition board member reported that the real reason behind the high figure was that the board feared a 'public outcry' over the 30 gram figure." I believe that we can now understand that we do not have a 'margin of safety' when it comes to protein. I do not believe they did this maliciously. They did not know the *danger* of excess protein. I am sure, however, that there were those who did not want to see the 30 gram figure published, and the pressure must have been great. However, I do not believe they would have done it if they had known what we know today.

E-4. *Excess Protein--Will Damage Kidneys*

4.1. Dr. Ralph Burcher, in the September 1975 edition of the *Bike World Magazine* states: "Excess protein can't be stored, it must be quickly metabolized. Acceleration of metabolism does, in fact, deliver an extra shot of energy . . . like flooring the gas pedal of metabolism . . . Excess protein overstresses the kidneys with an enormous amount of useless decomposition by-products which must be quickly eliminated. Post competition studies of athletes have discovered nearly 100% instance of kidney damage and even occasional kidney collapse--this, among young men who thought themselves to be in glowing health . . . .

E-5. *What Dr. Paavo Airola--Says About Protein*

5.1. Quoting Dr. Paavo Airola, Ph.D., N.D., from his book, *How to Get Well*, pp. 192-4: "In this era . . . you have been brought to believe that a high protein diet is a must if you wish to attain a high level of health and prevent disease. Health writers and 'experts' who advocated high protein diets were misled by slanted research, which was financed by dairy and meat industries, or by insufficient and outdated information. Most recent research, worldwide, both scientific and empirical, shows more and more convincingly that our past beliefs in regard to high requirements of protein are outdated and incorrect, and that the actual daily need for protein in human nutrition is far below that which has long been considered necessary.

5.2. Researchers, working independently in many parts of

the world, arrived at the conclusion that our actual daily need of protein is only 25-35 grams..." (raw proteins, being utilized twice as well as cooked). "Independent researchers, not associated with or paid by dairy or meat industries, also point out that, contrary to past beliefs, proteins from many vegetable sources are superior or equal to animal proteins in their biological value." If you don't believe this, ask any gorilla, and he will tell you. Where does he get all the protein for his body? Chiefly from vegetation. And what is amazing, as we said before, his digestive system is almost identical to a man's. The digestive tract of a meat-eating animal is two-thirds shorter than ours. The reason being that it must get rid of the toxic waste quickly.

5.3. We are not designed to eat very much meat. Excess protein will putrefy in our colon and the colon is loaded with lymphatics which try to pull the poisons out. From the science of Iridology we know that many problems in the body can be traced directly to the colon. Things are beginning to snowball, aren't they?

5.4. Here is some interesting and revealing information. The most reliable and respected nutrition research organization in the world, The Max Planck Institute for Nutritional Research, in Germany gives this list of Complete Proteins: "Almonds (Eat all nuts sparingly. They are a good source of protein, but are too high in fat.), sesame seeds, soybeans, buckwheat, peanuts, (Boil peanuts first.), sunflower seeds, pumpkin seeds, (All seeds and grains are better sprouted.), potatoes, (baked to make them easier to digest), and all leafy green vegetables." All of these "contain complete proteins, which are comparable in quality to animal proteins."

E-6. Praise--The Potato

6.1. In the December, 1976, issue of the *Reader's Digest Magazine*, the article, "Praise the Potato," p. 205, we find that, "Maligned and misunderstood, this homely tuber is, in fact the world's most important vegetable." The article further states, "We would have to eat *eleven pounds* of potatoes to gain one pound of weight . . . if a person's diet consisted entirely of potatoes, he would get all the Riboflavin (B2), 1-1/2 times the iron, 3 to 4 times the Thiamin (B1) and Niacin (B3), and more than 10 times the amount of Vitamin C that the body needs...a good source of essential amino acids...high in potassium--a valuable aid in treating digestive disorders...Potatoes are *valuable* in a balanced reducing diet... Thus, this humble vegetable from Peru, may soon leave its homeland on its second most important journey--to wipe out hunger--so praise the potato!"

E-7.   *Disease Results From High Protein--Well Documented*

7.1.   Back to Dr. Airola and excess protein, "But, what is even more important, the worldwide research brings almost daily confirmation of the scientific premise...that proteins, essential and important as they are, CAN BE EXTREMELY HARMFUL WHEN CONSUMED IN EXCESS OF YOUR ACTUAL NEED." Dr. Airola says this. Now do *you* understand it? With a knowledge of the lymphatic system, I believe you will be able to understand these next statements of Dr. Airola's:

7.2.   "The metabolism of proteins consumed in excess of the actual need leaves toxic residues of metabolic wastes in tissues, causes autotoxemia, overacidity and nutritional deficiencies, accumulation of uric acid and purines in the tissues, intestinal putrefaction, and contributes to the development of many of our most common and serious diseases, such as; arthritis, kidney damage, pyorrhea, schizophrenia, osteoporosis, arteriosclerosis, heart disease, and cancer. A high protein diet also causes premature aging and lowers life expectancy."

7.3.   All the above-mentioned results of high-animal protein diet are well documented by reliable scientific research.

7.4.   A recent American research done under the direction of Dr. Lennart Krook, (as reported in Dr. Paavo Airola's book, *How To Get Well,* shows that overindulgence in meat leads to a mineral imbalance in the system--(too much phosphorus and too little calcium) which leads to severe calcium deficiency and resultant loss of teeth and pyorrhea.

7.5.   Dr. Paavo Airola says: "A recent study, made at the U.S. Army Medical Research and Nutrition Laboratory in Denver, Colorado, demonstrated that the more meat you eat, the more deficient in Vitamin B_6, Magnesium, Calcium and Niacin (B_3). Mental illness and schizophrenia are often caused by Niacin deficiency and have been recently successfully treated with high doses of Niacin. Russian researcher, *Dr. Uri Nikolayev,* has been extremely successful in treating schizophrenic patients with a low protein diet."

7.6. *Dr. Airola* continues: "Extensive studies made in England showed a clear connection between a high protein diet and osteoporosis. And doctors at the Vascular Research Laboratory in Brooklyn conducted research which indicates that excessive meat-eating can be a cause of widespread arteriosclerosis and heart disease. To the same conclusion, came researcher *Dr. C. D. Langen,* from Holland, and *Dr. A. Hoygaard,* from Denmark.

7.7. Dr. Schwarz, of Frankfurt University, in Germany, and *Dr. Ralph Bircher,* a famous biochemist from Zurich, Switzerland, report that the aging process is triggered by myloid, a by-product of protein metabolism; *which is deposited in all the connective tissues* and causes tissue and organ degeneration--thus leading to premature aging. This explains why people who traditionally eat low protein diets; Hunzakuts, in Pakistan, Bulgarians, Russian Caucasians, Yucatan Indians, East Indian Todas--also have the highest average life expectance in the world, 90 to 100 years! And, why the people who live on high animal protein diets, such as Eskimos, Greenlanders, Lapplanders, Russian Kurgis tribes, etc., have the lowest life expectancy in the world, 30 to 40 years. Americans lead the industrialized world in per capita meat consumption--and they also are in 21st place in life expectancy among unindustrialized nations!

7.8. Recently, *Dr. Willard J. Visek,* of Cornell University, implicated a high protein diet in the development of cancer. "Ammonia, which is produced in great amounts as a by-product of meat metabolism, is highly carcinogenic and can cause cancer development. A high protein diet also breaks down the pancreas and lowers resistance to cancer as well as contributes to the development of diabetes."

E-8. The Following Testimonials Are An Additional Witness To The Truth Of Eating Right

8.1. Arnold Ehret charged medical doctors $100 to hear him. One foggy night after a lecture in California, he slipped on an oil slick and hit his head. Fred Hirsh was with him but Professor

Ehret died before they could get him to the hospital.

8.2. Had Arnold Ehret lived, he would have saved millions of lives. Many have misunderstood him. He did things most people could never do because they do not have the self-discipline.

E-9.   Arnold Ehret--"The Daddy of Transition"

9.1. Professor Arnold Ehret in his book *Mucusless Diet and Healing System,* taught these things over 60 years ago. He taught that excess protein would kill you. He had Bright's disease and went through 24 physicians and $6,000 to prove that he was going to die. He felt like committing suicide until he met someone who gave him a desire to live. Then he went all over the world trying to find a way to get well. He noticed how people were eating in different parts of the world, and he began to change his way of life, and this is what he said happened to him: "An indescribable feeling never known before of better health, more vital energy, better efficiency, and more endurance and strength came to me and gave me great joy and happiness just to be alive. This was not only the physical, but there was a great change in my mental ability to perceive, to remember, greater courage and hope...my faculties were improved far surpassing their best during my healthiest and best youth. My physical efficiency and endurance became wonderfully increased. I took a bicycle trip of about 800 miles, accompanied by a trained bicyclist who lived on an ordinary diet--I was never behind him, but often ahead toward night, when endurance became the test. Keep in mind that I was formerly a candidate for death, so declared by the doctor...." *From what came the energy for this efficiency?*

E-10.   Ehret Proved--Strength Comes From A Clean System

10.1. Professor Ehret taught, believed, and proved that strength and vitality does *not* come directly from food, but through a clean system. He taught that poisons and toxins would drain the body of energy. We now know that a poison is a poison because it short-circuits the electrical system of the body and drains the body of energy. The article published by Paul Harvey in The Phoenix Gazette, April 9, 1976, entitled "Body Electricity

Offers New Hope" brings out that "the foods which fuel our body are converted chemically to electricity which makes you function."

10.2. These new discoveries help us understand this in detail. As you free your body from poisons, your generators turn on. Therefore, the cleaner our system is, the less food will be required for energy. The *more toxic your body* is, the *greater will be your desire* for food. The sad thing is that the excess food you eat turns into toxic waste, which compounds the problem and will continue to keep you from getting well.

10.3. Most health writers say--Here's a good food, come and eat! Professor Ehret says---Here's good food, watch out, it can kill you! He taught that nothing needs more supervision than when a person begins to eat good food. Fruit is a relentless house-cleaner. If we try to eat a fruit too fast, it can pull the excess sodium out, dissipate the clustered proteins and release too much fluid with the build-up of toxic waste into the blood stream, and we can become sick.

10.4. Now we know why fruit may make you sick while it heals you. If this should begin to happen, eat a hamburger or something that will "trap" the proteins. The cleansing action would be slowed down, and you will feel better immediately. Fruit can make you *feel* sick while it heals you; a hamburger can make you *feel* better while it kills you.

E-11. Arnold Ehret Lived On Straight Fruit--For Two Years

11.1. Once Professor Ehret got his body clean enough, to *complete the cleansing action,* he went on straight fruit for two years. The result was that he had *endless strength* and boundless energy. He would fast for 7 days, eat 2 pounds of cherries, and then march for 56 hours continuously without sleep or rest or food, only drink. This was a living testimony of the things he taught. He believed in fasting, but with safeguards for the person who did it. To further prove his belief, he fasted four months out of fourteen---49 days at a time. This he did under supervision, performing feats of strength as he did so. The question that he continued to ask was, "From what comes the energy for this efficiency?" He proved that energy did not come directly from food, but from a clean system. He proved that as you "untrap" enough of your blood proteins and turn enough of your generators on, the body is able to maintain its energy for long periods of time.

11.2. Ehret had a sanitarium in Switzerland where thousands of people came and received help. Then he came to America to convert the doctors. He believed that if he could convert doctors, everyone would benefit. He charged them $100 for the lectures that are contained in his little orange book, *The Mucusless Diet Healing System*. This is not a novel. These are lectures that he gave, and he repeats himself many times.

E-12. *Teresa Mitchell Follows Ehret--No Fatigue In Body*

12.1. There are two other little books that give some insights and lend testimony to what Professor Ehret taught. One is *Roads to Health and Happiness* and the other is *The Definite Cure of Chronic Constipation*. In the first, Teresa Mitchell gives her own story. She wanted the strength, the vitality, and the endurance that Arnold Ehret received. She thought her body was in good enough condition to go on nothing but fruit for the final cleansing; therefore, she ate only fruit for nine months. In this little book she tells her story.

12.2. At the end of the 9 months this is what she says: "Then the first great event happened. One night, after a supper of grapes, I was awakened by a sensation of fullness in my throat. I had no particular feeling of nausea or pain, but upon reaching the bathroom I threw up large quantities of a thick, clear substance. After this ordeal was over I felt a new sense of well-being come over me. New strength and power seemed to fill my whole being. I thought this must be the great final cleansing that Professor Ehret taught us to expect. However, it was only a forerunner of two more similar experiences before the long expected day arrived."

12.3. "During this period of cleansing and elimination many interesting things took place--in fact, too many to enumerate here. One of the most outstanding facts, I think, was the complete absence of fatigue. My work required that I remain constantly on my feet for eight hours, and yet after a full day's work I felt just as fresh as though I had not worked at all. The only way I knew that rest was required by my body was a feeling of drowsiness." (How would you like that? Let anyone else produce the same results eating any other kind of food!) "Upon arriving home I usually took a short nap, after which I was ready for my vocal studies at the studio. My rest at night was complete and undisturbed, for I seldom dreamed. Upon awakening there was that indescribable clear-headedness which must be experienced in order to be understood and appreciated. No stimulants, such as coffee or tea, were needed to get me in good humor for the days work. Thinking became increasingly easier and I was actually becoming witty. In fact, I had never been aware of this gift in my adopted English language. I felt proud of my ability to give back a quick answer, as well as a ready come back to 'small' talk. My powers of concentration had become more acute. In fact, neither noises or confusion could distract my thinking. My shyness and reticence were being replaced by poise."

12.4. "My residence was close to the restaurant so that I could walk to and from work. There was one exceptionally steep hill to climb which would invariably cause me to puff and pant. One afternoon on my way home I felt inspired to create a poem. As the sentences took form I became deeply engrossed in thought when suddenly I noticed I had climbed more than half way up the hill, yet I had felt no exertion whatever. It was as though I had been walking on level ground and I could scarcely believe what was happening. I concluded that I must have been so engrossed in the poem that I forgot about my body. This, then, was the opportune time to make a test, so I decided to return to the bottom of the hill and walk up again, this time giving no thought to the poem. What I discovered was unbelievable. I felt as though my body had no weight at all. Here was I, ascending this steep incline, which in all probability is at least 69% grade, without the slightest feeling of fatigue whatsoever. I am sure that I could have easily run all the way up, and I would have tried it too, except I feared I would cause consternation among the puffing and panting pedestrians and telling them all about it. 'I must be at the gates of Shangri La,' I thought to myself,'To think that diet could do all this.'" (It should be noted that diet alone did not do all this.)

12.5 Both Arnold Ehret and Teresa Mitchell went on straight fruit for a long time but both were physically active and both had good mental attitudes. Compare this to The Art of Lymphasizing. They both did what they did just to prove that it could be done—not that everyone could or should do it! Both taught the importance of a 'transition' program for most people.

E-13. Testimony of Teresa Mitchell

13.1. At the end of part one, Teresa gives this outstanding testimony:

13.2. "Today, after a span of twenty-seven years, my faith in the efficacy of Ehret's Mucusless Diet Healing System is stronger than it ever was during my younger days of experimenting. At the age of fifty-three, I am proudly begining to admit my age. For years, I fibbed about it, especially to my employers. Now, my co-workers and neighbors look at me with great surprise. I am told that I should never admit to being more than thirty-six or seven at the most. My skin (I must admit, at the risk of seeming to brag) still has the unwrinkled smoothness of a much younger woman. My hair is in excellent condition. I have retained a youthful, streamlined figure. My voice, which I use a great deal as a soloist, is still young and vibrant. I keep up an extensive vocal repertoire. I still enjoy the zest, capacity and strength for work. I do all my own housework and carry on a seven or eight hour job, outside my home. I take care of such duties as two growing sons and a husband. In my spare time I try my hand at writing. I am completely without aches or pains of any kind, although I have been going through the difficult period of menopause. However, the generally accepted symptoms that plague the average woman during this period of life, have had very slight effects on me. I have not had 'shots', pills or tonics---in fact, I have had no need to seek the advise of a physician. My medicine cabinet is still free of pills, physics, or tonics, nor do I use creams and beauty preparations."

13.3. "Needless to say, I do not wander off the straight and narrow path as laid down by Professor Ehret in his wonderful book which, I am sure does not need my testimonial for it has stood on its own merits for many years. Over a hundred thousand persons have already read the book and many must believe its teachings just as I do. But, may I emphasize just one point, and it is this: Whoever desires to become a disciple of Ehret's teachings should himself attain a complete healing. Then, and then only, is he competent to teach the principles of "How to Control One's Health" through fasting and diet, without fear of unknown disease that might be lurking in the tissues and bloodstream of the body."

13.4. "Only this can give man's soul and mind the freedom Nature intended us to possess."

13.5. In Part II of that little book she gives a section entitled, "Build Your Own Road to Health." There are not very many pages in that little section, but they are priceless! She tells some of the things to expect, and the cautions in eating when a person tries to eat the right kind of food. Here are some of them:

13.6. "It is much better to take your time about this business of healing; it is the most important step you can take in this life."

13.7. "Persist until complete healing takes place."

13.8 "Whatever you do, DON'T give up too soon for you may well be just in sight of success . . . ."

13.9. Professor Ehret taught that it can take from one to three years to cleanse your system. On a transition program, the cleansing process may take longer.

E-14. *Eight Basic Rules For a Disease-Free, Healthy Life*

In the other book, *The Definite Cure of Chronic Constipation,* pp.24-25, Arnold Ehret presents eight basic rules for a disease-free, healthy life. We give them to you with the idea that you may understand transition. They are:

14.1. TO LENGTHEN YOUR LIFE, SHORTEN YOUR MEALS! Eat slowly and relish your food, for food must be appetizing and thoroughly masticated in order to digest properly. *The first stage of digestion takes place in the mouth;* hence the necessity of thorough mastication. To avoid overeating it is a good rule to leave the table while still hungry! Avoid eating between meals!

14.2. AVOID DRINKING ANY LIQUIDS WITH MEALS. This includes water, tea, milk, coffee, fruit juices and even soups. Wait at least 15 minutes after drinking before you start eating solid foods. And wait at least the same length of time after eating before you drink liquids. Liquids interfere with digestion of your food when taken together.

14.3. AVOID ALL HARSH CONDIMENTS AND SPICES. This includes salt, pepper, mustard, catsup, vinegar, pickles, etc. They may stimulate jaded appetites but digestion is retarded. (Use capsicum, Jensen's vegetable seasoning, kelp, bee pollen, and Bio-salt.)

14.4. AVOID USING BUTTER, MARGARINE, AND MOST COOKING OILS. Use pure olive oil where necessary to prevent sticking to baking dish. Starchy vegetables should be steamed or boiled until soft enough to insert a fork into easily, then baked for at least thirty minutes or until thoroughly dextrinized. (500°for twenty minutes for potatoes.) You will find added flavor through baking; also the food becomes more easily digestible.

14.5. AVOID ALL DENATURED AND OVER-PROCESSED FOODS (such as white flour and 'ready to use' cake mixes.) Prepared 'TV' frozen dinners should be avoided also. All nourishing content has been dissipated through the processor's use of food preservatives and chemical additives. A more nutritional meal would consist of a salad of fresh greens, cottage cheese, tomatoes and one or two cooked vegetables. Or better still a fruit salad with Yogurt or cottage-cheese. Dried figs, dates, apricots or raisins chewed together with a few nuts until thoroughly masticated, furnish the necessary protein content and are rich in polyunsaturated fat; but eat sparingly.

14.6. AVOID CONSTIPATING FOODS SUCH AS MASHED POTATOES WITH GRAVY, HOT BUNS, CAKES AND PASTRIES. Sprout seeds and grains and eat nuts and meat sparingly. Poultry and fish are best; make a mild barley drink-- as well as other grains. Soak 24 hours and drink the new mineralized distilled water. Dairy products--eggs, milk, cheese and butter, are constipating and form toxic waste poisons in the body and should be eaten sparingly. Make your own cheese with Bio-salt--see the sample recipes at the end of the transition program. Also millet is good with a little Bio-salt and cayenne pepper.

14.7. AVOID ALL FROZEN DESSERTS SUCH AS ICE-CREAM, SHERBET, ETC. Frozen desserts 'shock' the digestive apparatus, and have a high acid content. They rob the system of valuable vitality. The too liberal use of eggs and milk can cause putrefaction in the digestive tract; normal functioning is impeded and poisons which should have been eliminated are retained.

14.8. SINCE MAN IS A "CREATURE OF HABIT", IT IS

WISE TO TAKE ADVANTAGE OF THIS FACT. Make it a daily "habit" to visit the bathroom the first thing in the morning or immediately after eating. Allow yourself ample time; concentrate on elimination taking place. Be willing to spend fifteen or twenty minutes if necessary during the "experimental stage". It may require some time before Nature accepts the suggestion! You may use a bulb syringe--with luke warm water, not hot, when necessary, retaining the fluid at least ten minutes before rejecting. You will eventually be rewarded with permanent regularity, particularly if a corrective diet, proper physical exercises and deep breathing have been followed.

14.9. Incidentally, I have been in the home of Mr. Hirsch, and as of March, 1977, he was still running the Ehret Publishing Company at 86 years of age. He was a sparkling, rosy-cheeked example of Ehret's teachings and was still driving a car and reading without glasses. He was President and Vice-President of the Arnold Ehret Health Club of America.

E-15. Dr. Max Warmbrand, M.D., D.O. Confirms Above Research and Findings

15.1. Additional information to confirm these teachings is coming from doctors all over the world. For example: Dr. Warmbrand, M.D., D.O., author of *Encyclopedia of Natural Health; Living Without Pain; Eat Well to Keep Well,* makes these following statements:

(a) The body has the power to heal itself.

(b) To allow for self-healing we must never use anything harmful to the body. (Harmful are drugs like antibiotics, cortisone, the sulfas, fever and pain-killing pills.)

(c) The whole body needs treatment--not just symptoms like fever, pain, a cough, diarrhea, etc.

In his program for keeping well, Dr. Warmbrand lists:

(a) Eat healthy natural foods. Forget the myth about a *high protein diet* of meat, fish, or eggs, which in excess are hazardous to your health. WE CAN GET PROTEIN IN ABUNDANCE FROM NATURAL BROWN RICE, GREEN LEAFY VEGETABLES, THE ROOT VEGETABLE, AND LEGUMES LIKE CHICK-PEAS, AND LENTILS.

(b) Learn how to eat. Use the teeth in your mouth, there are none in the stomach. To benefit from food it has to be chewed well, and must be food your body can digest.

(c) Learn when to eat. The clock or dinner bell should not be your guide. *Eat only when you are hungry.*

(d) Keep away from coffee, alcohol and drugs.

(e) Get enough sleep and physical activity.

15.2 To understand why Professor Ehret was able to live on straight fruit for two years and why Teresa Mitchell was able to obtain such tremendous results, we will go to U.S. Department of Agriculture Circular No. 549, 1940. Keep in mind that mother's milk is 2.38% protein at birth and reduces down to 1.2-1.6% in 6 months. Remember also that the foods with low percentages of protein, which are low in fat but high in carbohydrates, are *good foods* (See chart page 225).

E-16. Complex Carbohydrates -- A Protein Sparer

16.1. The *Textbook of Medical Physiology* by Dr. Arthur C. Guyton gives priceless information concerning the ability of the carbohydrates in fruits and vegetables to prevent weakness and reduce your need for protein. "Consequently, carbohydrates appear to be essential to prevent weakness. This is especially true when the body undertakes a considerable workload. Finally, as already discussed, *carbohydrates are a protein sparer.*"

16.2. It goes on to say that carbohydrates are burned in "preference" to the burning of protein for energy, which "is very important for preserving functional proteins in the cells." Now isn't that interesting? *Carbohydrates preserve the proteins in the body!* THEY ARE PROTEIN SPARERS. This helps us to more fully understand why we should eat more fruit, vegetables and whole grains (sprouts) and eat meat sparingly.

PROTEIN, FAT, AND CARBOHYDRATE CONTENT
OF DIFFERENT FOODS

Food	Protein %	Fat %	Carbo-hydrates %	Fuel Value per 100 Grams, Calories
Apples	0.3	0.4	14.9	64
Asparagus	2.2	0.2	3.9	26
Bacon, fat	6.2	76.0	0.7	712
broiled	25.0	55.0	1.0	599
Beef, medium	17.5	22.0	1.0	268
Beets, fresh	1.6	0.1	9.6	46
Bread, white, milk	9.0	3.6	49.8	268
Butter	0.6	81.0	0.4	733
Cabbage	1.4	0.2	5.3	29
Carrots	1.2	0.3	9.3	45
Cashew nuts	19.6	47.2	26.4	609
Cheese, Cheddar, Am.	23.9	32..3	1.7	393
Chicken, total edible	21.6	2.7	1.0	111
Chocolate	(5.5)	52.9	(18.0)	570
Corn (maize), entire	10.0	4.3	73.4	372
Haddock	17.2	0.3	0.5	72
Lamb, leg intermediate	18.0	17.5	1.0	230
Milk, fresh whole	3.5	3.9	4.9	69
Molasses, medium	0.0	0.0	(60.0)	240
Oatmeal, dry, uncooked	14.2	7.4	68.2	396
Oranges	0.9	0.2	11.2	50
Peanuts	26.9	44.2	23.6	600
Peas, fresh	6.7	0.4	17.7	101
Pork, ham, medium	15.2	31.0	1.0	340
Potatoes	2.0	0.1	19.1	85
Spinach	2.3	0.3	3.2	25
Strawberries	0.8	0.6	8.1	41
Tomatoes	1.0	0.3	4.0	23
Tuna, canned	24.2	10.8	0.5	194
Walnuts, English	15.0	64.4	15.6	702

Extracted from data compiled by Chatfield and Adams, U. S. Department of Agriculture Circular No 549, 1940. (12)

As you can see from this table, it is amazing how much protein there is in fruits and vegetables. They are the primary source of protein, glucose, and minerals for humans and all long coloned animals.

E-17. Protein in the Body Stays High --- Even During Starvation
(Fasting)

17.1. Here is another chart from the medical text dealing
with starvation that is invaluable to help you really understand
that what we are teaching is true. The following graph indicates
what happens to carbohydrates, fats, and proteins during
fasting.

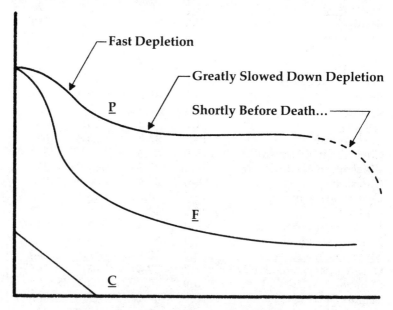

CHART ON STARVATION

(Adapted from *Textbook of Medical Physiology* by Arthur C.
Guyton, M.D., fifth edition, January 1976, p. 977.) (11)

1. Carbohydrates go immediately.
2. Fats go next.
3. Protein - The medical research states that protein
   undergoes three phases of depletion during starvation.
        Phase 1: There is a "fast depletion of protein at first",
        Phase 2: then a "greatly slowed down depletion";
        Phase 3: protein falls off "just shortly before death".

17.2. Now let us see if we can understand these three phases of protein depletion in the body during starvation.

17.3. *What is the fast depletion at first?* First, I would like to go to Dr. Airola's book, *How To Get Well* pages 215 and 216, section entitled "Why is Fasting so Effective?" where it states that: "During a prolonged fast (after the first three days on juice or fruit), your body will live on its own substance. When it is deprived of needed nutrition, particularly of proteins and fats, it will burn and digest its own tissue by the process of autolysis, or self-digestion. *But our body will not do it indiscriminately!* . . . and here lies the secret of the extraordinary effectiveness of fasting as curative and rejuvenative therapy! Your body will *first* decompose and burn those cells and tissues which are *diseased, damaged, aged* or *dead.* In fasting, your body feeds itself on the most impure and inferior materials, such as dead cells and morbid accumulations, tumors, abscesses, fat deposits etc."

E-18. What Dr. Otto Buchinger, M.D. Says About Fasting In How To Get Well, By Dr. Paavo Airola

18.1. In short, Dr. Otto Buchinger, M.D. who is perhaps the greatest fasting authority in the world, says, "Fasting is a "burning of rubbish." So, during starvation, the fast depletion at first is a "burning of rubbish", and this is why we believe people die during the first stages of starvation. They do not die from lack of food. They die because fasting (like fruit) can pull out the "pockets" of excess fluid, excess sodium and poisons too fast. The generators are turned on dissipating other "pockets" of clustered proteins which will release a tremendous amount of fluid (along with the toxic waste) into the blood stream. (Exercise can do the same thing if you are not accustomed to it.) When excess poisons and toxins are dumped into the blood stream too fast, it shocks the entire system and causes "trapped" proteins all over the body, and death can take place in just a few hours. This is why it is said, if you do not die from a snake or black widow bite within 24 hours you will probably live. Therefore, if you can survive the shock factor of starvation, you would not die during the first phase.

E-19. Vital Organs and Glands are Not Damaged From Fasting

19.1. *Why is there a greatly slowed-down depletion?* Again quoting from Dr. Airola, (*How To Get Well*, p. 215) "The essential tissues and vital organs, the glands, the nervous system, and the brain are not damaged or digested in fasting."

19.2. It is interesting that Professor Ehret taught this same thing 60 years ago. He taught that the body would not burn one cell that is in a healthy condition, and he proved it with the *many fasts that he was able to accomplish.*

19.3. This was again proven and demonstrated during *the famous Swedish fast marches* where eleven (and then nineteen) men who were accustomed to exercise, walked the road from Gothenburg to Stockholm (a distance of over 325 miles) in 10 days while on a total food fast. *It was observed that their protein level remained constant. Why did it remain constant?* Because as Dr. Airola states in his book, "The proteins in your body are in a dynamic state being constantly decomposed and re-synthesized and reused for various needs within the body. When old or diseased cells are decomposed, the amino acids are not wasted, but are released and used again in the process of building new vital young cells."

19.4. This explains why Ehret and Teresa Mitchell could go so long on only fruit. Knowing this, think of how much protein a person needs while he is trying to lose weight! Interesting, isn't it? What is more important, on the above Swedish fast marches, "their health only improved and they felt stronger and had more vigor and vitality after the fast than before it" as expressed by Dr. Karl Otto Aly, M.D., one of the participants in the marches.

19.5 With the knowledge of *THE SEVEN GOLDEN DISCOVERIES* and *THE BASIC FORMULA* we know why this happened. Exercise and fasting pulled out the "trapped" proteins, excess fluid, excess sodium and poisons which turned the generators on! This proves again that strength and vitality does *not* come directly from food---but from a clean system. On a transition program, as you stop doing the things that cause "trapped" proteins, your energy level will go up! Isn't that exciting?

19.6 *How about Phase Three?* Having this understanding, suppose you were to starve. If you could live through Phase One, come to the greatly slowed-down depletion of protein in your body, and then start eating fruits and vegetables---you would not die, but would obtain better health, strength and vitality. Isn't that beautiful? This research can bring you to a "new way of life" that will help you conquer disease and live in peace. (The information quoted in this session from *How To Get*

Well is quoted with permission. This is an excellent book-- a true classic on nutrition science by Paavo Airola. *How To Get Well* is published by Health Plus Publishers, Phoenix, Arizona 85028).

F. SPECIAL RECOGNITION GOES TO THE FOLLOWING LYMPHASIZER MANUFACTURES, OTHER COMPANIES AND INDIVIDUALS FOR HELPING TO FINANCE THE FIRST EDITION OF THIS BOOK

LYMPHASIZER MANUFACTURERS

J. B. Marketing, Inc.
Manufacturers of the GYM MASTER
   3200 S. Zuni
   Englewood, CA 80110
   Judith Burk

Trimway Corp.
Manufacturers of THE REBOUNDER
   P.O. Box 771B
   Seattle, WA 98133
   Jerry and Maple Hinkle

Olympus Distributors Corp.
Manufacturers of the SUNDANCER
   P.O. Box 969
   St. George, Utah 84770
   Carol and Delmont Truman

Natures Sunshine
Manufacturers of the ENERGIZER
   P.O. Box 1000
   Spanish Fork, UT 84660
   Kerry Asay

Natures Sunshine of CANADA
Distributors of the ENERGIZER
   Orangeville, Ontario, Canada L9W 2Z1
   Gordon Morten

Trampoline World
Manufacturers of the GLOBE JOGGER

P.O. Box 466
Hwy. 85 North
Fayetteville, GA 30214
John Williams

New Products International, Inc.
Manufacturers of the AEROBIC BOUNCER
2323 Woodlawn Street
Harrisburg, PA 17104
Chuck Stoner

Trimflex Manufacturing, Inc.
Manufacturers of the PACER MAT
1208 Missouri Ave.
South Houston, TX 77587
Victor and John Green

OTHER COMPANIES

C. C. Pollen Co.
Manufacturers of HIGH DESERT BEE POLLEN
7000 E. Camelback Rd.
Scottsdale, AZ 85251
Royden Brown

INDIVIDUALS

Sam and Afton Dunbar - California

Peary Barker - Utah

Vaughn Larsen - Utah

Miriam Jones - Ohio

Dean Black - Utah

Tom and Geanne Burgess - Oregon

Ray and Elva Danly - Washington

Joan Emery - Calgary, Canada

Phillip Ellert - Indiana

Margeret Kopi - Calgary, Canada

Mary's Natural Foods- Arkansas

Eric and Dorothy Nelson

Dorothy J. Nord - California

Lorentz and Fern Opdahl- South Dakota

John and Lucille Presnell - Arkansas

Rev. Derald K. and Anna Marie Rice - Nebraska

Jack and Verlin Ritchason - California

Bette & Al Schenkey - British Columbia, Canada

Emanuel Schlaback - Ohio

Rudy Schroch - Missouri

Bud & Violet Shuster - Pennsylvania

William & Margart Small - Illinois

Elmer Smith - Washington

David T. Stuck - Michigan

Henry & Mary Swantz - Missouri

Joyce & Earl Weisinger - Michigan

Frank and Kathy Angelo - Pennsylvania

Ralph and Norma Schaffer - Pennsylvania

David and Sarah Glick - Pennsylvania

G. *MY STORY BEHIND THE GOLDEN SEVEN PLUS ONE*

1. Many people have asked me, or have wondered how I came to know about the blood protein research, the seven golden discoveries and this formula, and how I got started lecturing on a full time basis. Well, the answer to these questions is my personal golden seven plus one, and is the story behind this book.

2. I love my family; and I want everyone to know that without the help of my angel wife, my 10 children, and all those who have been willing to help throughout the United States and Canada, it would have been impossible for me to have stayed with this program long enough to get the information needed to write this book. No one likes to leave their family for weeks at a time on a continued basis for even a few months, let alone what is now going on 6 years. However, with the knowlege of what is causing the death of over 240,000 men, women and children every two months in the United States, how could I put my life or even the lives of my family above theirs?

G-1. *Not To Tell Others About This Research--Is To Cause Their Destruction*

1.1. If you see a person drowning and you have a life-line in your hand, and you have the ability and strength, and the knowledge and the power to save his life; if you let something of less importance keep you from throwing that life-line, you are guilty of murder, just as sure as if you would have shot him in cold blood. This is why I have said many times if someone put a gun to my head and said, "Stop or I'll shoot", I would have to say, "Shoot"! Little did I realize at the start that this message would become as great or as important as it is today.

1.2. In 1974 I knew that proteins could cause death in the body within 24 hours if the lymphatic system did not function properly, but it took over a year to know that the protein spoken of was the proteins that make up a part of the blood stream. It also took that long for me to realize and understand the "trapped" protein concept. (I coined the term "trapped" protein in 1977 in San Diego, Ca.) Medical research does not refer to it as "trapped," only as *excess*. This is what threw me off for a long time. I was used to relating protein to the food we eat. This made it very difficult to teach during the first few years. All I really knew was that protein could cause death within 24 hours. Talking with the best surgeons and doctors that I knew, including people in Washington, D.C., showed that not one person I talked to knew anything about the relationship between protein, the lymphatic system, disease and death.

1.3. After seven years and continuous searching, I now know that there are only a handful of people in the world who know about the relationship between the lymphatic system and the blood proteins. As of November, 1979, there were approximately 300 lymphologists in the world, and only about 65 in the United States. My chances of knowing or talking with one of them was pretty slim even though the knowledge of blood proteins causing death in the body had been in medical research records for approximately 20 years. The fact that death due to traumatic or surgical shock is caused by loss of blood proteins and water from the blood stream was published in the 1953, 1956, and the 1960 edition of the *Encyclopedia Americana;* however it is not in the 1970 or later editions. This knowledge has been buried.

1.4. The International Society of Lymphology, of which I am now the 379th member, has been in existence for only about 16 years. I believe this Society will become one of the most important scientific societies in the world. However, as of today, this book represents the only health education program on the face of the earth that is designed to teach the public the blood protein research story. *And without THE SEVEN GOLDEN DISCOVERIES and THE ONE BASIC FORMULA,* it would be impossible for us to be teaching the knowledge that will enable us to raise up a golden posterity who will be able to conquer disease and live in peace.

1.5. Thus, we have our name, *The World-Wide Golden Family Self-H.E.L.P. Program.* The H.E.L.P. stands for Health Education for Longevity and Peace. This program is also referred to as *The Golden Family Health Education Program.*

1.6. May the Lord bless and inspire you to join with us in a burning and relentless desire to help get the message contained in these seven golden discoveries and this one basic formula to the nations of the earth. This message will not only enable you to save them from destruction, but you will also bring them the knowledge that will help them establish peace in their homes, in the nation, and throughout the world.

1.7. "Greater love hath no man than this, that a man lay down his life for his friends." If someone knew what would cause your death and cause a spirit of unrest in your home and you didn't-- would you want them to tell you? All we ask is this-- that you *"do unto others as you would have them to do unto you!"*

1.8. During my 1980 lecture tour I was staying in the home of Willard & Catherine Hunter in Heath, Ohio. On their wall I saw a plaque that said: *"Love has been defined as the desire to give everything you have to bless the lives of others."* I believe this about sums up how people feel who get involved and understand the purposes and the goals of this Golden Family Health Education effort. I would like personally to thank all of those who have been instrumental and will yet be instrumental in any way in helping to get this message to those who would like to become Golden Families.

G-2. Why I Learned About This Research

2.1. Especially, at this time, I would like to express my deep love and apreciation to a man without whose help this work would have been impossible. His name is Billy G. Gonzales. Without his help and the help of his wonderful, courageous and magnificent wife, Gennis, I would never have been able to go back to college full-time with six children, for there was no money in sight. This happened some time after I had received knowledge from Stanley Burroughs, Ina Bryant, Dr. Huls, D.O., and others. The Lord gave me a burning uncontrollable desire in my heart to go back to school to teach people how to take care of themselves.

2.2. Stanley Burroughs taught me how to bring my darling wife from a condition where she would have migraine headaches so bad she could hardly get out of bed, to a condition where she was up and around within about 5 minutes. (Using the Self-Help Pain Relief Techniques given in this book, we teach how you can do this by yourself in just a few minutes.)

2.3 I went through "steel walls" to teach people how to take care of themselves. The desire to become a doctor, to help people to take care of themselves was so great that not to fulfill this desire would have been the same as asking me not to live. I felt that if I could not fulfill this goal that my purpose for existence was over. Therefore, I prayed day and night unto my Father in Heaven that this desire would be granted. As I walked, I prayed; as I drove down the road, I prayed; and finally one morning I awoke with a start as the words came into my heart, "The money is going to come; you will be able to go to school."

G-3. *"Steel Wall" Number One*

3.1. My desire was to become an Osteopathic Physician. In order to fulfill that goal, I had counted the cost and I knew that with my six children, it would take a minimum of $10,000 a year plus all I could borrow for five years. So when I prayed that I might be able to go back to school, I also prayed for the $50,000 that it would take for me to do so. You see when the answer came--, "The money is going to come; you will be able to go back to school" it was not just a little thing. When the answer came that morning, I turned to my wife, woke her up and said, "Honey, the money is going to come, I'm going back to school."

She said, "I believe you."

3.2. Well, I looked and looked for the $50,000. I went to everybody I knew who might have it. They had the money, but it was all tied up and they couldn't get it loose. I had searched everywhere, and had run out of places to look. Where would it come from? This was my condition when all at once, out of the "clear blue sky" through my front door came Billy G. Gonzales and his wife, Gennis. I hadn't seen them for a long time and as far as I knew, they should have been a long way from Mesa, Arizona.

3.3. The first thing Bill said to me as he came through the door, was, "What are you doing?"

3.4. I said, "I want to go back to school."

3.5. "Great!" he answered, "I've been wanting you to go back for a long time."

3.6. "I know, Bill, but I don't know where the money is going to come from."

3.7. "Well, I know," said Bill.

3.8. "So do I," added Gennis.

3.9. "What do you mean?" I asked in total amazement.

3.10. Then Gennis said, "I wasn't going to teach school this year, but now I am going to teach and put you through school."

3.11. My reply was, "No way! You are my best friends and

you would end up being my worst enemies. Forget it! You don't realize what you are talking about. It wouldn't take very long before you would be sorry."

3.12. They would not take "NO" for an answer. They stayed with me for a week. Finally, one day, Gennis said to me, "Bill is where he is today because of you. And *you* are going to school!" (Ten years earlier Bill went back to school and became a coach because of my encouragement and counseling.)

3.13. Finally, I gave in and said, "All right! If that is the way you really feel about it, I will sell my home and let's go!"

3.14. Before they left, Bill and I made a miraculous one-week trip to Missouri as I thought that I would go to the Kansas City College of Osteopathy and Surgery for my Pre-Med. While there, Bill was interviewed by three schools; we had his car overhauled; I helped him find and buy a farm (which was another miracle in itself), and we were back home in Mesa in one week's time. To travel 2,400 miles and do all of this in a mere week is a story that few people would believe, even if I told them all the details; but this is nothing new for Bill and me. From that day to this, many things have happened in our lives that would seem like a miracle to many people.

3.15. All I can say is that we sacrificed to the "hilt." Some of my children still tell me they have nightmares from the little house that we moved into which had almost dirt floors. We had sold our beautiful "dream home" without getting the money we expected, so things were just plain "tough!"

G-4. *"Steel Wall" Number Two*

4.1. Bill and Gennis sent me between $150 and $200 a month for about a year. At the bottom of each check it said, "Gift, we love you." Johna May was able to work in a children's nursery where she could take care of our small children and help earn what money she could which was about $200 a month. I went back to school full time with six children on $400 per month. From that time on, miracles have taken place in our lives. We went through other seemingly "steel walls" before I was able to finish my Pre-Med program at Arizona State University in Tempe, Arizona.

G-5. *"Steel Wall" Number Three*

5.1. Then, as it came time for me to go on to the College of Osteopathy and Surgery at Kirksville, Missouri, I got hit with what I thought was a *bomb*. A letter came which said in essence, "We are accepting very few over twenty-five years of age, and none over 30. You are now 36 years old and our enrollment is full. If we accept you at this time, we would have to turn down a man ten years younger and we just can't do it."

5.2. What a blow! I went to the Lord and said, "What do I do now? You've taken me this far. Now what do I do?" The answer came. "Go into Chemistry." I said to myself, "Chemistry? If I did something else, I wanted to be either a seminary teacher or a lawyer."

5.3. I was on my way to becoming a lawyer *before* I got the burning desire to become a doctor. When I had only 4 children I had been going to school part-time in the evenings to become a lawyer. Now I had the six children, and I was struggling to go to school full-time; to try to live on a beginning teacher's salary with a family the size of mine would be rough. Besides, I did not have any desire to be a school teacher. However, the answer came so strongly to go into Chemistry that I changed my major and started in although I did not completely know why.

G-6.   *"Steel Wall" Number Four*

6.1 About this time, Johna May got the idea of getting a job at Motorola where she could get better pay. I really didn't think she would be able to do it, but told her to go ahead and try. She did and to my surprise, she made it. This happened at a very critical time. Gennis had become pregnant, and she was having problems. At the very time that Johna May was accepted at Motorola, where she could make about $400 a month net, we heard from Gennis; she told us that they were sorry but they would not be able to continue to help us any more financially.

G-7.   *"Steel Wall" Number Five*

7.1. Some people may think all of this was just coincidence. Well, it didn't stop there. Johna May was expecting and the very month that they told her she would have to quit at Motorola, I received my first check from teaching Chemistry at Westwood High School in Mesa, Arizona. We did not miss one check from the time I started to school until I began to teach Chemistry.

G-8. *"Steel Wall" Number Six*

8.1. For those who think this was a coincidence, when I went into Chemistry, as I was instructed to do, Dr. Edward Burgoine, one of the head people in the Chemistry Department, said to me one day, "What are you going to do in Chemistry?"

8.2. To this question I replied, "I am going to teach Chemistry in Mesa, Arizona." (I did not know at this time that in order for me to teach Chemistry, having Business as my minor, I would have to find a school where I could teach five full classes since the Business classes were handled by Business majors or related fields.)

8.3. "Forget it!" he said. I asked, "Why?" He answered, "Because there has not been an opening in Chemistry in Mesa for years. And even if a position would open up in Chemistry, there is a list a mile long of people who are trying to get into Mesa, as that is a choice area."

8.4. I looked him in the eye and without hesitation said, "Dr. Burgoine, if I teach Chemistry anywhere, it will be in Mesa." How I knew this is a miracle. I never questioned or had any doubts as to where I was going to teach.

G-9. *"Steel Wall" Number Seven*

9.1. When it came time for me to teach Chemistry in September, 1969, five full classes of Chemistry just happened to open up at Westwood High School where I just happened to be doing my student teaching. It is another story, too long to tell here, of how I chose to do my student teaching at this high school and how I was chosen to be the teacher of those five classes of Chemistry, but to me, that was a miracle. My "Plus-One" is this. Those five classes of Chemistry were only available for seven years. I learned about the blood protein research during the fifth year. During the seventh year the door opened to teach this research all over the United States, and I obtained a leave of absence to lecture full-time on these new discoveries. On the eighth year when I started to lecture full-time, the five classes I was teaching came to an end. Another high school opened in the area and the enrollment was split. Even if I had wanted to teach another year, they would not have had a place for me. The opportunity to teach the blood protein research had to come when it did. I will explain later how the door was opened for me to lecture full-time on this research.

G-10. *How I Learned About Protein and Death*

10.1. In September, 1969, I didn't understand what in the world I was doing teaching Chemistry, because I still had a burning desire to become a doctor to teach people how to take care of themselves. As I said earlier, it wasn't until 1974 during the fifth year of teaching that I learned protein could cause death within 24 hours. And this is how it happened.

10.2. I had a theory that pain was due to blocked circulation. So one day, I went across the hall to Mr. Chase who taught Biology, and said, "Mr. Chase, do you have a book that tells about circulation? I've just got to get into it." He said, "Here's a medical text; somebody gave it to me. Take it and see if you can use it."

10.3. When I opened the *Textbook of Medical Physiology* by Dr. Arthur C. Guyton, there it was! *We shall see that the removal of protein from the tissue spaces by our lymphatic system is an absolutely essential function without which we would die in about 24 hours.*

10.4. I couldn't believe my eyes! In my Pre-Med program, they talked a little about the lymphatic system, but nothing was ever said about protein causing death in our body if our lymphatic system couldn't remove it. I called the best surgeon in the area. When I talked to him to see if he could give me some information about this subject, he told me that he didn't know enough about the lymphatic system to carry on an intelligent conversation with me. My head was spinning! I went back to my office, The Naprapathic Clinic of Mesa. (From 1971 to 1974 I had gone to The American College of Natural Healing Sciences at night to become a D.N. [Naprapathic physician]). This is another amazing story. Also, in 1971, Bill and I had obtained a Master's Degree in Public School Administration at the University of Arizona. This had required driving six hours a day for 2 summers which is also another marvelous story. My office at the clinic was where I worked in the evenings to supplement my teaching salary.

10.5. It was hard to believe what was taking place! I was reading a well-known medical textbook published in 1961 which talked about death in the body due to protein, and I couldn't find anybody who had any knowledge whatsoever about what I was reading. This was thirteen years after the information was published! The more I found that nobody knew anything about protein and death, the greater I felt the responsibility coming upon me to teach this information to others. This feeling kept building up until it began to take hold of me just like the desire I had felt to go back to school and become a doctor. To obtain the knowledge concerning the blood proteins was the reason I went back to school. This was the knowledge that would enable me to "teach people how to take care of themselves." I soon realized my responsibility was to teach all who would listen about this discovery. This knowledge concerning life and death had been given to me, and I felt in my heart, even at that time, that this knowledge had to go to the nations of the earth.

G-11. *I Began To Teach About Protein Causing Death*

11.1. My teaching through lectures began in the home of Mr. and Mrs. Gurr, who owned a produce market west of Mesa. From then on, I did not lack for people to teach. They all had families, and loved ones; and everyone who heard it became as excited as I was about getting it to others. Finally, I got on the radio. Wow! The doors opened, and I began teaching in bigger halls everywhere.

G-12. *How The Door Opened To Lecture Full-Time*

12.1. Again, I went to the Lord and asked for help. I knew this message had to go to the nations of the earth, and I told him that if He wanted me get the message to all who would listen, it was going to be up to Him to make it possible for me to do so. In 1976, during my seventh year of teaching Chemistry, I saw some new scientific films. One of these films showed a person with electrodes from his brain to an electric train. He was able, by magnifying his thought waves, to stop, start, and speed up the electric train just by thinking about it. This film, along with one more which showed that electric energy was produced by the eyes opened my mind to a brand new concept. If there was constant electricity coming out of our bodies by way of our thought waves and the energy from our eyes, there *MUST* be electric generators inside the body producing that electricity. I found that discovery later, and it is now one of the SEVEN GOLDEN DISCOVERIES which establishes the fact that every living cell is an actual electric generator!

12.2. These films opened the door to the discovery which I made in about March, 1976, on how to use what I now call a LYMPHASIZER to convert mechanical energy into electric energy. This makes it possible for anyone to mentally direct the thought wave, to magnify electric energy into any area of the body to dissipate the clustered proteins to relieve pain and cause healing to take place. (This is similar to what Dr. Waltz is doing in N.Y. with electrodes.) This discovery is now called, the Bio-Electric "Gentle Bounce for Health." This is the discovery that I showed to the manufacturers in my office at the Naprapathic Clinic in Mesa, Arizona, in about May of 1976. And this is how the door opened to lecture full-time, beginning the end of my seventh year of teaching Chemistry. I believed with all my heart that the Lord gave me this discovery to help get the BLOOD PROTEIN RESEARCH to the nations of the earth. In the writing of this manuscript, I did not know that I would be telling this story. However, I feel to testify that the Lord has helped me to write this book. It is not just "my doings"

G-13. How I Was Given Help To Write This Book

13.1. Many times I have tried to write this book, but I could not do it! By myself I could not write this material! Many people have tried to get me to write this book for a long time. Mainly, Al Carter, Jerry and Maple Hinkle, Jerome Cook, Frank Angelo, Dr. Morton Walker, Anna Short, Sarah Glick, Scott Forsyth, Karol and Delmont Truman, Dean Black, Kim Asey, Stan Malstrom and many others. I knew I had to have someone to help me to write the educational materials for The World-Wide-Self H.E.L.P. Program. I kept thinking of my very dear friend, Billy, who was head basketball coach at the Franklin High School in West Virginia, so I called him, telling him that I needed his help to write the educational material for this program.

13.2. He told me if I had called him at any other time he

would not have been able to come. He then told me that he had to write the story of his life before he could come. He also told me that he felt the Lord had instructed him to write a book called "The Golden Seven Plus One"; but that the name of this book meant nothing to him.

13.3. I told him at that time about the seven major discoveries that I had been lecturing on, and we sort of laughed about this at the time. When I called him later, it was after I realized that I had THE FORMULA for the Cause of Loss of Energy and Death at the Cell Level. I had been talking about it for a long time but it wasn't until the day that I was to lecture in Seattle, Washington, on June 19, 1980, that the importance of what I have been saying was opened to my understanding.

G-14. *The Day I Knew I Had "The Formula"*

12.1. It came to me in a flash. All at once, I knew that I had the scientific formula for the Cause of Loss of Energy and Death at the Cell Level, and that it was as important if not greater than $E = MC^2$, which is the Theory of Relativity discovered by Einstein. $E = MC^2$ means Energy equals Mass times the Speed of Light Squared. The formula which I had developed showed that Trapped Plasma Protein around the cells produces excess fluid and excess sodium around the cells which reduces the Electric Energy produced by the cells and damages or kills the cells.

12.2. That presentation in Seattle was one of the most exciting lectures I have ever given. I became so excited that I had to change my entire lecture to center around the FORMULA. There were almost 200 people in the audience. Jerry and Maple Hinkle, who have done a great deal to promote the BLOOD PROTEIN RESEARCH, were my sponsors. After the lecture was over, Jerry was excited, and so was I! All the people, even those who had heard me before, were enthused about this FORMULA.

G-15. *How This Book Was Named*

15.1. The next time I called Bill to check with him about coming out to help me write, I told him that I had the FORMULA for the Cause of Loss of Energy and Death at the Cell Level. He turned to Gennis and explained to her what I had said and she replied to Bill, "There's your Golden Seven Plus One." Bill then passed on to me what Gennis had said, "Maybe that's The Golden Seven Plus One." There was a big question in my mind for a second, and then I thought and exclaimed for joy!

15.2. "WOW! The Golden Seven Plus One. That's it, Bill! That's it!"

15.3. After Bill arrived on June 30, 1980, we talked about this for quite a while. We couldn't get over what was taking place. Bill was given instructions to write a book called The Golden Seven Plus One, and now here he was writing this all down on paper, acting as my scribe.

15.4. The principles and concepts contained in this book are the foundation upon which preventive medicine must be based. They are the keys to health; the principles and concepts which must be obeyed if we are to establish peace throughout the world!

G-16. *What Happened When I Tried To Write The Original Manuscript*

16.1. Since Bill had been writing as my scribe, we came to know beyond a shadow of a doubt that he was meant to be here at that time and act as scribe in doing exactly what he was commissioned to do.

16.2. On one occasion, Bill left to go for a walk at the end of a very tiring day. I decided I would write a few more pages, as I didn't feel I was finished yet. I wrote about three pages which I thought were pretty good. The next morning, we got up to begin our day's work as usual. I was to dictate the original manuscript and Bill was to act as the scribe. We looked over the three pages that I had written the night before. They were terrible! In fact, so terrible, that I took them and tore them into pieces, saying to Bill, "This is what happens every time I try to write this book. I have been able to dictate it to you, but I can't write it. Bill, no wonder the Lord told you to write this book."

16.3. This story is almost impossible to believe. I do not believe anyone could have taken Bill's place. He acted as a true scribe, sitting for hours not saying a word, giving me time to concentrate and ponder until I knew what should come next.

The story of The Golden Seven Plus One began when Bill came into my home in 1958 and I inspired him to go back to school to become a coach; and it hasn't ended yet. Bill is writing a history of his life in a book that gives his story behind this book.

16.4. This is a true story of his life. Even though he was born with what some would call serious physical handicaps--he became a coach who is respected nationwide. His story is almost impossible to believe, also.

16.5. All I can say now is, if you believe the principles and concepts that are given in this book, you've got to believe the story of how and why it was produced. Bernard Tanner later played a big role in making this book possible.

16.6. May I end this story by saying that I do not take credit for the writing of this book, for I am only doing what I feel the Lord wants me to do, and I am willing to give my life, if necessary, to get the BLOOD PROTEIN RESEARCH to you. I hope and pray you now have a desire to help get it to others.

H. "SPECIAL" ACKNOWLEDGMENT AND APPRECIATION TO OTHERS WHO HAVE HELPED TO MAKE THE GOLDEN SEVEN PLUS ONE POSSIBLE

1. As many of you have heard me say in the lectures I have given, it is a great priviledge and honor for me to be able to share The Blood Protein Research which I know, beyond a shadow of a doubt, I have been able to learn only with the help of my Father in Heaven. Therefore, all the honor and glory must be given to Him.

2. I can testify that without the help of my family, it would have been impossible for me to spend weeks at a time away from home lecturing in city after city for a period which is now going on six years.

3. First goes appreciation to my angel wife, Johna May, who has supported me without complaining. Thanks also to my ten children, eight of which are still at home, for their support. A special thanks goes to the older children because theirs was the greater sacrifice. I also have a great appreciation for the fact that I have been able to teach the principles and concepts pertaining to "The Art of Lymphasizing" to my family, as I have learned them. This total experience has been a great blessing

to all of us; for I know that my children as well as my wife count the understanding of the principles and the concepts contained in this book as one of the greatest blessings they have ever received.

4. I also must acknowledge other members of my family, especially my mother, Irma Hansen West, and my father who died from an automobile accident when he was 82 years of age. Without the example of their lives and the things that they taught me, I would not be here; my sister, Mildred, and her husband Roland Wiseman; and Bernard and Jo Tanner, who provided us finances and with a home where Billy G. Gonzales and I could have privacy in writing the original manuscript.

5. To give personal recognition beyond this would be impossible, for I would have to give recognition to the teachers, the schools, the colleges; all the scientists and medical doctors for their knowledge and discoveries in this area; to all of the companies who manufacture the LYMPHASIZERS and to all the distributors who have labored long and hard. Many have taken me from city to city, for a week and sometimes two at a time, providing me with a place to eat and sometimes, even arranging for the payment of lecture halls and at their own expense doing a great deal of publicity by way of fliers, newspaper ads, and setting up radio talk shows and T.V. appointments.

6. Without the help of all the people who have been and are continually being involved in helping to get this message to others, and also without the help of thousands of others, who have been willing to donate to make it possible to take this World-Wide Family Health Education Program from its infancy to where it is today; yes, without the help of all these people and the others who helped in the very beginning, this book, *The Golden Seven Plus One*, which contains the principles and concepts which, if followed, will help people conquer disease and bring health and peace to the nations of the earth, could not have been written.

7. We therefore call upon all who have the opportunity, to help get this book into the homes of families throughout the world; that they will put the principles and concepts that are taught in this book above all prejudices they may have towards any race, color, creed, or religion; and this they will do, if they truly believe in the principles and concepts that are presented herein.

8. Let us all join together with one goal in mind as far as this

work is concerned; and that is to bring health and establish peace throughout the world.

9. I would like to end this book by again giving you the words of the song, "Let There Be Peace on Earth", which I believe were inspired by our Father in Heaven; and we hereby offer this book with the hope and faith that these words will become a reality in the not-too-distant future.

> *Let there be peace on earth,*
> *And let it begin with me.*
> *Let there be peace on earth,*
> *The peace that was meant to be.*
> *With God as our Father,*
> *Brothers all are we.*
> *Let me walk with my brother*
> *In perfect harmony.*
> *Let peace begin with me,*
> *Let this be the moment now,*
> *With every step I take,*
> *Let this be my solemn vow.*
> *To take each moment,*
> *And live each moment in peace*
> *Eternally.*
> *Let there be peace on earth,*
> *And let it begin with me.*
> > *--Sy Miller and Jill Jackson*

I offer this book to the world with the desire to help make the words of this song come true.

> *Sincerely, Dr. C. Samuel West, D.N., N.D.*
> *Chemist & Lymphologist*

APPENDIX A

Excerpts From
The Dietary Goals For The United States

Dr. West's Statements Regarding
The Three Page Forward

Senator Percy's Three Page Forward To The
Second Edition Of The Dietary Goals

95th Congress
1st Session   COMMITTEE PRINT

DIETARY GOALS FOR THE UNITED STATES

PREPARED BY THE STAFF OF THE
SELECT COMMITTEE ON NUTRITION
AND HUMAN NEEDS
UNITED STATES SENATE

FEBRUARY 1977

Printed for the use of the Select Committee on Nutrition
and Human Needs

U.S. GOVERNMENT PRINTING OFFICE
WASHINGTON, D.C.: 1977

For sale by the Superintendent of Documents, U. S. Government Printing Office
Washington, D.C. 20402

Stock No. 052-070-03913-2 /Catalog No. Y 4.N95:D 63/3

**(Italics added by this author to emphasize certain
statements in this report.)**

FOREWORD

The purpose of this report is to point out that the eating patterns of this century represent as critical a public health concern as any now before us.

We must acknowledge and recognize that the public is confused about what to eat to maximize health. If we as a Government want to reduce health costs and maximize the quality of life for all Americans, we have an obligation to provide practical guides to the individual consumer as well as set national dietary goals for the country as a whole.

Such an effort is long over-due. Hopefully, this study will be a first major step in that direction.

I would like to thank Mr. Nick Mottern of the Committee staff for his extraordinary effort and the high degree of professionalism he used in the preparation of this publication.

GEORGE McGOVERN,
Chairman.

In addition to acting as a practical guide to promote good eating habits, this report, hopefully, will also serve as a catalyst for Government and industry action to facilitate the achievement of the recommended dietary goals. *Without Government and industry commitment to good nutrition, the American people will continue to eat themselves to poor health.* Government and industry have a responsibility to respond to the findings of the report. Action is needed to determine how changes can be made regarding the content of nutritional information provided to the public; the kinds of foods produced; how foods are processed and advertised; and the selection of foods offered by eating establishments. *Our national health depends on how well and how quickly Government and industry respond.*

CHARLES H. PERCY,
Ranking Minority Member.

(v)

SELECT COMMITTEE ON NUTRITION AND HUMAN NEEDS

GEORGE McGOVERN, South Dakota, *Chairman*

HERMAN E. TALMADGE, Georgia	CHARLES H. PERCY, Illinois
EDWARD M. KENNEDY, Massachusetts	ROBERT DOLE, Kansas
GAYLORD NELSON, Wisconsin	HENRY BELLMON, Oklahoma
ALAN CRANSTON, California	RICHARD S. SCHWEIKER, Pennsylvania
HUBERT H. HUMPHREY, Minnesota	MARK O. HATFIELD, Oregon

ALAN J. STONE, *Staff Director*
MARSHALL L. MATZ, *General Counsel*

(II)

1 & 2
[Press Conference, Friday, January 14, 1977, Room 457, Dirksen Senate Office Building]

STATEMENT OF SENATOR GEORGE McGOVERN ON THE PUBLICATION OF DIETARY GOALS FOR THE UNITED STATES

Good morning.

The purpose of this press conference is to release a Nutrition Committee study entitled *Dietary Goals for the United States,* and to explain why we need such a report.

I should note from the outset that this is the first comprehensive statement by any branch of the Federal Government on risk factors in the American Diet.

The simple fact is that our diets have changed radically within the last 50 years, with great and often very harmful effects on our health. These dietary changes represent as great a threat to public health as smoking. *Too much fat, too much sugar or salt, can be and are linked directly to heart disease, cancer, obesity, and stroke, among other killer diseases.* In all, *six of the ten leading causes of death* in the United States *have been linked to our diet.*

Those of us within Government have an obligation to acknowledge this. The public wants some guidance, wants to know the *truth,* and *hopefully today we can lay the cornerstone for the building of better health for all Americans, through better nutrition.*

Last year every man, woman and child in the United States consumed 125 pounds of fat, and 100 pounds of sugar. As you can see from our displays, that's a formidable quantity of fat and sugar.

The consumption of soft drinks has more than doubled since 1960–displacing milk as the second most consumed beverage. In 1975, we drank on the average of 295 12 oz. cans of soda.

In the early 1900's almost 40 percent of our caloric intake came from fruit, vegetables and grain products. Today only a little more than 20 percent of calories comes from these sources.

My hope is that this report will perform a function similar to that of the Surgeon General's Report on Smoking. Since that report, we haven't eliminated the hazards of smoking, nor have people stopped smoking because of it. But the cigarette industry has modified its products to reduce risk factors, and many people who would otherwise be smoking have stopped because of it.

The same progress can and must be made in matters of nutritional health, and this report sets forth the necessary plan of action:

    1. Six basic goals are set for changes in our national diet:

    2. Simple buying guides are recommended to help consumers attain these goals; and

    3. Recommendations are also made for action within Government and industry to better maximize nutritional health.

I hope this report will be useful to millions of Americans. In addition to providing simple and meaningful guidance in matters of diet, it should also encourage all those involved with growing, preparing, and processing food to give new consideration to the impact of their decision on the nation's health. There needs to be less confusion about what to eat and how our diet affects us.

With me this morning are three of the country's leading thinkers in the area of nutritional health. They have very graciously assisted the staff of the Select Committee in the preparation of this report. They will explain in greater detail its purpose and goals.

First, Dr. Mark Hegsted, Professor of Nutrition from the Harvard School of Public Health. Dr. Hegsted has a long and distinguished career in science, bringing conscience as well as great expertise to his work. Dr. Hegsted has worked very closely and patiently with the committee staff on this report, devoting many hours to review and counseling. He feels very strongly about the need for public education in nutrition and the need to alert the public to the consequences of our dietary trends. He will discuss these trends and their connection with our most killing diseases.

Following his presentaiton, Dr. Beverly Winikoff of the Rockefeller Foundation will discuss the changes necessary in food marketing and advertising practices if the consumer is to make more healthful food choices. Dr. Winikoff, who with Dr. Hegsted and Dr. Lee testified at our hearings in July, has also been extremely helpful in assisting the committee staff in preparing this report.

Dr. Philip Lee, the Director of the Health Policy Program at the University of California in San Francisco, and a former Assistant Secretary for Health, will conclude our presentation with a discussion of the costs of our current dietary trends. Dr.

Lee has also consulted with the committee staff on this report and has offered much encouragement.

Before Dr. Hegsted begins, I would also like to note that the staff has also received valuable assistance from Dr. Sheldon Margen, a nutritionist with the University of California in Berkeley, who is traveling outside the country today.

I want to thank each of these people personally for their help and their spirited concern for the public interest.

The Committee will continue its investigation into the connection between diet and health on February 1 and 2, when hearings will be held concentrating on problems of diet and heart disease and obesity.

After the presentation today we will be glad to answer questions.

3

[Press Conference, Friday, January 14, 1977, Room 457, Dirksen Senate Office Building]

STATEMENT OF DR. D.M. HEGSTED, PROFESSOR OF NUTRITION, HARVARD SCHOOL OF PUBLIC HEALTH BOSTON, MASS.

The diet of the American people has become increasingly rich --rich in meat, other sources of saturated fat and cholesterol, and in sugar. There will be people who will contest this statement. It has been pointed out repeatedly that total sugar use has remained relatively constant for a number of years. We would emphasize, however, that our total food consumption has fallen even though we still eat too much relative to our needs. Thus, the proportion of the total diet contributed by fatty and cholesterol-rich foods and by refined foods has risen. We might be better able to tolerate this diet if we were much more active physically, but we are a sedentary people.

It should be emphasized that this diet which affluent people generally consume is everywhere associated with a similar disease pattern--high rates of ischemic heart disease, certain forms of cancer, diabetes, and obesity. These are the major causes of death and disability in the United States. These so-called degenerative diseases obviously become more important now that infectious diseases are, relatively speaking, under good control. I wish to emphasize that these diseases undoubtedly have a complex etiology. It is not correct, strictly speaking, to say that they are caused by malnutrition but rather that an inappropriate diet contributes to their causation. Our genetic make-up contributes--not all people are equally susceptible. Yet those who are generally susceptible, most of us, are those who would profit most from an appropriate diet. Diet is one of the things that we can change if we want to.

There will undoubtedly be many people who will say we have not proven our point; we have not demonstrated that the dietary modifications we recommend will yield the dividends expected. We would point out to those people that the diet we eat today was not planned or developed for any particular purpose. It is a happenstance related to our affluence, the productivity of our farmers and the activities of our food industry. The risks associated with eating this diet are demonstrably large. The question to be asked, therefore, is not why should we change our diet but why not? What are the risks associated with eating less meat, less fat, less saturated fat, less cholesterol, less sugar, less salt, and more fruits, vegetables, unsaturated fat and cereal products--especially whole grain cereals. There are none that can be identified and important benefits can be expected.

Ischemic heart disease, cancer, diabetes and hypertension are the diseases that kill us. They are epidemic in our population. We cannot afford to temporize. We have an obligation to inform the public of the current state of knowledge and to assist the public in making the correct food choices. To do less is to avoid our responsibility.

5 & 6

[Press Conference, Friday, January 14, 1977, Room 457, Dirksen Senate Office Building]

STATEMENT OF DR. BEVERLY WINIKOFF, ROCKEFELLER FOUNDATION, NEW YORK, N.Y.

What are the implications of these dietary goals?

The fact that the goals can be stated in nutritional terms first and then mirrored in a set of behavioral changes impels a closer look at why Americans eat the way they do. What people eat is affected not only by what scientists know, or by what doctors tell them or even by what they themselves understand. It is affected by Government decisions in the area of agricultural policy, economic and tax policy, export and import policy, and involves questions of good production, transportation, processing, marketing, consumer choice, income and education;, as well as food availability and palatability. Nutrition, then, is the end result of pushes and pulls in many directions, a response to the multiple forces creating the "national nutrition environment."

Even "personal dietary preferences" are not immutable but interact with other forces in the environment and are influenced by them. People learn the patterns of their diet not only from the family and its sociocultural background, but from what is available in the marketplace and what is promoted both formally through advertising and informally through general availability in schools, restaurants, supermarkets, work places, airports, and so forth.

It is generally recognized with regard to the overall economic climate that both what the Government does do and what it does not do shape the arena in which other forces interact. This is also true with regard to nutrition. In determining the parameters of the socioeconomic system. Government also determines the nature of the national buffet. Government policy, then, must be made with full awareness of this responsibility.

It is increasingly obvious that if new knowledge is to result in new behaviors then people must be able to act, without undue obstacles, in accordance with the information that they learn. The problem of education for health as it has been practiced is that it has been in isolation, not to say oblivion, of the real pressures, expections, and norms of society which mold and constrain individual behavior. There must be some coordination between what people are taught to do and what they can do. Part of the responsibility for this coordination rests with the Government's evaluation and coordination of its own activities. Effective education must be accompanied by Government policies which make it easier, indeed likely, that an individual will change his or her lifestyle in accordance with the information offered.

At present, we see a situation in which the opposite is often the case. Nutrition and health education are offered at the same time as barrages of commericials for soft drinks, sugary snacks, high-fat foods, cigarettes and alcohol. We put candy machines in our schools, serve high-fat lunches to our children, and place cigarette machines in our work places. The American market-place provides easy access to sweet soft drinks, high sugar cereals, candies, cakes, and high-fat beef, and more difficult access to foods likely to improve national nutritional health.

This trend can be reversed by specific agricultural policies, pricing policies, and marketing policies, as well as the recommendations outlined in these "Dietary Goals for the United States."

In general, Americans have quite accurate perceptions of sound nutritional principles, as was demonstrated recently by a Harris poll conducted for the Mount Sinai Hospital in Chicago. However, people do lack understanding of the consequences of nutrition-related diseases. *There is a widespread and un-founded confidence in the ability of medical science to cure or mitigate the effects of such diseases once they occur. Appropriate public education must emphasize the unfortunate but clear limitations of current medical practice in curing the common killer diseases. Once hypertension, diabetes, arteriosclerosis or heart disease are manifest, there is, in reality, very little that medical science can do to return a patient to normal physiological function.* As awareness of this limitation increases, the importance of prevention will become all the more obvious.

But prevention is not possible solely through medical interventions. It is the responsibility of government at all levels to take the initiative in creating for Americans an appropriate nutritional atmosphere—one conducive to improvement in the health and quality of life for the American people.

7 & 8

[Press Conference, Friday, January 14, 1977, Room 457, Dirksen Senate Office Building]

STATEMENT OF DR. PHILIP LEE, PROFESSOR OF SOCIAL MEDICINE AND DIRECTOR, HEALTH POLICY PROGRAM, UNIVERSITY OF CALIFORNIA, SAN FRANCISCO, CALIF.

The publication of *Dietary Goals for the United States* by the Senate Select Committee on Nutrition and Human Needs is a major step forward in the development of a rational national health policy. The public health problems related to what we eat are pointed out in *Dietary Goals*. More important, the steps that can and should be taken by individuals, families, educators, health professions, industry and Government are made clear.

As a nation we have come to believe that medicine and medical technology can solve our major health problems. The role of such important factors as diet in cancer and heart disease has long been obscured by the emphasis on the conquest of these diseases through the miracles of modern medicine. Treatment not prevention, has been the order of the day.

The problems can never be solved merely by more and more medical care. The health of individuals and the health of the population is determined by a variety of biological (host), behavioral, sociocultural and environmental factors. None of these is more important than the food we eat. This simple fact and the importance of diet in health and disease is clearly recognized in *Dietary Goals for the United States.*

The Senate Select Committee on Nutrition and Human Needs has made four recommendations to encourage the achievement of the very sound dietary goals incorporated in the report. These are:

1. a large scale public nutrition education program involving the schools, food assistance programs, the Extension Service of the Department of Agriculture and the mass media;

2. mandatory food labeling for all foods;

3. the development of improved food processing methods for institutional and home use; and

4. expanded federal support for research in human nutrition.

It is important that *Dietary Goals for the United States* be made widely available because it is the only publication of its kind and it will be an invaluable resource for parents, school teachers, public health nurses, health educators, nutritionists, physicians and others who are involved in providing people with information about the food they eat.

The recommendations, if acted upon promptly by the Congress, can help individuals, families and those responsible for institutional food services (schools, hospitals) be better informed about the consequences of present dietary habits and practices. Moreover, they provide a practical guide for action to improve the unhealthy situation that exists.

The effective implementation of the Senate Select Committee recommendations and the proposed dietary goals could have

profound health and economic benefits. Not only would many
people lead longer and healthier lives but the reduced burden of
illness during the working lives of men and women would
reduce the cost of medical care and increase productivity.

What can be done to assure sustained and effective action on
these recommendations? First, the Congress can act to
appropriate the needed funds for the proposed programs. In
some instances, such as mandatory food labeling, it must also
enact the authorizing legislation. Second, the new Secretaries of
Agriculture and Health, Education, and Welfare can act as soon
as they take office to create a joint policy committee to address
the issues raised by the Senate Select Committee and provide a
means to assure that health considerations will no longer take a
back seat to economic considerations in our food and agriculture
policies. *Finally, our greatest bulwark against the interests that
have helped to create the present problems is an informed public.*

9, 10 & 11

Part I

DIETARY GOALS FOR THE UNITED STATES

INTRODUCTION

During this century, the composition of the average diet in the
United States has changed radically. Complex carbohydrates--
fruit, vegetables and grain products--which were the mainstay
of the diet, now play a minority role. At the same time, fat and
sugar consumption have risen to the point where these two
dietary elements alone now comprise at least 60 percent of total
calorie intake, up from 50 percent in the early 1900's.

In the view of doctors and nutritionists consulted by the Select
Committee, these and other changes in the diet amount to a wave
of malnutrition--of both over-and under-consumption--that may
be as profoundly damaging to the Nation's health as the
widespread contagious diseases of the early part of the century.

The over-consumption of fat, generally, and saturated fat in
particular, as well as cholesterol, sugar, salt and alcohol have
been related to six of the ten leading causes of death: Heart
disease, cancer, cerebrovascular disease, diabetes, arterio-

sclerosis and cirrhosis of the liver.

In his testimony at the Select Committee's July 1976 hearings on the relationship of diet to disease, Dr. D. Mark Hegsted of Harvard School of Public Health, said:

I wish to stress that there is a great deal of evidence and it continues to accumulate which strongly implicates and, in some instances, proves that the major causes of death and disability in the United States are related to the diet we eat. I include coronary artery disease which accounts for nearly half of the deaths in the United States, several of the most important forms of cancer, hypertension, diabetes and obesity as well as other chronic diseases.

In 1924, Marc LaLonde, Canada's Minister of National Health and Welfare said:

Even such a simple question as whether one should severely limit his consumption of butter and eggs can be a subject of endless scientific debate.

Faced with conflicting scientific opinions of this kind, it would be easy for health educators and promoters to sit on their hands; it certainly makes it easy for those who abuse their health to find a real "scientific" excuse.

But many of Canada's health problems are sufficiently pressing that action has to be taken even if all scientific evidence is not in.

Based on (1) the Select Committee's July 1976 hearings on the relationship of diet to disease and its 1974 National Nutrition Policy hearings, (2) guidelines established by governmental and professional bodies in the United States and at least eight other nations (Appendix B), and (3) a variety of expert opinions, the following dietary goals are recommended for the United States. Although genetic and other individual differences mean that these guidelines may not be applicable to all, there is substantial evidence indicating that they will be generally beneficial.

[2]Statistics from reports and testimony presented to the Select Committee's National Nutritional Policy hearings, June 1974, appearing in National Nutrition Policy Study, 1974, Pt. 6, June 21, 1974, heart disease, p. 2633; high blood pressure, p. 2529, diabetes, p. 2523.

12

U.S. DIETARY GOALS

1. Increase carbohydrate consumption to account for 55 to 60 percent of the energy (caloric) intake.
2. Reduce overall fat consumption from approximately 40 to

30 percent energy intake.

3. Reduce saturated fat consumption to account for about 10 percent of total energy intake; and balance that with poly-unsaturated and mono-unsaturated fats, which should account for about 10 percent of energy intake each.

4. Reduce cholesterol consumption to about 300 mg. a day.

5. Reduce sugar consumption by about 40 percent to account for about 15 percent of total energy intake.

6. Reduce salt consumption by about 50 to 85 percent to approximately 3 grams a day.

13

The Goals Suggest the Following Changes in Food Selection and Preparation

1. Increase consumption of fruits and vegetables and whole grains.

2. Decrease consumption of meat and increase consumption of poultry and fish.

3. Decrease consumption of foods high in fat and partially substitute poly-unsaturated fat for saturated fat.

4. Substitute non-fat milk for whole milk.

5. Decrease consumption of butterfat, eggs and other high cholesterol sources.

6. Decrease consumption of sugar and foods high in sugar content.

7. Decrease consumption of salt and foods high in salt content.

71 & 72

APPENDIX A

BENEFITS FROM HUMAN NUTRITION RESEARCH

[By C. Edith Weir]

This report is part of a study conducted at the direction of the Agricultural Research Policy Advisory Committee, U.S. Department of Agriculture. A joint task group representing the State Agricultural Experiment Stations and the U.S. Department of Agriculture was assigned the responsibility for making the study. Task group members were:

Dr. Virginia Trotter, co-chairman, dean, College of Home Economics, University of Nebraska; Dr. Steven C. King, co-chairman, associate director, Science and Education Staff, U. S. Department of Agriculture; Dr. Walter L. Fishel, assistant professor, Department of Agriculture and Applied Economics, University of Minnesota; Dr. H. Wayne Bitting, program planning and evaluation staff, Agricultural Research Service, U. S. Department of Agriculture; Dr. C. Edith Weir, Assistant Director, Human Nutrition Research Division, Agricultural Research Service, U. S. Department of Agriculture.

Better health, a longer active lifespan, and greater satisfaction from work, family and leisure time are among the benefits to be obtained from improved diets and nutrition. Advances in nutrition knowledge and its application during recent decades have played a major role in reducing the number of infant and maternal deaths, deaths from infectious diseases, particularly among children, and in extending the productive lifespan and life expectancy. Significant benefits are possible both from new knowledge of nutrient and food needs and from more complete application of existing knowlege. The nature and magnitude of these benefits is estimated in Table 1. Potential benefits may accrue from alleviating nutrition-related health problems, from increased individual performance and satisfactions and increased efficiency in food services. A vast reservoir of health and economical benefits can be made available by research yet to be done on human nutrition.

Major health problems are diet related.--Most all of the health problems underlying the leading causes of death in the United States (Fig.1) could be modified by improvements in diet. The relationship of diet to these health problems and others is discussed in greater detail later in this report. Death rates for many of these conditions are higher in the U.S. than in other countries of comparable economic development. Expenditures for health care in the U.S. are skyrocketing, accounting for 67.2 billion dollars in 1970--or 7.0 percent of the entire U.S. gross national product.

The real potential from improved diet is preventative.--Existing evidence is inadequate for estimating potential benefits from improved diets in terms of health. Most nutritionists and clinicians feel that the real potential from improved diet is preventative in that it may defer or modify the development of a disease state so that a clinical condition does not develop.

SOURCE. Human Nutrition Research Division, Agricultural Research

Service, U. S. Department of Agriculture. Issued August 1971 by Science and Education Staff, United States Department of Agriculture, Washington, D.C.

The major research thrust, nationwide, has been on the role of diet in treating health problems after they have developed. This approach has had limited success. USDA research emphasis has been placed on food needs of normal, healthy persons and findings from this work contributed much of the existing knowledge on their dietary requirements.

Benefits would be shared by all.--Benefits from better nutrition, made possible by improved diets, would be available to the entire population. Each age, sex, ethnic, economic, and geographic segment would be benefited. The lower economic and nonwhite population groups would benefit most from effective application of current knowledge.

These savings are only a small part of what might be accomplished for the entire population from research yet to be done. Some of the improvements can be expressed as dollar benefits to individuals or to the nation. The social and personal benefits are harder to quantify and describe. It is difficult to place a dollar figure on the avoidance of pain or the loss of a family member; satisfactions from healthy, emotionally adjusted families; career achievement; and the opportunity to enjoy leisure time.

Major health benefits are long range.--Predictions of the extent to which diet may be involved in the development of various health problems have been based on current knowledge of metabolic pathways of nutrients, but primarily of abnormal metabolic pathways developed by persons in advanced stages of disease. There is little understanding of when or why these metabolic changes take place. The human body is a complex and very adaptive mechanism. For most essential metabolic processes alternate pathways exist which can be utilized in response to physiological, diet, or other stress. Frequently, a series of adjustments take place and the ultimate result does not become apparent for a long time, even years, when a metabolite such as cholesterol accumulates. *Early adjustment of diet could prevent the development of undesirable long-range effects. Minor changes in diet and food habits instituted at an early age might well avoid the need for major changes, difficult to adopt later in life.*

END OF FIRST EDITION

Dr. West's Statement Regarding The Following Three-Page Forward Of The Second Edition Which Attempted To Destroy The Dietary Goals For The United States.

There were five positive forwards and one negative forward in the front of the second edition of The Dietary Goals. The five positive ones were written by Senator Robert Dole, Senator George McGovern, Dr. D. M. Hegsted, Dr. Beverly Winikoff, and Dr. Phillip Lee. The one negative forward was written by Senator Charles H. Percy. How Richard Schweiker and Edward Zorinsky got their names on Percy's forward is a mystery. This whole forward was written in first person by Percy. Maybe it's because he needed some moral support. Read Percy's statement in the first edition again.

In reading the second edition we find that Senator George McGovern, Dr. Hegsted, Dr. Beverly Winikoff, and Dr. Philip Lee did not change their statements. Charles Percy is the only member of the committee who did. The question is — Why?

Senator Percy starts off good in the second edition but in selecting a few opinions to supposedly give both viewpoints, for some reason Percy cleverly tries to completely discredit The Dietary Goals for the United States. Notice who's viewpoints he emphasizes.

This government document does not speak kindly of the American Medical Association. And the statement by the A.M.A. in Percy's report proved the statements made in this government document, concerning the inability of current medical science to deal with the crippling and killer diseases, to be correct.

Also, as this book proves, Percy made a very misleading statement when he said, *"...science cannot at this time insure that an altered diet will provide protection from certain killer diseases such as heart disease and cancer."* That statement was not only unwise; it was also foolish.

SUPPLEMENTAL FOREWORD BY SENATORS PERCY, SCHWEIKER, AND ZORINSKY

In my Foreword to the first edition of "Dietary Goals for the United States," I stated that Government and industry have a responsibility to respond to the findings of the report. They have done just that. The response has been vigorous and constructive. The original "Dietary Goals" report, though controversial, has helped focus public and professional attention on the need for continuous assessment of the current state of the art in the nutrition field. Furthermore, the report has stimulated debate and research on unresolved issues, and has helped us progress toward the formulation of a national nutrition policy based on sound dietary practices.

The second edition of "Dietary Goals," the product of commendable staff work, greatly improves upon earlier efforts by refining some of the original dietary goals, by adding sections on obesity and alcohol consumption and by more fully representing the scientific controversies which exist both with respect to the setting of dietary guidelines and to the substance of the goals themselves. I am most grateful for the help we have received in connection with this edition. I have long believed in the merits of dietary moderation, maintaining ideal body weight and avoiding excess, especially so called empty calories. To me this emphasis, taken together with regular physical exercise, are as sound public health measures as I know.

Despite the many improvements reflected in this second edition, however, I have serious reservations about certain aspects of the report. After hearing additional testimony from witnesses, discussing these goals with a number of experts and reading rather convincing correspondence from a variety of informed sources,, I have become increasingly aware of the lack of consensus among nutrition scientists and other health professionals regarding (1) the question of whether advocating a specific restriction of dietary cholesterol intake to the general public is warranted at this time, (2) the question of what would be the demonstrable benefits to the individual and the general public, especially in regard to coronary heart disease, from implementing the dietary practices recommended in this report and (3) the accuracy of some of the goals and recommendations given the inadequacy of current food intake data.

The record clearly reflects extreme diversity of scentific opinion on these questions. Many such conflicting opinions are included in the Committee's recent publication, "Dietary Goals for the United States—Supplemental Views." Since it is possible that this diversity might be overlooked simply because few people will be able to take the time to read through the voluminous (869 pages) "Supplemental Views" publication, I have selected a few opinions representative of both viewpoints on the issues in controversy.

On the question of whether or not a restriction of dietary cholesterol intake for the general populace is a wise thing to recommend at this time, the Inter-Society Commission for Heart Disease Resourses (1972), the American Heart Association (1973), and several other expert panels suggest a reduction of dietary cholesterol to less than 300 mg per day.

Yet, in October 1977 the Canadian Department of National Health and Welfare reversed its earlier position and concluded in a National Dietary Position that:

> Evidence is mounting that dietary cholesterol may not be important to the great majority of people.... Thus, a diet restricted in cholesterol would not be necessary for the general population.

A similar conclusion was drawn in 1974 by the Committee on Medical Aspects of Food in its report to Great Britain's Department of Health and Social Security.

Between these points of view are groups such as the New Zealand Heart Foundation which recommends a range of daily cholesterol intake, the maximum of which roughly equals the current average American intake.

Because of these divergent viewpoints, it is clear that science has not progressed to the point where we can recommend to the general public that cholesterol intake be limited to a specified amount. The variances between different individuals are simply too great.

A similar divergence of scientific opinion on the question of whether dietary change can help the heart illustrates that science can not yet verify with any certainty that coronary heart disease will be prevented or delayed by the diet recommended in this report.

For example, Dr. Jeremiah Stamler, chairman of the Department of Preventive Medicine, Northwestern School of

Medicine, strongly believes thousands of premature coronary heart disease deaths can "probably be prevented annually through dietary change." However, Dr. E. H. Ahrens, Jr., Professor of Medicine at Rockefeller University, told the Select Committee in March:

Advice to the public on changing its dietary habits in hope of reducing the rate of new events of coronary heart disease is premature, hence unwise.

The same polarity is evidenced when one compares the view of William Kannel, Framington Heart Study's Director, the Dietary Goals, "could have a substantial effect in reducing" coronary heart disease, with the opinion of Vanderbilt University's Dr. George Mann that "no diet therapy has been shown effective for the prevention or treatment" of that disease.

The American Medical Association in an April 18, 1977, letter to the Nutrition Committee states:

The evidence for assuming that benefits to be derived from the adoption of such universal dietary goals as set forth in the report is not conclusive and ... potential for harmful effects ... would occur through adoption of the proposed national goals.

This impressive lack of agreement among scientists on the efficacy of dietary change was also noted by the National Heart, Blood and Lung Institute's Dr. Robert Levy, when he observed that there are "bona fide scientific people coming out on both sides of the issue." and by Health Undersecretary Theodore Cooper's remarks last year to the Committee that a "great deal more nutrition work (is needed) ... before one can speak with greater certainty concerning large-scale application" of dietary change. Because of this continuing debate, I feel great care must be taken to accurately inform the public about the benefits of the diet proposed in this report.

In fact, because I recognize many will read or hear only about the Dietary Goals and Food Selection pages (pp, 4 and 5) of this Second Edition, I feel the American public would be in a better position to exercise freedom of dietary choice if it were stated in bold print on the Goals and Food Selection pages that *the value of dietary change remains controversial and that science cannot at this time insure that an altered diet will provide improved protection from certain killer diseases such as heart disease and cancer.*

Finally, I want to emphasize the limitations, acknowledged in this edition, in setting goals and food selection recommendations on the basis of food disappearance data, because of the difference between disappearance data, household food consumption data and intake data, which are discussed in the Preface. These data were used because they are the best available at this time. However, in some cases they may not accurately reflect actual food intake. For example, the recommendations to reduce animal fat intake from the present level shown by food disappearance data must be viewed with some reservation because food disappearance data does not adjust for fat loss from retail preparation of meat, fat trimming before and after cooking, fat loss during cooking and tablewaste. The same case could be made for vegetable fat because many vegetable oils used in cooking are discarded and not consumed. Better food intake information, expected shortly, may produce more reliable and perhaps altered recommendations.

In conclusion, I recognize the desirability of providing dietary guidance to the public and in helping the consumer become more responsible for every day health status. In my judgment, however, the best way to do this is to fully inform the public not only about what is known, but also about what remains controversial regarding cholesterol, the benefits of dietary change, and the reliability of current food intake data. Only then, will it be possible for the individual consumer to respond optimally to the Dietary Goals in this report.

After the Nutrition Committee staff is transferred to the Senate Agriculture Committee's Subcommittee on Nutrition, I hope they will, in cooperation with the Human Resourses Subcommittee on Health and Scientific Research continue to review the science and revise Dietary Goals in order that we may continue to progress toward the formulation of national dietary guidelines based on sound dietary practices.

CHARLES H. PERCY,
Ranking Minority Member.
RICHARD SCHWEIKER.
EDWARD ZORINSKY.

APPENDIX B

Food Shopping List

Sample Lunch And Dinner Menu

Recipes To Help With Transition

Directions For Dehydrating Foods

Also

How Hypoglycemia Can Turn
Into Diabetes, High Blood Pressure
And Heart Disease

Suggested FOOD SHOPPING LIST to feed a family of three
for one week. (Adjust for your family)

FOOD SHOPPING LIST

VEGETABLES
>   2 lbs. carrots (juice or grate and eat raw)
>   2 lbs. beets (grate and eat raw)
>   6 lbs. spinach (for salad)
>   2 lbs. ruffled kale
>   2 lbs. collard greens
>   3 lbs. string beans
>   1 head romaine lettuce
>   3 lbs. pole beans
>   2 lbs. brussel sprouts
>   4 medium butternut squash
>   or 2 large butternut squash
>   12 ears yellow corn (sweet) (eat some raw)
>   3 large egg plant
>   4 large sweet potatoes (raw or baked)
>   4 yams (raw in salads)
>   7 large tomatoes (raw in salads)
>   1 or 2 green peppers
>   2 bunches scallions
>   3 lg. reg. onion
>   1 bunch celery
>   2 cucumbers
>   2 bags radishes
>   2 lbs. yellow squash
>   1 head cabbage
>   5 lbs. potatoes (bake or eat raw)
>   2 lbs. turnips (yellow)

FRUIT
>   12 oranges
>   12 red apples
>   12 yellow apples
>   12 tangerines
>   6 lemons
>   12 bananas

FOR TRANSITION

1 doz. eggs
Nuts (Almonds and eat sparingly)
1 qt. real mayonnaise
2 lbs. salt free soybean margarine
   (obtain at health food store)
Bio-salt, Vege-Salt, kelp, Jensen's broth or
   seasoning.
1 small bottle apple cider vinegar--Giant
3 lbs. honey
Cheese (homemade if possible)

SAMPLE LUNCH OR DINNER VEGETABLE MENU

Mon.	Spinach
	Butternut Squash
	Eggplant
	Salad
	Soybean Patties or baked
	  potato
		Fri.	String Beans
			Rice
			Squash (yellow)
			Salad
			Sweet Potatoes
			  (raw or baked)

Tues.	Kale Potato Brussel Sprouts Whole Wheat Muffins	Sat.	Turnips Corn Green Vegetable Salad Baked Potato
Wed.	Collard Greens Sweet Potatoes (baked or raw) String Beans Salad Whole Wheat Rolls	Sun.	Soup Baked Potatoes Tomatoes Celery Onion Carrots String Beans Yams
Thur.	String Beams Rice Squash (yellow) Salad		

NOTES:

   1. Fast one day out of the week to clean out your system.
Try 1-3 T. unsulphured Grandma's Molasses, or pure maple
syrup, with 1/2 lemon in 8 oz. warm water first thing in the
morning. You can also fast for 1-3 weeks on this drink.

SUGGESTED RECIPES TO HELP WITH
THE TRANSITION PROGRAM

   1. Here is a sample of recipes that some people enjoy. Most
are good, but some of them are meant to be used only when you
want to "have a ball." Also it is best not to cook with salt. If
necessary, be sure you use a salt that has potassium in it. Use a
vegetable salt, a natural seasoning or Bio-salt when you eat.

SPROUTS: Almost any seed, grain or legume can be sprouted.
   Try alfalfa, mung bean, lentil, soy bean, chickpea,
   sunflower seeds, wheat, radish, etc.
   1. Soak seeds about 8 hours in warm water.
   2. Rinse and place in sprouter tray (jar covered with
      cheesecloth or nylon stocking remnant works fine.)
   3. Rinse 2 or 3 times a day and drain. Soy beans must be
      rinsed real often.)
   4. In 3 to 5 days sprouts are ready to eat. Rinse and store in
      refrigerator. Seeds sprout better in a dark place, but
      don't forget they are there and neglect rinsing them.

REJUVELAC - a mild barley or wheat drink: Better than
   yogurt. Puts enzymes back into the body that cooked foods
   do not have. Helps colon get rid of disease producing
   bacteria. Proteins are broken down into Amino Acids.

   1. Take 1 cup wheat kernels (or barley) and place in 2 cups
      Spring Water.
   2. Discard dead seeds that float on top.
   3. Soak the wheat berries or barley for 24 to 48 hours.
   4. Pour off water and use it for drinking or store in frig for
      later use.
   5. Drink the water that becomes fermented, REJUVELAC,
      for 4 days, than discard wheat berries or barley.

PINK SAUERKRAUT:

red cabbage   l tsp thyme 3-4 ground juniper berries
1 white cabbage 1 tsp dill   1 tsp kelp

Shred cabbage and grind spices. Pound cabbage for 10-15 minutes with wooden mortar until each piece appears translucent. Put cabbage in crock layering with mixed ground spices. Cover cabbage with large outer leaves of cabbage head. Cover with plate with a heavy weight on it. Let it sit for one week to naturally ferment.

HOMEMADE GRAPENUTS: *by Fannie Schrock*

1½ cups honey
10 cups whole wheat flour
1 teaspoon (Bio-salt)
¾ cup melted butter
7 cups buttermilk
3 (rounded) teaspoons soda, added to milk
1 tablespoon vanilla
   Mix dry ingredients, then buttermilk and soda, honey, last butter and flavoring. Mix well. Dough should be fairly thick. Bake at 325°F. for 1½ hours.

The URIAS AND MARRIETTA MILLER HOMEMADE CHEESE RECIPE:

1. Obtain cheese rennet tablets from Family Health Foods, R. Rt., Authur, Illinois, 61911, 10 tab., for $2.13.
2. Put three gal. of milk in stainless steel container.
3. Put container in hot water until film forms on top.
4. Dissolve 1/4 tab. in water and stir into milk. (Keep container in hot water)
5. Let sit until milk gets thick while container is still in hot water.
6. Cut with knife into small pieces and stir so whey can come to the top.
7. Dip as much whey out as possible.
8. Toward the end, work with your hand, break it apart, so more whey comes out and starts to get hard.

9. Add ¼ cup *Bio-Salt and mix with your hands (DO NOT SQUEEZE, just break it up as you mix.
10. Put in a cheesecloth.
11. Place in your homemade press. (A cut off chlorox bottle with holes punched from inside to outside so cheese can drain).
12. Put a plate on top with a weight on it.
13. If it ends up too wet, the water was too cold. If it is too dry, the water is too hot.
15. Practice makes perfect.
16. *For more information on Bio-salt, contact: The Biochemic Center, R.R. No. 1, Anola, Manitoba, Canada ROE OAO.

ETHEL'S MEATLESS PATTIES:

Mix cooked brown rice, soaked alfalfa seed (not sprouted), eggs, onions, cayenne and a little Bio-salt or Jensen's veg. broth.

BASIC SEED SAUCE:

½ cup Sunflower Seeds (ground in blender or nut grinder)
½ cup Sesame Seed
2 cups REjuvelac or water

To the mixed ground seed, add water a little at a time in a blender or Vita-Mix until smooth. Add:

1 tsp basil   1 beet (puréed in blender)
1 tsp thyme   1/8 tsp capsicum (or to taste)
2 T Dr. Bronner's Soya-   ½ tsp garlic powder
Bouillon Sauce.

Put in bowl and cover with a plate or lid. Allow it to ferment to taste 4-8 hours. Stir before serving. Sauce may also be eaten without fermentation.

BASIC SEED LOAF

Same as above except reduce water (or REjuvelac) to 1/3 cup. Form into a loaf and let sit 24-30 hours. Other vegetables can be grated and added such as carrots, onions, peppers, parsley, celery, mushrooms, etc.

CRACKED WHEAT SAUSAGE

1 c. cooked cracked wheat	1 tsp. Worchestershire sauce
1 tsp. sage	1 egg
2 dashes onion salt	1 tsp. honey
2 dashes garlic salt	dash cayenne pepper
1 tsp. beef flavor base	5 drops liquid smoke

Combine all ingredients, form patties and fry in small amount of oil. Patties are best if not over ½ inch thich.

POPPED WHEAT

Wash 1 cup wheat and soak overnight in 2 cups of water. In same water bring to boil, turn heat low and simmer to tender about 1 to 1½ hours. Drain.

or

Wash 1 cup wheat, place in quart jar with 2 cups of water. Let set in refrigerator about ten days. Drain.

Water must be drained from wheat completely. Heat 2 to 4 inches of cooking oil in deep sauce pan or deep fryer to very hot 285° F. to 400° F. Pop about ¼ C. wheat at a time. Cook only until the kernels start to brown. Remove with perforated spoon. Kernels may be popped in a sieve lowered in hot oil. Kernels should be very light.

ROLLED WHEAT

Roll cooked wheat with rolling pin. Dry flakes in oven. Use in cookies or as a cold cereal. (350° F. until dry.)

SPROUTED WHEAT CEREAL

Makes a good cold cereal just by adding a sliced banana, milk and honey. Toast sprouted wheat in the oven and use as a cold cereal.

VERSATILE WHOLE WHEAT BREAD

5 c. warm water	2/3 c. cooking oil
12 - 13 c. whole wheat flour	2/3 c. honey (part molasses)
2 Tbsp. dry yeast	2 Tbsp. Bio-salt

With dough hook combine water, 7 c. of flour and yeast. Add remaining flour or enough flour until dough cleans from side of bowl. Knead ten minutes, form loaves and place in pans, let rise to near double. Bake 350° F. 30-35 minutes.

If mixed by hand, knead 10 minutes. Cover and let rise to double. Punch down, let rest 15 minutes. Second rising in bowl makes finer textured bread. Form loaves and bake.

Use this versatile bread dough for many kinds of bread:

Some of these recipes are from: Magic Mill Center, 7065 So. State, Midvale, UT 84047.

CRACKERS, CEREALS AND SNACK FOODS

GRANOLA

4 cups rolled oats (old fashioned)	1 cup whole wheat flour
½ cups wheat germ	1 cup almonds, cashews or your choice of nuts (raw)
1 cup coconut	

Mix all ingredients together in Magic Mixer Bowl. Combine together in a saucepan: 1 cup honey, ½ cup vegetable oil, ½ cup margarine, 2 tbsp. milk and 1 tsp. Bio-salt. Heat until margarine melts. Pour over oatmeal mixture. Spread onto 2 large cookie sheets. Bake at 275 ° F. for 1 hour. Stir occasionally. Store in air-tight container when cool. You can also add pumpkin seeds or change your mixture to suit your family. After it has baked, add 2 cups raisins. Delicious for breakfast with milk or just plain for snacks.

WHEATNUTS (GRAPENUTS)

3 cups whole wheat flour	½ tsp. salt (Bio-salt)
½ cup wheat germ	1 cup brown sugar or

2 Tbsp. malted milk   try ½ cup honey
    powder, natural flavor   1 cup sour milk or buttermilk
2 Tbsp. baking powder

Combine all ingredients in Magic Mixer Bowl. Dough should be sticky. Press onto greased cookie sheet to ½ inch thickness. Bake at 350° F. for 30 - 35 min. It should be firm but not crisp. Turn off oven. Cut into 1" x 2" strips. Turn the strips over on the pan and return to oven until dried out. Grind in Meat Mincer, using coarse disc. Sift through a wire strainer to separate the course from the fine crumbs. Use the coarse for cereal and the fine for cracker crumbs, like graham cracker crumbs.

WHEATIES

    1 cup whole wheat flour
    1 Tbsp. wheat germ
    1 Tbsp. malt powder
    1 Tbsp. honey
    1 1⅓ to 1½ cups water

Mix all ingredients together. Pour onto oiled cookie sheet (½ cup). Tip sheet back and forth to cover entire surface. Bake at 375° F. for 10 minutes. Peel off the cookie sheet and turn over and return to oven. Check every couple of minutes and break off the dried, browned pieces and continue to let rest bake, checking the same as before. Store in air-tight container.

WHEAT FLAKES

    2 cups whole wheat flour
    2 cups water (or more)
    1 Tsp. salt (Bio-salt)

Pour onto a greased cookie sheet (½ cup). Tip sheet back and forth to cover entire surface. Follow directions same as for WHEATIES.

CRACKED WHEAT

Toast leftover cracked wheat which has been cooked. Roll it fine and serve as cold cereal.

CROCK POT WHEAT CEREAL

2 cups whole wheat kernels
4 cups water
1 tsp. salt (Bio-salt)

Place all ingredients in 3-3½ quart size crock-pot. Cover and cook on low 8 - 9 hours. If possible stir once at the end of first hour. Put on night before and it will be ready for breakfast. Makes very fluffy wheat. Refrigerate unused portion and reheat before serving again. This cooked wheat may also be used in bread and casserole recipes. It can also be used for the following recipe.

VELVET WHOLE WHEAT CAKE

8 eggs, separated
1 tsp. cream of tartar
1 c. cold water
1 1/3 c. honey
2 c. whole wheat flour

½ c. cornstarch
  sifted into flour
1½ tsp. vanilla or
  almond extract
½ tsp. Bio-salt

Beat egg whites with cream of tartar until stiff, set aside. Beat egg yolks until light, add cold water and whip until light and airy then slowly, very slowly add honey. Add flour, cornstarch, vanilla and salt and beat 4 minutes on fast speed.

Very gently fold egg whites into flour and egg yolk mixture. Pour into greased and floured 9 X 12 inch pan and 12 cup cupcake pan. Bake 350° F. 1 hour and 15 minutes.

For French Pastries: Freeze cakes, then cut while frozen into squares, triangles, diamonds or with cookie cutter. Keep cake frozen at all times as cake will cut easier and there will be less crumbs.

FRESH CORN CHIPS

2 Cups (3 lg. ears) cut fresh corn (about 1 1/3 cups puréed)
1/4 tsp. dried powdered onion
1/4 tsp. dried powdered garlic
Dash Bio-salt
3 Tbsp. chopped green pepper
3 Tbsp. chopped tomato, with seeds and peels
   Purée corn and seasonings in blender. Prepare tray as for leather. Sprinkle with tomato and peppers. Dry overnight until crispy and crinkled. Break into chips and serve with dip, if desired.
Yield: 1 or more cups of chips.

TEMPTING WHEAT SALAD

1 c. cooked cracked wheat	1 c. ground gluten
1/2 c. tomato soup sauce or	1/4 c. green pepper, chopped
French dressing	2 Tbsp. green onion, chopped
2 c. mayonnaise or	2 Tbsp. green onion, chopped
salad dressing	3/4 c. celery, chopped
1-1 1/2 c. tuna, flaked	

Combine ingredients. Chill several hours or over night.

COOKED CRACKED WHEAT

Combine 1 c. wheat, 3 c. water, bring to boil and simmer covered 20 minutes.

MILLET SOUP

2 cups millet
1 quart stock (1 1/2 Tbsp. chicken base in water)
1/2 cup chopped onions
1/2 cup chopped parsley
1/2 cup chopped celery
2 Tbsp. butter
1 cup cabbage
Sauté vegetables in butter. Add water. Cook until tender. Combine all, add cabbage. Cook 10 minutes. Stir in parsley.

POPPED WHEAT

Put ½ cup of whole wheat kernels into a heavy skillet or pan (hot) and stir with a spatula until all the wheat is popped. Pan should be dry. Eat just as it is or add salt and butter or your favorite seasoning. Can also be made in a dry popcorn maker.

MILLET RECIPES   Rose Michels

Millet has the ability to pick up the trace minerals from the soil when these minerals are available. This fact makes millet very nutritious. Millet is also one of the few grains which has an alkaline ash. These recipes were submitted by a grower of organic millet and flax. Mr. A. Scheresky, Saskatchewan.

MILLET PATTIES

1½ c. precooked millet	1 med. onion, finely chopped
1 c. wheat germ	¼ tsp. celery seeds
½ c. rolled oats	1 tsp. garlic powder
2 tbsp. oil	1 tsp. Bio-salt
½ c. water	

Combine ingredients. Shape into round patties on oiled cookie sheet. Brown in oven (hot) approx. 25 to 30 min. If patties are too dry, add more water, if too moist, decrease the amount.

MILLET PUDDING

1 c. hulled millet	1 tsp Bio-salt
4 c. water	1 c. chopped apples
1 c. raisins	

Combine millet, water and salt in kettle, bring to boil. Turn down heat and cook approx. 45 min. Then add chopped apples and raisins, continue cooking over low heat for approx. 15 min. more. Serve with honey or a little butter, cayenne pepper, spike or Jensen's vegetable seasoning.

MILLET CASSEROLE

Precook: 1 cup hulled millet, 4 cups water
Add: 2 finely chopped onions, 1 clove finely chopped garlic, 2 cups tomato purée, 2 c. wheat germ, 2 tbs. oil, 2 tbsp. sweet basil more or less. 1 tbsp. dried parsley flakes, ½ tsp. Bio-salt.
Bake: In loaf tins or casserole dish at med. heat for approx. If loaf seems too dry add more tomato purée, if too thin, add more wheat germ before baking.

MILLET'N VEGETABLES

1 c. chopped fresh carrot	½ c. hulled millet
½ c. chopped fresh onion	2 tbsp. parsley flakes
1 c. chopped uncooked potato	1 tsp. Bio-salt
½ c. chopped parsnips or turnips	2½ c. water (approx.)
	1 c. chopped fresh cabbage

Place vegetables in large covered stainless steel saucepan. Add millet and seasoning and add water. Bring to boil, then turn down heat and cook approx. 45 min. over low heat. If mixture seems too thick, add a little more water and continue cooking for 15 min. Dribble 1 tbsp. oil over the top before serving.

MILLET   (By Johna May West)

4 cups water
1 cup millet

Cook in double boiler for approximately 20 minutes. Let sit with lid on for approximately 15 minutes. Add a little butter, Bio-salt, cayenne, or Jensens Vegetable broth and *eat*.

I like to precook millet and keep it in the refrigerator for use.

TOFU "EGG SALAD"

1 lb. Tofu	½ tsp tumeric
½ tsp basil	½ tsp curry powder
2 T mayonaise	1 green pepper (chopped)
	or you may prefer celery

Mix all ingredients well and serve on greens, sprouts or sandwiches.

TOFU BURGER

Mash 2 lbs. Tofu and mix well with the following ingredients:

2 T rice flour	½ tsp basil
½ tsp cumin	½ tsp curry powder
2 T Dr. Bronner's protein seasoning powder to taste	1 T olive (or mixed oils) oil

Form patties and sauté.

TOFU CASSEROLE:

Mash Tofu and mix with sprouts, carrots, celery, onion, green peppers, etc. Add spices (as in Tofu Burger) and bake in oven until firm. Add tomato sauce and capsicum after cooking if desired.

TOFU "SLOPPY JOES"

Same as above except omit sprouts and simmer in tomato sauce. Add capsicum after cooking.

TOFU "BANANA NUT SURPRISE":

1 lb. Tofu diced into cubes. Soak for 30 minutes in a mixture of ¼ cup honey and the juice of one lemon. Cut up over the soaked tofu any combination of fruits such as: bananas, dates, apples, raisins, etc.

Dressing: 2 bananas, 10 dates, ½ cup coconut milk, ½ tsp cinnamon. Place these ingredients in blender (add nuts if desired) and purée. If dressing is too thick, add water. Pour dressing over tofu and fruit.

*** Tofu is very versatile and an excellent protein source. Use as dressing, entrée, or dessert. Sauté in place of scrambled eggs. Make your own recipes. You may even want to try it as a pizza, sliced and baked with various toppings.

HUMUS:

2 cups chick-pea sprouts	¼ cup fresh lemon juice
¼ cup soy oil	¼ cup Tahini
1 cup water	¾ T Tamari Soy Sauce

Purée sprouts in the blender and then add other ingredients. Add garlic to taste. Use sauce for 'burgers', salads, or sandwiches.

BANANA ICE CREAM

Peel very ripe bananas (brown spots or brown skin). Mash and put in plastic bag and freeze. Any other fruit can be used, by blending it up thoroughly or using a juicer such as Champion.

RAW ENCHILADA:

Mix wheat, lentil and alfalfa sprouts together with salad dressing of choice. Put on corn tortilla - sprinkle with cayenne and/or tabasco over dressing of your choice. Roll up and enjoy. (May use any fresh vegetables also)

FRUIT CRISP:

Slice fruit of your choice (apples, apricots, cherries, plums, or any combination) to fill half way pan of choice.

Dribble honey and cinnamon or nutmeg over fruit.
Cover with a generous covering of whole grain bread crumbs mixed with a bit of honey, oil and spice.
Bake in the oven at 350° F. until topping is crisp and fruit is tender-crisp.

SEVEN GRAIN CEREAL:

1 cup cracked cereal blend*
4 cups boiling water
¼ tsp. Bio-salt

Boil water and salt. Remove from heat. Add cereal and cover. Let stand 20-25 min.

*Note: Cereal blend: equal parts wheat, millet, brown rice, rye, oats, barley, and flax seed. Crack through wheat grinder.

SEVEN GRAIN BREAD:

5 cups cereal blend (See recipe for Seven Grain Cereal)
8 cups whole wheat flour
5 ½ cups water
3 Tbsp. yeast
⅓ cup honey
⅓ cup molasses
2 Tbsp. Bio-salt
¼ cup oil (olive, safflower, corn)

Grind all grains together on fine. Mix water, honey, molasses, Bio-salt, oil and yeast in bowl. Add 1/3 flour. Mix well. Add remaining flour. Knead 10 min. in mixer (Address for Bio-salt stated in Homemade Cheese Recipe)

RYE BREAD

¼ recipe of dough   ½ tsp. Anise seed
1 Tbsp. Caraway seed

Knead together until mixed, in bread mixer or by hand. Form in two long rolls. Place in greased rye bread pans or on cookie sheet. Let rise and bake as bread. Makes two loaves.

DILL BREAD

¼ recipe of dough   2 Tbsp. dill seed
1 Tbsp. lemon juice   1 Tbsp. dry onion soup
Knead together just until mixed well. Form into loaves.
Bake with rest of bread. Makes 1 large or 2 small loaves.

SWEET ROLLS: NUTS AND CINNAMON FROSTING

2 Tbsp. butter or margarine 2 tsp. cinnamon
¾ c. powdered sugar   ½ c. nuts, chopped
¼ c. light cream or
    evaporated milk
In 9 inch square pan melt butter. Stir in sugar, cream and
cinnamon. Sprinkle with nuts. Using ¼ of the dough roll to
⅓ inch thickness and to a rectangle. Sprinkle with brown
sugar and cinnamon. Roll dough from long side, seal ends
and place with seam side down. Slice crosswise about 1
inch or less slices and arrange over frosting mix. Bake
400°F. about 25 minutes.

MUSHROOM AND WHEAT CASSEROLE

4-6 cups wheat
1 can mushroom soup
½ can milk
1 onion sautéed
Mix in casserole. 350° F. for 20-30 min. For variety add
celery, green onions, and green peppers.

WHEAT CRISP

2 cups wheat
2 Tbsp. butter
1 cup cheese
Meat grind fine. Roll into balls and put on greased cookie
sheet. Bake for 15 minutes at 350° F. temperature.

WHEAT SALAD

6 cups cracked wheat
1 ¾ cup miracle whip

1 ¾ cup Miracle Whip
1 ¾ cup French dressing
4 Tbsp. green peppers
½ cup green onions
1 cup chopped celery
1 cup tuna (2 cans)
½ tsp. Bio-salt
Mix together and enjoy.

FRESH PEACH JAM

3½ cups peaches puréed in blended. Taste for sweetness. Prepare tray as for leather, and spread mixture ⅜ thick. Place in dehydrator. Dry 3 to 3 ½ hours. Mix up and re-spread about once an hour. (if any of it dries, it will even out when stored.) When mixture is thickness of jam, pour into a glass jar and refrigerate. (Will keep a few weeks in refrigerator or 3 months to 1 year in freezer).
Yield: Little over ½ cup. To make one cup double this recipe. You can use strawberries, apricots, or almost any fruit or berry you desire. If you get it too sweet, add a little more fresh lemon juice.
Great on toast, pancakes, waffles, ice cream, cheesecake and crepes.
Tastes fresh......without white sugar!!!!!

"FOR MORE RECIPES ORDER *EYDIE MAE'S NATURAL RECIPES* WHERE SHE GIVES THE DIET SHE LIVED ON TO CURE HER CANCER. THE DIET THAT HELPED HER CURE CANCER SHOULD HELP PREVENT ALL DISEASES.

(See Bibliography for address)

DIRECTIONS FOR DEHYDRATING FOODS

APPLES: Slice with or without peel, into ¼ inch-thick slices. Arrange in a single layer on trays. Dry 8 to 10 hours or overnight, until beyond the bendable and leathery stage. The sweeter the fruit the longer the drying time. For apple rings, remove core with apple corer and dry as above.

RHUBARB: Sliced. Cut in ½ inch slices and dry about 18 to 20 hours, until hard.

BEANS, SNAP: Slices. For quickest drying, slice beans lengthwise and then across in ½ to 1 inch pieces. Place on trays and dry 5 to 7 hours, until hard. If not sliced lenthwise, they require 7 to 9 hours to dry.

BEETS: lice ¼ inch thick. Dry about 9 hours until rather hard but spongy. They may be dried to a crisp chip if sliced ⅛ inch thick and dried for 6 to 7 hours. Grated. Wash and blot dry and grate onto tray. Dry about 3 hours, until hard and slightly spongy.

BROCCOLI: Quartered. Wash, blot dry, and cut into quarters lenthwise. Place on trays. Dry 6 to 10 hours, until hard but slightly spongy.

BRUSSELS SPROUTS: Sprouts may be shredded, cut in squares or pieces. For shredded, spread evenly about ⅝ inch thick and dry 4 to 6 hours. If broken apart in loose leaves, dry 6 to 10 hours.

CABBAGE: Shredded. Same as brussels sprouts. Squares or pieces. Cut washed cabbage in ½ to ¾ inch pieces. Spread on trays about ⅝ inch thick. Dry 6 to 8 hours until almost crispy but still chewable.

CARROTS: Wash and grate and arrange evenly on trays about ⅝ inch thick. Dry about 4 to 6 hours. Slices. Slice ¼ inch thick and arrange in single layers on trays and dry about 6 to 8 hours until hard.

CAULIFLOWER: Slices. Remove leaves, wash, blot dry and break into flowerettes. Cut flowerettes into ¼ inch slices. Dry about 9 hours in single layers until rather hard but still spongy.

CELERY: Slices. Cut slices across stalks about ¼ to ½ inch thick. Dry in single layers 5 to 10 hours until very hard and dry. It will be about 1/10th of its original size.

CHINESE CABBAGE: Dry same as cabbage.

CORN: Cut kernels from cob and arrange in layers 2 or 3 kernels thick on tray. Dry 6 to 10 hours, until crispy. The sweeter the corn the longer the drying process and the better tasting.

CUCUMBERS: Slices. Wash and dry and peel if waxed. Cut into ⅛ to ¼ inch slices. Dry in single layers 6 to 10 hours, depending on thickness. They should be crisp and snap when broken or rattle if stored in glass jar.

GREENS: Cut same as for cabbage and dry in one or two layers for 3 to 6 hour, until crisp. (endive, escarole, kale, collards, turnip tops, beet greens, chard, mustard greens, broccoli leaves, chicory, dandelion greens, watercress, sorrel, spinach, etc.)

MUSHROOMS: Small ones may be dried whole in single layers for 5 to 7 hours, until leathery and spongy. Slices. Cut clean, dry mushroms in ¼ inch slices. Dry 3 or 4 hours.

ONIONS: Cross-cut slices or rings. Cut into ⅛ to ¼ inch slices. Dry in single layers 8 to 12 hours. Chopped. Cut in medium to coarse pieces and dry 5 to 8 hours.

PEAS: Place young, shelled peas in single layer and dry 14 to 16 hours until hard and dry.

PEPPERS: Slices, strips or cross-cut rings. Cut in ¼ inch slices or length-wise strips. For cross-cut slices, cut into ¼ inch slices across pepper. Dry 6 to 8 hours, until dry but bendable. Chopped. Same as for chopped onions.

RADISHES: Same procedure as for beets.

SQUASH (SUMMER(: Crookneck, yellow straightneck, zucchini, etc. Slices. Wash and cut into ⅛ to ¼ inch slices and dry in single layers until crisp and hard, about 6 to 8 hours. Will rattle in container or bag if dry.

TOMATOES: Slices. Slice ¼ inch thick. Dry approximately 12 hours.

APRICOTS: Cut into ¼ inch slices; arrange in single layers and dry 7 to 10 hours or until fairly hard but chewable. For halves, place halves skin side down on trays and dry approximately 16 to 18 hours.

BANANAS: Dry when skins are solid yellow and specked with brown. Use over-ripe fruit for fruit leather. Slice ¼ inch thick and arrange in single layers. Dry 12 to 16 hours. For chips, slice ⅛ inch thick and dry until very crisp; about 8 to 12 hours.

CHERRIES: Remove pits and dry in single layers. Halves of sweet or Bing cherries take approximately 24 to 30 hours. Whole; dry until similar to large raisins. Drying time depends on sweetness of fruit.

GRAPES: Halves. Wash any variety. Seeds may or may not be removed. Dry out side up on trays 24 to 48 hours.

PEACHES & NECTARINES: Slices. Wash. Cut into ¼ inch slices, with or without peel. Arrange in single layers. Dry 8 to 12 hours, depending on sweetness of fruit, until it is between a brittle and bendable stage.

PEARS: Slices. Wash. Slice with or without peel, ¼ inch thick. Dry in single layers 10 to 14 hours or until rather dry but chewy. Rings do same as for apple rings and dry 10 to 14 hours.

PINEAPPLE: Slices. Wash pineapple. Cut off green top, and cut in half lengthwise. Cut each half in four wedges. Using a sharp knife, remove core from each wedge. Next, run knife between bottom skin and fruit. Slice down on fruit at ¼ intervals, from where core was removed to pineapple peel on bottom. Place on trays and dry 24 hours or more, until dry but chewy. Fruit will always be a little sticky but shouldn't stick together when dry.

PLUMS: Slices. Do no peel. Wash and cut into ¼ inch slices. Arrange in single layers and dry 8 to 10 hours until fairly hard but chewable. Halves, dry 36 to 40 hours.

How Hypoglycemia Can Turn Into Diabetes, High Blood Pressure And Heart Disease

The following chart describes what happens in your body if you don't get enough glucose from fruits, vegetables, whole grains and sprouts to supply the demand for glucose required by your cells. See explanation on pages 116-120.

High Protein Diet (H.P.D.)

Poisons

LIVER

KIDNEY

ADRENAL

H.P.D.

CELL

Glucose

Poisons

Poisons will damage the Liver and Kidneys

Improper Diet (I.D.)
Refer to chart on page 130

Glucose

Cortisol

I.D.

Protein

Glucose

Growth Hormone

Insulin

Excess Glucose

BLOOD STEAM

PITUITARY

PANCREAS

Excess glucose in the blood stream will cause diabetes and will also rob oxygen from the red blood cells, which will cause them to stick together, dilate the blood capillaries and cause trapped blood proteins which can produce high blood pressure and heart disease.

288

APPENDIX C

"The Basic Formula For Life"

And

"The Basic Formula For Death"

Definition Of Terms
And Charts

DEFINITION OF FORMULA TERMS

(– Chg.)	Means negative charge;
(–)	Means negative charge;
(+)	Means positive charge;
(=)	Means equals or produces;
( )	Means yields or produces;
(TPP)	Means trapped plasma proteins around the cells;
(EX Fl)	Means excess fluid around the cells;
(EX Na +)	Means excess sodium (single positive ions around the cells;
(▲)	Means alter, change or upset;
(EE)	Means the electrical energy produced by the cells. The "electric generator." The body works electrically. The food that we eat is converted chemically into electricity which enables us to function. The thought waves are electrical, the energy which comes from the eyes is electrical, and muscles work by electrical impulses from the brain. The nervous system is electrical.
(▲EE)	Means any loss of energy that is produced or experienced in the body. If there is no ▲EE we could run 150-200 miles without rest.
(☐)	Means perfectly healthy cells.
(☒)	Means damaged or dead cells.
(O$_2$)	Means oxygen.
(K +)	Means the potassium single positive ion.
(Na +)	Means the sodium single positive ion.

K +
Na +
This represents a cell in the body. The concentration of K + inside the cell must remain high, and the concentration of Na + inside the cell must remain low.

(◯)   This represents the Na – K Pump which = EE. The main purpose of this pump is to bring potassium, calcium, iron, glucose, and other minerals and nutrients into the cell and to pull any excess sodium out of the cell. The rotation of minerals in and out of the cell creates the EE.

(GLUCOSE)   Is the main fuel for the cell. The primary source of glucose is fruits, vegetables and sprouts. High protein foods are a very poor source of glucose because the poisonous by-products produce TPP.

(A.T.P.)   Stands for adenosine tri-phosphate. Glucose plus oxygen = A.T.P. (A.T.P. is pure energy which the cell must have in order for the Na – K Pump to produce the EE.) A.T.P. is the energy needed to maintain the life process of the cell. The life process has been found to generate electrical fields in every organism that has been examined. And it is the delicately balanced distribution of minerals in and around a living cell, whether plant or animal, which accounts for its electrical properties.

290

"The Basic Formula for Life" and "The Basic Formula for Death"

by C. Samuel West, D.N., N.D.
Chemist and Lymphologist

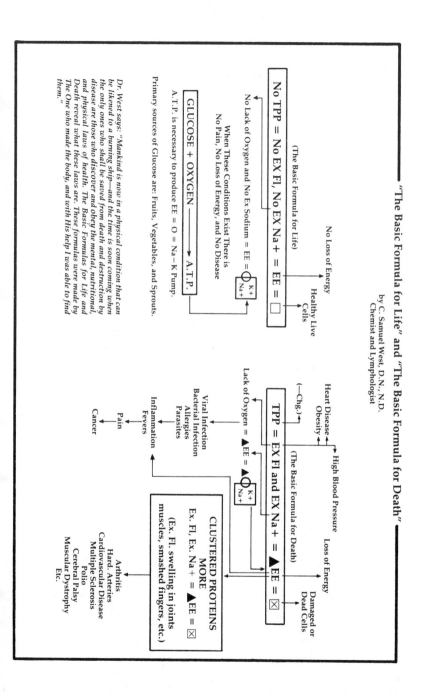

No TPP = No EX Fl, No EX Na + = EE = ☐

(The Basic Formula for Life)

No Lack of Oxygen and No Ex Sodium = EE = (K+/Na+) = ☐

When These Conditions Exist There is
No Pain, No Loss of Energy, and No Disease

No Loss of Energy → Healthy Live Cells

GLUCOSE + OXYGEN ——→ A.T.P.

A.T.P. is necessary to produce EE = O = Na–K Pump.

Primary sources of Glucose are: Fruits, Vegetables, and Sprouts.

Dr. West says: "Mankind is now in a physical condition that can be likened to a burning ship—and the time is soon coming when the only ones who shall be saved from death and destruction by disease are those who discover and obey the mental, nutritional, and physical laws of health. The Basic Formulas for Life and Death reveal what these laws are. These formulas were made by The One who made the body, and with His help I was able to find them."

TPP = EX Fl and EX Na + = ▲EE = ☒

(The Basic Formula for Death)

(—Chg.)
Heart Disease
Obesity
High Blood Pressure
Loss of Energy
Damaged or Dead Cells

Lack of Oxygen = ▲EE = (K+/Na+)

Viral Infection
Bacterial Infection
Allergies
Parasites
Inflammation
Fevers
Pain
Cancer

CLUSTERED PROTEINS MORE
Ex. Fl, Ex. Na + = ▲EE = ☒
(Ex. Fl. swelling in joints muscles, smashed fingers, etc.)

Arthritis
Hard. Arteries
Cardiovascular Disease
Multiple Sclerosis
Polio
Cerebral Palsy
Muscular Dystrophy
Etc.

THE BASIC FORMULAS FOR LIFE AND DEATH SUMMARIZED

The Tree of Life	SERVED	The Tree of Death
Good	F	Evil
Love	O	Hate
Peace	R	War
Health	C	Sickness
Life	E	Death
	S	

PREVENTION OF TPP

CAUSE OF TPP

MENTAL

Love, Bless
Do Good
Desire to Give
All to Bless Others

MENTAL

Shock, Stress, Anger
Fear, Loss of Temper,
Holding Grudges
Resentment, Greed

NUTRITIONAL

More
Fruits
Vegetables
Grains
Fish
(No Thirst—
Energy High)

NUTRITIONAL

Tea, Coffee, Liquor,
Tobacco, Soft Drinks
Drugs, Salt, Sugar, Fat
High-Cholesterol Foods
Too Much Meat
(Thirst and
Loss of Energy)

PHYSICAL

Breathe Deeply
and
Exercise Properly
(Lymphasize)
(Energy High)

PHYSICAL

Shallow Breathing
and
Improper Exercise
(Loss of Energy)

APPENDIX D

Bibliography

Additional Reading Material

BIBLIOGRAPHY

Books

Airola, Paavo, Ph.D., N.D. How to Get Well, Phoenix, Arizona: Health Plus Publishers, 1976.

Campbell, Giraud W., D.O. A Doctor's Proven New Home Cure For Arthritis. New York: Island Park Publishing Inc.

Culburt, Michael L. and Harold W. Harper, M.D. How You Can Beat The Killer Diseases. Connecticut: Arlington House Publications, 1977.

Guyton, Arthur C., M.D. Textbook of Medical Physiology. 5th Ed. Pennsylvania: W. B. Saunders Co., 1976.

Holy Bible, The. "Genesis, 3:17-19", "Matthew 5:43-44", "Isaiah 40:31", and "Luke 23:34", Authorized King James Version published in The United States of America.

Mansell, Tom. Cancer Simplfied. Aliquippa, Pennsylvania: Woodlawn Press, 1977.

Mendelsohn, Robert S., M.D. Confessions of A Medical Heretic. Illinois: Contemporary Books, Inc., 1979 and Ontario, Canada: Beaver Books, Ltd.

Van Aaken, Ernst, M.D. The Van Aaken Method. Mountainview, California: World Publications, 1976.

Wade, Carlson. Miracle Protein: Secret of Natural Cell, Tissue Rejuvenation, West New York: Parker Publishing Co., Inc.

Periodicals

Benditt, Earl P. "Origin of Atherosclerosis." Scientific American, February, 1977.

Harvey, Paul. "Body Electricity Offers New Hope." Los Angeles Times Syndicate, April 9, 1976.

Lavine, Leroy S., Dr. and Morris H. Shamos. "When Bones Heal, Is Electricity the Key?" Science World, January, 1973.

Mayerson, H. S., M.D. "Lymphatic System." Scientific American, June, 1963.

McClellan, Bill. "The World's Toughest Runners." Runners World, October, 1979.

Parker, Lester, Dr. and James R. Smith. The Medical World News, October, 1974.

Scott, Bruce L. H. "Electricity in Plants," Scientific American October, 1962.

Warburg, Otto, Dr. Director, Max Planck-Institute for Cell Physiology, Berlin-Dahlem (Nobel Prize 1931); "On the Origin of Cancer Cells," Science Magazine, February, 1956.

West, C. Samuel, N.D. Trapped Plasma Proteins, August 1978 and The Lymphatic Exercise Home Study Program, July, 1978.

Wigmore, Ann, N.D. "Spiritual Physical Survival Sprouting." Health Digest, 153:16

Witte, Charles L., M.D.; Marlys Hearst Witte, M.D.; Allan E. Dumont, M.D.; William R. Cole, M.D.; and John R. Smith, M.D. "Protein Content in Lymph and Edema Fluids in Congestive Heart Failure," Circulation, Vol. XL, November, 1969.

Wood, W. Barry, Jr. "White Blood Cells V. Bacteria." Scientific American, February, 1951

Other

Film. Shields, Jack, M.D. "The Central Propulsion of Human Thoracic Duct Lymph," Santa Barbara, California.

Film. "The Incredible Machine."   Arizona University Film
Library. Tempe, Arizona.

Film. "Coronary Counter Attack" Brigham Young
University Library. Provo, Utah

Pamphlet. Olney, Robert C., M.D. "Blocked Oxidation."
Lincoln, Nebraska.

Pamphlet, United States Government, Dietary Goals For The
United States, Stock No. 052-070-03913-2, Washington,
D.C.: U.S. Government Printing Office, February, 1977.

Personal Conversation. Plog, Fredrick M., Ph.D.   "The Lasar
Acupuncture Machine,"   February 1980.

Personal Conversation. Walker, Norman, Dr. Sc. "Walker-
West-Walk," June, 1978.

Personal Conversation. Waltz, Joseph M., M.D. "The
Spinal Cord Stimulator," July, 1980.

Song. Miller, Sy and Jill Jackson. "Let There Be Peace On
Earth."   Jan-Lee Music, Beverly Hills, California.

ADDITIONAL READING MATERIAL

Airola, Paavo, Ph.D., N.D.,:
1. How To Get Well
2. The Airola Diet and Cook Book
3. Are You Confused
4. Hypoglycemia, A Better Approach

Health Plus Publishing
P.O. Box 22001
Phoenix, Arizona 85028

Alsaker, Rasmus, M.D.   Victory Over Arthritis,
Groton Press, Inc. 74 Third Ave.
Brooklyn, N. Y. 1966.

Boyd, Nathaniel Welsher, III, D.O.   Stay Out of The Hospital
 Boyd Clinic
 Loganville, York Co., PA 17343

Burroughs, Stanley.   The Age of Enlightenment.
 P.O. Box 260
 Kailua, HAW 96734

Carter, Al.   The Miracles of Rebound Exercise, National
 Institute of Reboundology and Health; Bothell,
 Washington 98011; Snohomish Publishing Co., P.O.
 Box 687, Snohomish, WASH 98290.

Caum, Suzanne.   Cancer Cures Crucified   Caumsette Press
 Box 132 Pilgrim Gardens Station
 Drexel Hill, PA 19026 1968.

Christopher, John R.   (Master Herbalist), The School of
 Natural Healing and Childhood Diseases.
 Christopher Publications
 P.O. Box 412
 Springville, Utah 84663

Clark, Linda.
 1. The Ancient Art of Colon Therapy
 2. Know Your Nutrition
 3. Stay Young Longer

 Keats Publishing Inc.
 Box 876,
 36 Grove St.
 New Canaan, CONN

Cooper, Kenneth H., M.D.   The Aerobics Way,
 Bantom Books
 666 5th Ave., New York, New York 10019.

Davison, Jaquie.   Cancer Winner (How I Purged Myself of
 Melanoma Cancer.)
 Pacific Press
 P.O. Box 219
 Pierce City, MO 65723

Ehret, Arnold.
1. Mucusless Diet Healing System
2. Roads to Health and Happiness
3. Thus Speaketh the Stomach
4. Definite Cure of Chronic Constipation

Ehret Publishing Co., Beaumont, CA
and Ehret Literature Publishing Co., Cody, WY:

Eydie Mae, Eydie Mae's Natural Recipes from How I Conquered
Cancer Naturally.
Production House
4307 N. Euclid Ave.
San Diego, CA 92115

Fredericks, Carlton, Ph.D.   Eat Well, Stay Well, Get Well.
Grosset & Dunlop, Publisher, a Filmways Company
New York, New York

Gerson, Max.   A Cancer Therapy (Results of Fifty Cases).
Totality Books Publishers
P.O. Box 1035
Del Mar, CA 92014

Griffin, LaDean.
1. Is Any Sick Among You?
2. The Return To Herbal Medicine With No Side
Effects,
Bi-World Publishers
Provo, UT 84601

Heinerman, John.   The Science of Herbal Medicine.
Bi-World Publications
Provo, Utah 84601

Hurd, Frank J., D.C., and Rosalie Hurd, B.S., A Good Cook and
Ten Talents.
Published by Authors
Box 86A Rt #1
Chisholm, MINN 55719

Jensen, Bernard, D.C.
    1. Blending Magic Bernard Jensen Products,
       Publishing Division P.O. Box 8, Solana Beach,
       California 92075
    2. Health Magic Through Chlorophyll from Living
       Plant Life Bi-World Publishers Inc. P.O. Box 62
       Provo, Utah 84601 1973.

Kadans, Joseph M., Ph.D.   Encyclopedia of Fruits, Vegetables,
      Nuts and Seeds For Healthful Living
      Parker Publishing Company, Inc.
      West Nyack, New York 1973.
Kelley, William Donald, D.D.S; M.S.   One Answer to Cancer
      The Kelley Research Foundation P.O. Box 89
      Grapevine, Texas 76051 1971.

Kervran, Louis C.   Biological Transmutations   Swan House
      Publishing Co. 1972   P.O. Box 170
      Brooklyn, N.Y. 11223

Kirban, Salem.   How to Keep Healthy and Happy by Fasting
      Salem Kirban, Inc. Kent Road,
      Huntingdon Valley, PA 19006 1976.

Kirschner, H. E., M.D.   Live Food Juices, 1957 - Nature's
      Healing Grasses, 1960 - Nature's Seven Doctors, 1962
      H. C. White Publications
      P.O. Box 8014
      Riverside, CA 92505

Kloss, Jethro.   Back to Eden.
      P.O. Box 1439
      Loma Linda, CA 92354

Kulvinskas, Viktoras H.   Survival Into the 21st Century.
      Mango Press
      P.O. Box 64
      Woodstock Valley, CONN 06282

Landgrebe, Gary.   Tofu Goes West--Recipes.

Fresh Press
774 Allen Court
Palo Alto, CA 94303

Malstrom, Stan, N.D.   Own Your Own Body.
Keats Publishing Co.
36 Grove St.
New Canaan, CONN 06840

Manner, Harold W., Ph.D.   The Death of Cancer.
Advanced Century Publishing Co.
4908 N. Lincoln
Chicago, ILL 60625

Mansell, Thomas H.   Cancer Simplified.
Woodlawn Press
604 Briar Cliff
Aliquippa, PENN 15001

Mendelsohn, Robert S., M.D.
        1.   Confessions of a Medical Heretic
        2.   Malepractice
Contemporary Book Inc.
180 N. Michigan Ave.
Chicago, ILL 60601

        Also in Canada
        Beaver Books Ltd.
        150 Lesmil Rd.
        Don Mills, Ontario M3B 2T5 CANADA

Natenberg, Maurice.   Forward by Robert D. Bernard, M.D.,
        The Cancer Outbreak   History of Denial and
        Supressed Remedies and the Methods to Discredit
        Independent Cancer Research and Treatment. 1959.
        Regent House, Chicago

Nittler, Alan, M.D. A New Breed of Doctor.
        Pyramid Communications Inc.
        919 3rd Ave.
        New York, New York 10022

Pritikin, Nathan.
    1. The Pritikin Program for Diet and Exercise,
    2. The Pritikin Permanent Weight Loss Manual.
    Today Press
    Grosset and Dunlap
    A Filmways Co. N.Y.

Ritchason, Jack.
    1. The Little Herb Encyclopedia
    2. The Little Vitamin and Mineral Encyclopedia.
    Bi-World Publishers
    Provo, UT 84601

Tobe, John H. Cancer--How To Prevent and Gain Remission
    From Cancer.
    The Provoker Press
    Lakeshore Rd.
    St. Catherines, Ontario, CANADA

Van Aaken, Ernest, M.D. Van Aaken Method.
    World Publications
    P.O. Box 366
    Mountainview, CA 94040

Wade, Carlson. Miracle Protein.
    Parker Publishing Co., Inc.
    West New York, New York

Walker, Morton, D.P.M. and Frank Angelo. Rebounding
    Aerobics,
    National Institute of Reboundology and Health
    Edmonds, WASH 98020

Walker, Norman, Dr. Sc.
    1. The Vegetarian Guide to Diet and Salad
    2. Colon Health
    3. Raw Vegetable Juices
    4. Become Younger
    5. Vibrant Health
    O'Sullivan Woodside and Co.
    2218 E. Magnolia
    Phoenix, AZ 85034

White, James R., Ph.D.   <u>Jump For Joy.</u>
      Nutri Books
      Box 5793
      Denver, COLO 80217

Wigmore, Ann, D.D., N.D.
      1. <u>Why Suffer</u>
      2. <u>Be Your Own Doctor</u>
      3. <u>The Answer? Wheatgrass, God's Manna</u>
      Hemisphere Press International Inc.
      263 9th Ave.
      New York, New York

Wood, H. Curtis, Jr., M.D.   <u>Over Fed But Under Nourished,</u>
      1959 <u>The Doctors Speak Out, 1965</u>
      Forward by Herbert Rainer, M.D.
      Rodale Press, Inc., Emmaus, Penn. 18049

Wood, J. Edwin, M.D.   "The Venous System,"
      <u>Scientific American,</u> January, 1968.
      W. H. Freeman & Co.
      660 Market Street
      San Francisco, CA 94104

<u>Additional Research By Several
United States Lymphologists</u>

Reprint, Marlys Hearst Witte, M.D., F.A.C.A.; Douglas Hanto;
      and Charles L. Witte, M.D., F.A.C.A. "Clinical and
      Experimental Techniques to Study the Lymphatic System,"
      Vascular Surgery, Vol. II, No. 3, May/June, 1977.

            Marlys H. Witte, M.D.
            Dept. of Surgery
            University of Arizona
            College of Medicine
            Tuscon, AZ 85724

Reprint.   Charles L. Witte, M.D.; Marlys Hearst Witte, M.D.;
      Kathleen Kintner, B.A.; William R. Cole, M.D., F.A.C.S.;
      "Colloid Osmotic Pressure in Hepatic Cirrhosis and
      Experimental Ascites,"

<u>Surgery, Gynecology and Obstetrics,</u> Vol. 133:65-71. July, 1971.

> Depts. of Surgery & Medicine,
> Cardiology
> University of Arizona
> College of Medicine
> Tuscon, AZ 85724
>
> Depts. of Surgery
> Washington University School of Medicine
> St. Louis, Missouri
>
> New York University School of Medicine
> New York, NY

Article.   Marlys Hearst Witte, M.D.; Allan E. Dumont, M.D.; Roy H. Clauss, M.D.; Bertha Rader, M.D.; Norman Levine, B.S.; Ernest S. Breed, M.D., "Lymph Circulation in Congestive Heart Failure," <u>Circulation,</u> Vol. XXXIX, June, 1969.

> Depts. of Medicine & Surgery
> New York School of Medicine
> New York, NY
>
> Dept. of Medicine (Cardiology Div.)
> Washington School of Medicine
> St. Louis, Missouri

Reprint, Special Article.   Charles L. Witte and Marlys Hearst Witte,* "Physiology 301, Clinical Correlation Lectures: Lymph Formation - Lymph Absorption: The Formula For Edema. A Second Experiment in the Teaching of Lymphology to Medical Students." <u>Lymphology,</u> Official Organ of The Internatioal Society of Lymphology, Vol. 6, No. 2, June, 1973.

> George Thieme Publishers
> P.O. Box 732
> D-7000
> Stutgart 1

*Dr. M. Witte is currently recipient of a U.S.P.H.S. Cancer Research Development Award and has just completed tenure as an established investigator of the American Heart Association.

Reprint.   C. L. Witte; M.H. Witte; A. E. Dumont, "Significance of Protein in Edema Fluids," <u>Lymphology,</u> Official Organ of the International Society of Lymphology, Vol. 4, No. 2, June, 1971.

Charles L. Witte   Depts. of Surgery
    and   University of Arizona
Marlys Hearst Witte: College of Medicine
                                   Tuscon, AZ 85724
Allan E. Dumont: New York School of
                                   Medicine New York, NY

INDEX

Addiction--How To Overcome 132
Ankle, Freshly Turned--To Help Relieve Pain In 65
Arms--To Help Relieve Pain In 63
Arthritis--The Cause Of 72

Basic Formula For Loss Of Energy, Disease
        And Death, The--Thirty One Steps 10
    Explained In Detail 42
Basic Formula For Perfectly Healthy Cells, The--
        In This Condition, The Cells Would
        Reproduce Forever 13
Basic Formula's For Life And Death--
        Charts, Definitions,The Tree Of Life
        And The Tree Of Death 290-292
Bio-Electric Energy--Definition 185
Bio-Electric Energy Field 204
    Reverses Injuries 204
Bio-Electric Eye Exercise, Special 195
Bio-Electric Gentle Bounce For Health, The--
        Dorothy Howard's Testimonial 190
Bio-Electric Gentle Bounce For Health, The--
        How To Do It 187
Bio-Electric Gentle Bounce For Health And
        Special Bio-Electric Eye Exercises--
        Story Behind 186
Bio-Electric Lymphasizing Techniques--Explanations
        With Pictures And Stories 185
Bio-Electric Pin-Point Technique 202
Bio-Electric Self-Help Pain Relief Techniques, Basic . . . 62
    Why And How They Work 54
    The Basic Details Of Energy Flow 203
Bio-Electric Techniques--A List Of Advanced
        Techniques Which Can Be Demonstrated By
        A Qualified Instructor 185
Bio-Electric Wheelchair Technique 198
"Bionic Arm"--Controlled By Thoughts--Developed
        By Dr. Daniel Graupe 174
Blood--Learn About To Save Your Life 85
Blood Protein And Death--How I Learned About 239
Blood Protein Causing Death--I Began To Teach About . . 240

Blood Protein Research--Teaches Cause Of Disease
    And Enables People To Take Care Of
    Own Problems 191
Blood Proteins--Can Cause Death 31
    Knowledge Of Will Restore Health And Peace 86
    Medical Research 29
Body Chart By Dr. West 188
Book, This--How It Was Named 242
"Bouncy, Bouncy Baby" (Poem by Johna May West) . 153, 193
Breathing And Directed Thinking Technique 195
Breathing--Breathe Deeply Everywhere You Go 133

Calcium Requirements, The Body's--Low, Not High . . . 114
Cancer--The Cause Of 70
Carbohydrates, Complex--A Protein Sparer 224
Catarrh (Mucous)--Cause Of 41
Cause, The College Of 70
Cells--How Fed 38
    Meant To Live Forever 39
Cholesterol, High--Why A Poison 103
Clustered Proteins--Electricity Can Dissipate 53
Colon--Techniques That Stimulate And Revitalize 64
Congestion--Cause Of 41

Death, Cause Of--Has Changed Since 19th Century, Why? . 98
Dehydrating Foods, Directions 284
Diabetes Mellitus 118
Diet--The Basic Transition 132
Diet Change--Article: "Top Doctors Reveal
        Simple Diet Change Can Prevent Breast
        And Colon Cancer" 208
Dietary Goals For The United States, The--
        A "Fifteen Page" Exerpt 248
    A.M.A., Food Processors And Others Tried To
        Discredit And Silence This Government
        Document 104
    Agrees With Medical Research--The Best Way To
        Treat Protein Deficiency 119
    Agrees With Medical Research--The Body's Calcium
        Requirements Are Low, Not High 114
    Agrees With Medical Research--The Body's

Protein Requirements Are Low, Not High 115
Asked For A Nation-Wide Health Education Program . 103
Explained Here In More Detail 110
Gives Good Nutritional Diagnosis For The
    Crippling And Killer Diseases 111
Gives Good Nutritional Prescription For The
    Crippling And Killer Diseases 113
How To Use This Document To Help Get The Blood
    Protein Research To Friends And Loved Ones . . 108
Lets You Diagnose And Prescribe 105
Says That Our Problems Cannot Be Solved By
    More And More Medical Care 106
Says Very Little Current Medical Practice Can Do
    For the Crippling And Killer Diseases 106
Tells What Foods Are Directly Related To The
    Death Of 240,000 Men, Women And Children
    Every Two Months 100
Why We Are Publishing A "Fifteen Page Excerpt"
    Of The First Edition Of This Document 105
Discoveries--Doors Opened To Other 190
Discoveries, The Seven Golden 4
Discovery By Dr. West--How To "Run And Not Be
    Weary, And Walk And Not Faint!" 136
Disease-Free Healthy Life--Eight Basic Rules For 221
Disease--Symptoms Of 45, 99
Doctor Friedrich M. Plog-- Gave Dr. West Discoveries
    Six And Seven 53
Doctors--Some Are Willing To Share 184
Dolorology--The Science Of Pain 172
Dr. Arthur C. Guyton--Published The Revolutionary
    Discovery--Blood Proteins Cause Death 30
Dr's Charles and Marlys Witte--Lymphology
    Laboratory 172
Dr. Daniel Graupe--Developed A "Bionic Arm" 174
Dr. Fuller Royal--Nevada Clinic Of Preventive
    Medicine 173
Dr. Joseph M. Waltz--St. Barnabas Hospital, N.Y.--
    Introducing His Discovery 55
    Uses Electrical Stimulation to Help Previously
        Helpless Cerebral Palsy, M.S. And Polio Patients . 174
    Pictures And Letter 177

Dr. Scribonius Largus--43 A.D.--Used Electric Fish To
      Cure Pain Of Gout And Migraine Headaches 172
Ehret, Arnold--Lived On Straight Fruit For Two Years . . . 217
      Strength Comes From Clean System 216
      "The Daddy Of Transition"   216
Eight Basic Rules--Dr. Max Warmbrand Confirms Them   . 223
Eighth International Congress--Basic Formula Presented   . 13
Electrical Secrets Of Life And Death At The Cell Level   . . 45
Electrically--How To Use A Lymphasizer   187
Electricity--Dr. Waltz Uses Electrical Stimulation
            To Help Cerebral Palsy, Multiple Schlerosis,
            And Polio Patients 174
      Eyes, Thoughts, And Muscles Work Electrically   . . . 173
      Used By Medical Doctors To Diagnose And Prescribe . 172
Excerpts To *Dietary Goals . . ., The*--Why Published . . . 105

Fasting--Dr. Otto Buchinger, M.D. Talks About
            Fasting In Dr. Paavo Airola's Book
            How To Get Well 227
      Vital Organs And Glands Not Damaged 227
Fingers, Smashed Or Cut--To Help Relieve Pain In 65
Fluid Retention--Cause Of   51
Foods--Directly Related To Six Of The Ten Leading
            Causes Of Death In The United States 100
      How To Combine 129
      Recipes To Help With Transition   170
      Sample Lunch Or Dinner Menu 269
      Shopping List 268
Forgive Them, For They Know Not 91
Formula For Death, The-- Charts And Definitions 289
Formula For Life, The--Charts And Definitions 289
Formula--Dr. West Writes The One Basic Formula
            Which Shows The Cause Of Disease And Death
            At The Cell Level   9
Formula, The One And Only--Explained In Detail   42
Formula, The--The Day I Knew I Had It 242

Gall Bladder--Techniques That Increase The Circulation . 63
Glycogen--Can Give You Super-Human Strength 152
      Miracle Of It 151
Golden Families--Will Be Established Who Will

Conquer Disease, Replace Hate With Love,
And Live In Peace And Harmony 169
Golden Family--How To Become One 134
What If No Support From Your Own Family 134
Golden Seven Plus One, The--Acknowledgement To
Those Who Helped Make It Possible 229
My Story Behind 232
How I Was Given Help To Write 241
How This Book Was Named 242
Special Recognition To Others Who Helped To Make
The Golden Seven Plus One Possible 244
Graduation From College Of Cause, College of Self-
Help Pain Relief, And College Of Prevention . . 167

Headaches And Sore Neck Problems--To Help Relieve . . 62
Headaches--Cause Of 57
Heal A Smashed Finger In Minutes 58
Healing--Activity Is "Magic" Healer 144
Healing Arts--How They Work 14
Healing In The Body 57
Healing Process--Examples 57
The Secret Of 61
The Secret To 46
Health Discovery--The Most Important On Earth 1
Health--Doctors And People Must Fight For Freedoms . . 88
Government Asks For A Nation-Wide Health
Education Program 103
Introduction To The Mental Laws And Trapped
Plasma Proteins 17
Introduction To The Nutritional Laws And Trapped
Plasma Proteins 19
Introduction To The Physical Laws And Trapped
Plasma Proteins 22
Health and Peace--Must Take The Offensive 109
Health Discoveries--Blood Protein Research And
the Art Of Lymphasizing 1
Health Freedoms--Doctors And People Must Fight For . . 88
Healthy Cells--Conditions To Produce 48
Hip Pain--To Help Relieve 63
How To Use Lymphasizing Electrically; Bio-Electric
Lymphasizing Techniques; Work Of Drs. Waltz,

Graupe And Royal; Story Behind Book; Special
  Acknowledgments; And Testimonials 171
Human Body--An Electric Being 44
Hypertension (High Blood Pressure)--The Cause Of 74
Hypoglycemia--Can Turn Into Diabetes, High Blood
  Pressure and Heart Disease 117
  Not Enough Fruits, Vegetables And Whole Grains . . 116

Inflammation--Cause Of 41,71

Kidneys--Techniques That Increases The Circulation . . . 64

Lecturing Full Time--Dr. West Tells How Doors Opened . 240
Legs--How To Help Relieve Pain 63
Let There Be Peace On Earth--History 81
  Song 83
  Poem 95, 246
Letter--From Dr. Joseph Waltz, St. Barnabas Hospital . . . 184
Life And Death--Now You Can Defend Yourself 169
Live Laws Of Peace--Like City Of Enoch 95
Liver--Techniques That Increase The Circulation 63
Loss Of Energy--Trapped Proteins, The First Sign Of . . . 45
Love--The Desire To Give Everything You Have To Bless . 112
Lower Back Pain--How To Help Relieve 63
Lower Back Problems--The Cause Of 45
Lymphasize--Babies Say, "If You Love Me
  Lymphasize Me" 145
  You Will Feel Like Soaring Through The Skies
    When You Learn To Lymphasize" 166
  "Don't Just Exercise, Lymphasize" 136
Lymphasizer--Definition 144
  Get One 147
  How To Use Correctly 154
  How To Use One Electrically 187
  Why Miracle Take Place On 154
Lymphasizing--Aerobic 165
  Aerobic, The Miracles Of 150
Lymphasizing--Complete List Of Terms 139
  Definitions And Explanations Of a To e Terms 140
  Golden Discovery Number V 7
  The Art Of, A New Science 16
  The Art Of, Definition 140

The Art Of, Those Who Master Will Raise Up A
    Posterity Who Will Conquer Disease And
    Live In Peace 167
The Art Of, Man Must Master 79
The Art Of, Reveals What Causes Trapped Proteins . 16
The Four Physical Laws Of 140
The "Run And Not Be Weary; Walk And Not
    Faint" Program 156
Why Concepts Of Are In This Book 137
Where It First Began 145
Lymphatic System, The--How It Functions In Detail . . . 40
Importance Of 32,37
Like A Tree, Figure 1 33
Lymph Fluid--What Is It 38

Man, The Natural--An Enemy To Himself 92
Manuscript, Original--What Happened When I
    Tried To Write 243
Medical Doctors--A.M.A. Keeps From Practicing
    Prevention 87
    Beginning to Fight for Freedom 88
    Why Some Are Afraid To Teach Blood
    Protein Research 86
Mental Attitudes--That Cause Death Also Cause War . . . 84
Message, This--Must Go To The Nations Of The Earth . . 96
Mitchell, Teresa--Follows Ehret--No Fatigue 218
    Her Testimony 220

Natural Laws, The--When Do We Begin To Break Them . 146
Nutrition--Prevention Through Proper 96
Nutritional Concepts And Transition Program--
    Scientific Evidence And Testimonies
    Lend Validity 208

Obesity--The Cause Of 73

Pain--Cause Of Most 48
Pancreas--Techniques That Increase The Circulation . . . 63
Peace And Health, An Age Of 90
Peace, The Laws Of--To Have Health We Must Obey . . . 81
Physical Exercise--Prevention Through Proper 136

Poem By Johna May West--"Bouncy, Bouncy Baby" . 153,193
Poison--How You Can Tell If You Eat A 98
    Why Fat Is A 102
    Why High Cholesterol Is A 103
    Why Simple Sugars Are 101
    Why Too Much Meat Is A 212
    Why Too Much Salt Is A 99
Potato--Praise The 213
Prevention, The College Of 79
    Through Proper Exercise 136
    Through Proper Mental Attitudes 80
    Through Proper Nutrition 96
Promise, A--To Those Who Learn The Principles And
        Apply The Concepts Contained In This Book . . 3
Protein Deficiency--How To Treat 119
Protein, Excess--Will Damage Kidneys 212
Protein, High--Disease Results From, Well
        Documented 214
    For Athletes? 212
    Makes You Feel Good While It Kills You 119
    What Dr. Paavo Airola Says About 212
Protein Requirements, The Body's--Low, Not High . . . 115

Recipes, Sample Menu, Shopping List Etc. 267
Research, This--Not To Tell Others Is To Cause
        Their Destruction 232
Research, This--Why I Learned About 234

Salt--Why It Is A Poison 99
Sciatic Nerve Pain--To Help Relieve 63
Sciatic Problems--Cause Of 57
Scientific Message For Health And Peace 13
Self-Help Pain Relief Techniques--Massage And
        Light, Fast Stroke 60
Self-H.E.L.P. Program, Introducing 93
Seven Golden Discoveries, The 4
Shopping List, Sample Menu, Recipes Etc. 268
Song--Let There Be Peace On Earth 83,95,246
Spleen--Techniques That Increase The Circulation . . . 63
Sprouts, How To Prepare 270
Starvation (Fasting)--Protein Stays High 226

Stress And The Death Process, Review Of 84
Stress--To Cause Willfully Is To Cause Destruction 92
Sugar--Why It Is A Poison 103

Tarahumara Indians--Information About Them 138
    Their Secret 138
Testimonial Letters--Approximately 30 Pages Not
        Numbered (Between 207-208) From Those Who
        Have Received Help From Applying The
        Self-Help Lymphasizing Concepts 207
Testimonials--Of Eating Right 215
Testimony Of Transition And The Art Of
        Lymphasizing--By Dr. West 135
Transition Concepts--In Condensed Form 131
Transition Diet--The Basic 132
Transition Process--Why It Works 128
Transition Program--Is Necessary 121
    Shopping List, Menu, Recipes, Dehydrating
        Techniques (Found In Appendix B) 267
Trapped Proteins--The Mental Laws 17,80
    The Nutritional Laws 19,96
    The Physical Laws 23,136

Walker-West-Walk, The--Introduction 24
    Definition 141
Water-Eight Glasses A Day If You Eat The Wrong
        Foods 120
Writing This Book--How Help Was Given 241

SPECIAL INDEX

Charts, Photographs And Special Items
In Order Of Appearance

SESSION 1

The Power Behind This Book   I
  Dr. West says, "The one who made the body made
  'The Basic Formula's For Life And Death At The Cell
  Level.' With His help we have finally found them.
  With this knowledge, the name of the problem or the
  name of the disease means nothing anymore."
The Certificate That Was Given At The 8th International
  Congress Of Lymphology To Certify That Dr. West
  Presented "The Basic Formula For Death" Which
  Shows How The Blood Proteins Produce The
  Conditions At The Cell Level Which Cause Loss
  Of Energy, Disease And Death   II
  (This Formula is what all those who are
  researching disease have been looking for.)
The Seven Golden Discoveries   4
"The Basic Formula For Death"   10
"The Basic Formula For Life"   13
  (This formula was also presented at the 8th Congress.
  Dr. Zelikovski, a surgeon from Israel told Dr. West,
  "If we got our body in this condition, we would have
  to close our hospitals.")
These Seven Golden Discoveries And This One Basic
  Formula Reveal What A Healing Art Must Do In
  Order To Work. The Miracles Of Science Are
  Now Revealed   14
Introducing A New Science Called, "The Art Of
  Lymphasizing" Which Reveals What Causes Trapped
  Plasma Proteins (TPP) Around The Cells   16
The Mental Laws Of Health And Trapped Proteins   17
The Nutritional Laws Of Health And Trapped Proteins . .   19
The Physical Laws Of Health And Trapped Proteins . . .   22

SESSION II

The Lymphatic System, Like A Tree (Fig. 1) 33
Healthy Cells & Unhealthy Cells (Fig. 2) 35
Energy From "Finger Tip" And "Leaf" (Fig. 3) 44
Healthy Cells - Unhealthy Cells (Fig. 4) 49
Water And Excess Sodium Retention Ability Of TPP
     To Cause Obesity, And/Or High Blood Pressure,
     Heart Disease, Cancer, Arthritis, M.S., Polio,
     Cerebral Palsy, Etc., Etc., (Fig. 5) 52
Electricity Heals Bones In Weeks, That Could Not Be
     Healed For Fourteen Years (Fig. 6) 54
Previously Helpless Patients Helped By
     Dr. Joseph Waltz, M.D. 55
Illustrations Showing The Basic Bio-Electric
     Self-Help Pain Relief Techniques 62
Headache And Sore Neck Problems (Fig. 7) 66
Sore Arms And Shoulders (Fig. 8) 66
Sore Knees And Legs (Fig. 9, 9A) 66
Lower Back And Sciatic Nerve Problems (Fig. 10, 10A) . . 67
Liver And Gall Bladder (Fig. 11) 67
Spleen And Pancreas (Fig. 12) 67
Colon: Descending, Tranverse, Ascending
     (Fig. 13, 13A, 13B) 68
Kidneys And Adrenals (Fig. 14) 68
Smashed Fingers (Fig. 15) 69
Turned Ankle (Fig. 16, 16A, 16B) 69

SESSION III

PREVENTION THROUGH PROPER MENTAL
     ATTITUDES 80
Song, "Let There Be Peace On Earth" 83
Introducing The World-Wide Golden Family
     Self-H.E.L.P. Program 93
Poem, "Let There Be Peace On Earth" 95
PREVENTION THROUGH PROPER NUTRITION 96
Testimonial Letters 1 & 2 From Christina Skidmore 122
Food Combining Chart (Fig. 1) 130
The Transition Concepts In Condensed Form 131
The Basic Transition Diet 132
PREVENTION THROUGH PROPER EXERCISE 136
The Secret Of The Tarahumara Indians 138

A Complete List Of Lymphasizing Terms 139
Dr. VanAaken, M.D. Proves The Lymphasizing
     Principle Works 143
Why Babies Love To Be Lymphasized 145
Ninety-Eight Year-Old Woman Saved From Death 148
Letter From Florence Franet Telling How Special
     Education Children Respond To Lymphasizing 148
The Miracle Of Glycogen 151
Poem, BOUNCY, BOUNCY BABY by John May West . . . 153
How To Use A Lymphasizer Properly 154
The Run And Not Be Weary - Walk And Not Faint
     Lymphasizing Program 156
Different Styles Of Lymphasizers (Fig. 2) 157
The Gentle Bounce (Fig. 2A) 157
The Soft Walk (Fig. 3) 157
Variation Of Soft Walk (Fig. 3A) 157
     (Stay on page 157 until you can go for at least
     30 minutes and "Keep Your Body Feeling Like You
     Are Sitting In A Chair.")
The Low Jog (Fig. 4) 158
The Front Kick (Fig. 5) 158
The Side Kick (Fig. 6) 158
The Seat Bounce (Fig. 7) 158
     (Fig. 7 could be used in the beginning for those
     who have a hard time standing. The others are
     more advanced.)
Turning The Other Cheek (Fig. 8) 159
The Pony Trot (Fig. 9) 159
The Bronco Buster (Fig. 10) 159
The Medium Jog (Fig. 11) 159
The High Jog (Fig. 12) 160
For Those Who Can't Stand Or Sit By Themselves -
     (Figure 13 and 15) 160
The Bio-Electric Wheel Chair Technique
     (Dr. West And His Wife) (Fig. 14) 160
Directions For Step One 161
Directions For Step Two 162
Directions For Step Three And Four 163
Directions For Step Five 165
Directions For Step Six and Seven 166

SESSION IV

Electricity Used By Medical Doctors To Diagnose
    And Prescribe 172
Eyes, Thoughts And Muscles Work Electrically 173
The Work Of Dr. Daniel Graupe: "Bionic Arm"
    Controlled By Thoughts 174
Dr. Joseph Waltz Uses Electrical Stimulation To Help
    Previously Helpless Cerebral Palsy, Multiple
    Sclerosis, And Polio Patients 174
Pictures From Dr. Joseph Waltz, M.D.:
    Cerebral Palsey (Fig. 1) 178
    Cerebral Palsey (Fig. 2) 179
    Dystonia (Fig. 3) 181
    Torticollis (Fig. 4) 183
Letter From Dr. Joseph Waltz 184
List Of The Advanced Bio-Electric Lymphasizing
    Techniques Which Can Be Demonstrated By
    A Qualified Instructor 185
Explanations With Pictures, And Stories
    Illustrating The Advanced Bio-Electric
    Lymphasizing Techniques 185
The Bio-Electric Gentle Bounce For Health 187
Body Chart-Exercise Sequence (Figure 5) 189
Dorothy Howard Reversed Her Sixty-Five Year Old
    Crippling Condition Caused By Polio, In Four
    Months By Using The Bio-Electric Gentle Bounce
    For Health 190
Why Different Products Work. This New Blood Protein
    Teaches Many People What To Do To Take
    Care Of Themselves 191
Poem, BOUNCY, BOUNCY, BABY By Johna May West . . 193
Bouncy, Bouncy Baby By Dr. West And Son (Fig. 6) 194
The Bio-Electric Eye Exercise (Fig. 7) 194
The Breathing And Directed Thinking Techniques:
    Master Position For All Body Parts (Fig. 8) 196
    For The Heart (Fig. 9) 196
    For The Thyroid (Fig. 10) 196
    For The Kidneys (Fig. 11) 196
    For The Whole Spine (Fig. 12) 197
    For the Lungs, Sinuses, etc. (Fig. 13) 197

(Note: Figure 13 is specifically for the lungs, but
it is the same as Figure 8.)
Bio-Electric Wheelchair Technique Demonstrated
By Dr. West And His Daughter (Fig. 14) 198
Paralized Young Man Uses A Lymphasizer 199
Bio-Electric Pin Point Technique (Fig. 15) 203
The Bio-Electric Energy Field Technique (Fig. 16,
16A, 16B, 16C) 205
Testimonial Letters (30 Pages) 207
Additional Scientific Evidence With Testimonies
Gives Validity To The Nutrition Program In
Session Three 208
Chart Showing Protein, Fat, And Carbohydrate
Content Of Different Foods 225
Chart On Starvation 226
Dr. West Says, "Pages 226-228 Are Priceless."
Special Recognition To Those Who Helped to Finance
The First Edition Of This Book 229
Dr. West's Story Behind "The Golden Seven Plus One". . 232
"Special" Acknowledgment And Appreciation To
Others Who Have Helped 244
The Dietary Goals For The United States (Excerpts
Of The First Edition) 247
Dr. West's Statement Regarding The Three
Page Forward In the Second Edition 262
Shopping List, Sample Lunch And Dinner Menu And
Suggested Recipes To Help With Transition 267
How Hypoglycemia Can Turn Into Diabetes, High
Blood Pressure and Heart Disease 288
"The Basic Formula For Life" And "The Basic Formula
For Death" With Definition Of Terms 289

To donate, send check or money order
To: The I.A.L. (International Academy of Lymphology)
P.O. Box 351, Orem, UT 84059
or call 1 (800) 975-0123 or (801) 226-0123 for Credit Card donations.

For donating to help get this priceless research to the world, you will receive the following:

			QTY.		
	1.	"THE GOLDEN SEVEN—PLUS ONE"		1 Book Only $30.00	$
		Conquer Disease with		2-9 @ 27.00 ea.	$
		Eight Keys to Health, Beauty and Peace		10-19 @ 24.00 ea.	$
		The only book of its kind in the world.		20-29 @ 21.00 ea.	$
				Inst. @ 18.00 ea.	$
QTY.		DONATE TO HELP PROMOTE THE GOLDEN FAMILY SELF-H.E.L.P. PROGRAM			
	2.	The Certified Course in "Applied Lymphology"			$
		Priceless Knowledge—Guaranteed!	$485.00	with Certification	$
		Includes: 6 two-hour videos ($50.00 each) . . .	$350.00	with Exam	$
		and items 1, 3, 11, and 12.			$
	3.	"The Special Pink Document" (approx. 50 pgs.)	$ 10.00	Inst. @ $5.00 ea.	$
	4.	Dietary Goals for the U.S.—Excerpts (15 pages)	$ 1.00	Inst. @ $ .50 ea.	$
	5.	NHG 27th Annual conv. (audio cassette)	$ 5.00	Inst. @ $3.00 ea.	$
	6.	Human Sacrifice in America (audio cassette)	$ 5.00	Inst. @ $3.00 ea.	$
	7.	Medical Research Proves (audio cassette)	$ 5.00	Inst. @ $3.00 ea.	$
	8.	Intro. To Pain Relief Tech. (audio cassette)	$ 5.00	Inst. @ $3.00 ea.	$
	9.	Intro. Brochure - Conquer Pain and Disease	$ 2.00	20 copies	$
	10.	The Golden Family Tapes (2 audio cassettes)	$ 20.00	Inst. @ $10.00 ea.	$
	11.	How to Heal and Purify (audio cassette)	$ 10.00	Inst. @ $ 5.00 ea.	$
	12.	Discover the Power Plants in Your Body	$ 20.00	Inst. @ $10.00 ea.	$

	SUBTOTAL	$
Add #2.50 per book (1-10 books) or $1.50 per book (11 + books) shipping/handling ($10.00 per course) ($3.00 minimum)		$
		$
	TOTAL DONATION (U.S. funds only)	$

Make Donations to the I.A.L. (A Non-Secular, Charitable, Educational Entity under Title 26, Section 508(c)(1)(A) of the United States Code.)

☐ I am interested in becoming an Area Coordinator.

☐ VISA/Master Card   Expiration Date _____ Add 4%

Account No. _____

Cardholder's Signature _____

NAME _____ PHONE (_____) _____

ADDRESS _____

CITY _____ STATE _____ ZIP _____

PLEASE PRINT

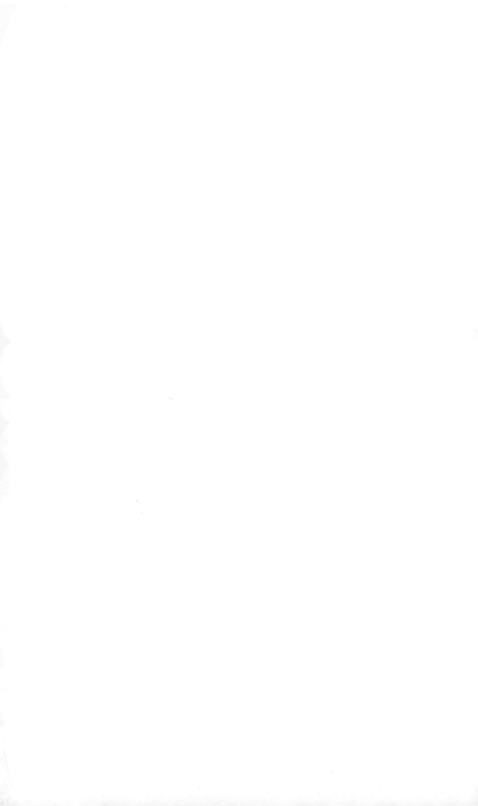